W9-CMS-898

WITHDRAWN

THE **BLACK** PRESS, U.S.A.

THE **BLACK** PRESS, U.S.A.

■

ROLAND E. WOLSELEY

WITH AN INTRODUCTION BY **ROBERT E. JOHNSON**, EXECUTIVE EDITOR, **JET**

■

THE IOWA STATE UNIVERSITY PRESS ● AMES, IOWA

233368

■ DEDICATED TO **ROBERT W. ROOT,** 1915–1970
FRIEND AND COLLEAGUE, EDUCATOR, AUTHOR, AND JOURNALIST
WHOSE BOOKS ON THE CHURCH AND RACE
ARE A CONTRIBUTION TO BETTER INTER-RACIAL RELATIONS

■

PN
4888
N4
W6

© 1971 The Iowa State University Press
Ames, Iowa 50010. All rights reserved

Composed and printed by
The Iowa State University Press

First edition, 1971

International Standard Book Number: 0–8138–0185–0
Library of Congress Catalog Card Number: 74–126160

H.D.S.U. LIBRARY

CONTENTS

∎

PREFACE

■

"THE NEGRO PRESS has become the most influential Negro business in the Twentieth Century. . . . Unfortunately, [it] has not received the scholarly research attention it deserves."

Erwin K. Welsch, author of *The Negro in the United States,* makes this observation at the outset of his discussion of the black press and the literature on it. He then notes that the only general book was published in 1922. *The Black Press, U.S.A.* was written to provide information about this ethnic press at a time when the black citizens and all their problems, interests, and enterprises have taken on a new importance. It is not a textbook about the techniques and methods of black journalism, which are similar to those of any other in this country, although some distinctions are drawn.

After an opening chapter discussing the validity of the entire concept of a black press and setting the stage in general come three chapters that briefly relate the history. Not all background is confined to these chapters, however; additional historical information appears in various other sections where it contributes to understanding of a particular facet. The history is followed by four chapters that examine the newspapers and magazines of today; another chapter describes types of material offered, although that is evident in many other sections as well. Next come chapters on reporters and editors of the present and past, followed by a chapter about the training and educational problems and possibilities for the journalist. From there the book considers the problems facing owners and publishers, the ideologies of the times and their impact upon the press, and a number of practical areas: advertising, circulation, and production. In another chapter syndicates, public relations, and black radio are treated. The attacks upon and defenses of the press then are reviewed, after which comes the evaluation of black journalism. Finally, the traditional and essential discussion of what may be ahead is provided.

The book attempts, therefore, to explore the nature of a heretofore neglected and subordinated press, depicting it today against its background. It seeks, also, to relate the press to the social movements now attracting many black or Afro-American people. Its objective is neither to put the black press in a necessarily positive light nor, on the other hand, to emphasize shortcomings, but simply to report on that press with understanding of how it came to be and why it is what it is.

As is customary at this point in a preface, the author invites readers to inform him of significant omissions. He is aware that many persons and publications have gone unmentioned, but this book does not pretend to be an encyclopedic record.

● ACKNOWLEDGEMENTS

The author is grateful to Wesley C. Clark, dean of the School of Journalism at Syracuse University; Frank P. Piskor, and William Pearson Tolley, the latter two then of the Syracuse University administration, for their encouragement to him in arranging a leave of absence and thus additional time for travel and research.

Scores of organizations, companies, and individuals aided in various ways. Extraordinarily helpful were Sheila Maroney, Ruth Kimball Kent, S. Jack Weissberger, and David Collington. Mrs. Elizabeth Gardiner, journalism librarian at Syracuse, and her staff cooperated cheerfully. The author also wants to credit the following for their aid:

E. Lance Barclay, Sherilyn Cox Bennion, Elwood Berry, Robert D. Bontrager, Bernice L. Borgeson, Sherman Briscoe, Philip Ward Burton, Rhea E. Calloway, Caroline Dillon Carpenter, James W. Carty, Jr., George M. Daniels, Lawrence Davis, Micheline Delgatto, K. E. Eapen, Rosemary Eng, Kent W. de Felice, Carlton J. Frazier, Bernard E. Garnett, W. Rick Garr, Gene Gilmore, Meg Hale, Sue Holaday, Betsy Homer, Everett Hullum, Geraldine Keating, Ida Phillips, Theodore Pratt, Armistead S. Pride, Lawrence Ragan, Lillian Reiner, Frank Render, Jay Riedel, Dan Ritey, Susan Rittenhouse, Patricia Roesch, the late Robert W. Root, Sue Shields Rosenberg, Linda Chiavaroli Rosenbloom, Kenneth Sparks, W. David Stephenson II, Nora Swindler, William Howard Taft, Margaret Troutt, Carolyn Watson, Eva M. Willard, and Valena Minor Williams.

Officers and staff members of numerous publishing firms, advertising agencies, and journalistic syndicates were helpful. Particularly so were Lionel C. Barrow, Jr., of Foote, Cone and Belding; Thomas J. De Bow, Jr., of Young and Rubicam, Inc.; W. Leonard Evans, publisher, *Tuesday;* Carlton B. Goodlett, publisher, San Francisco *Sun-Reporter;* J. Darnell Harvey, *New Lady* magazine; Mrs. Esther Jackson, *Freedomways;* John H. Johnson, editor and publisher, Johnson Publishing Company; Robert E. Johnson, executive editor, *Jet;* Ken Jones, publisher, *Soul* and *Soul! Illustrated;* Lewis A. Little, vice-president and general manager, Register and Tribune Syndicate;

Clarence H. Markham, Jr., editor and publisher, *New Negro Traveler and Conventioneer;* Louis E. Martin, vice-president and editor-in-chief, Sengstacke Newspapers; Ernie McMillan, president, Proud, Inc.; Henry Lee Moon, editor, *Crisis;* Mrs. Ethel M. Moore, Amalgamated Publishers, Inc.; Mrs. Elizabeth Murphy Moss, vice-president, Afro-American Newspapers; Herbert Nipson, executive editor, *Ebony;* Thomas Picou, managing editor, Chicago *Daily Defender;* Mimi Reimel, *Philly Talk;* John H. Sengstacke, president, Sengstacke Newspapers; Mrs. Barbara Winters, editor, *Star,* New Haven; and John Woodford, editor, *Muhammad Speaks.*

My wife, Bernice Browne Wolseley, always helpful, is thanked for having once again been willing to suffer through the writing stages of a book and for aiding with many details. ●

ROLAND E. WOLSELEY

INTRODUCTION
A JOURNEY OF JOURNALISTIC REFLECTIONS
BY **ROBERT E. JOHNSON,** EXECUTIVE EDITOR, **JET NEWSMAGAZINE**

■

WHEN PROFESSOR ROLAND E. WOLSELEY asked me to write an introduction to his book, *The Black Press, U.S.A.*, he said, "Your introduction can say what you wish, good and bad alike. Any observations about your own experience or views on the black press will be welcomed by readers and reviewers alike."

As a member of the black press establishment and an alumnus of Syracuse University's School of Journalism, I accepted this honor with misgivings because it casts me in the role of a student doing a critique of his teacher's writing.

After reading press proofs of *The Black Press, U.S.A.*, profound in its scholarship and significant in the scope of objectives, I was propelled on a journey of reflections.

This book had to be written. It asked me to write it in 1948 when I was a Morehouse College senior and editor of the *Maroon Tiger,* student newspaper whose 1938 editors V. Trenton Tubbs, Moss H. Kendricks, and Bernard Milton Jones founded Delta Phi Delta journalistic society which originated the celebration of "Negro Newspaper Week" in March each year. Nobody, I reasoned, would take seriously anything written by a student.

This book urged me to write it in 1950 when I was a "veteran" of two years of reporting for the Atlanta (Ga.) *Daily World*. At that time, my resources not only included the libraries of Atlanta's accredited black colleges—Morehouse, Spelman, Clark, Morris Brown, and Atlanta University—but included such World and Scott Newspaper Syndicate journalists as Emory O. Jackson, William Fowlkes, Marion E. Jackson, V. W. Hodges, Joel Smith, and William Gordon. Moreover, there were such *World* alumni veterans as Robert Ratcliffe, Lucius (Lou Jo) Jones, Ric Roberts, and the late Cliff W. MacKay. I didn't write the book then because I was convinced that no one would believe a good book on the black press could be written by a black reporter whose fingers were not yet saturated with printer's ink.

This book begged me to write it in 1952 when I was enrolled at Syracuse, studying for a master's degree in journalism. I declined, this time with distaste and disdain. This was a result of the fables of the 1950's. Integration was the "in" thing. It was the decade of the negro backlash when it was considered a put-down for a white professor to advise a negro student to select a black subject for his master's thesis or Ph.D. dissertation. It wasn't hip to be that black and proud. It was a time to be ashamed if your white classmates caught you reading a black newspaper. This was the decade when a negro student thought it to be more relevant to write a thesis on, say, "An Interpretative Analysis of John Milton's Areopagitica and Its Literary Impact "Upon the Liberty to Print Tracts without License" rather than, say, "The History of Black Journalistic Thought from John Russwurm to John H. Johnson."

At the end of the decade of the 1960's, I was executive editor of *Jet* with sixteen years of newsmagazine experience. Finally, in 1970, this book demanded that I write it. Immersed in administrative rather than writing responsibilities, I deferred again.

Blacks should plead their own cause since we know our condition better than anyone, the founders of the black press, Samuel E. Cornish and John B. Russwurm, tell us. But if we fail to do so, it behooves anyone to come forth, reminds Dr. Howard Thurman, former Howard and Boston universities theologian who was voted by *Ebony* magazine as one of the "Ten Best Preachers in America."

Professor Wolseley came forth to do this book because black journalists like myself could sleep at night rather than yield to the pressure of the unwritten manuscript of the 144-year journey of the black press in America.

The Black Press, U.S.A. is a redeeming document of black men and black media struggling to overcome chaos and establish community in a racist society against incredible odds. To whites who read this book, it may be described as a case for chauvinism. My reaction to this is contained in the conversation a group of black journalists and myself had in Tel-Aviv, Israel, November 21, 1969, with Foreign Minister Abba Eban. He observed, "You, as members of the black press, may be accused of being a selfish press. Everybody who looks after himself is said to be selfish by those who have already looked after themelves." Drawing a parallel of blacks and Jews, he allowed: "There is a beloved quality that men call patriotism if they possess it themselves, and chauvinism if they see it in others. It's obvious that those who have to fight for survival—whether as groups within the nation or nations within the 126 sovereign states of the world—they are obviously going to be more preoccupied than those whose survival is assured."

Similarly, Professor Wolseley offers this kind of empathy and insight in his book.

The only quarrel—and it's really not a quarrel—is that I prefer to speculate on the future of the black press. Nearly always, whites ask about the future of *Jet* or *Ebony* or the black press in an integrated society, but they don't ask about the future of *Life* or *Look* or the white press. I'm reminded of the response of Dr. Benjamin E. Mays, president-emeritus of 104-year-old Morehouse College, when a similar question was raised about the future of the black college. To paraphrase him, if we really get rid of white racism we will concede the fact that the black press has just as much right to exist as the white press. Nobody ever raises the question of what is the future of the white press, and they have been discriminating more than the black press all through the years. But when you ask about the black press, you want to know what's going to happen to it. This is a kind of discrimination which is abominable.

Professor Wolseley's book is an invaluable ally in helping the black press convince white America that blacks can mobilize their own talents, their own genius, and take fate into their own hands. That is the secret to black emancipation—black liberation!

Chicago, Illinois
April 30, 1971

THE **BLACK** PRESS, U.S.A.

1. IS THERE A BLACK PRESS?

WHEN A COURSE on the black press in the United States was launched at Syracuse University in the fall, 1968, several professors in other areas of knowledge raised doubts about the existence of such a press.

"How do you tell?" a political scientist asked.

"What determines it?" came from an historian, who went on to inquire: "Is it that the readers are blacked-skinned?"

Indeed, how does one tell? And is it important that there be a distinction?

This problem was one of the first presented to the students, as it has been in every offering of the course since. For in such a course, as in this book, it is a central point. If there is no black or Negro press there is no point in publishing books about it or scheduling courses concerned with it. The skepticism is not one that springs from ignorance only of this ethnic press; some black publishers also question such a distinction.

The conclusion by the class, at term's end, was that there is such a press and that it definitely is important that a distinction be made between it and other press groups. One graduate student, Kent W. de Felice, selected the problem for deeper investigation and obtained reactions from several leading black journalists.[1] His report concluded that there are certain qualifications which a publication must meet to be considered a unit of the black press. They are:

1. Blacks must own and manage the publication; they must be the dominant racial group connected with it. (In support of that requirement it can be said that if the publication is not black-owned and black-operated, its aims, policies, and programs can be altered by persons unsympathetic to the goals of black editors and publishers. An instance occurred in 1968 when an apparently black-owned newspaper supported George Wallace during the presidential campaigns. Investigation brought out the fact that the paper had been black-owned until shortly before the campaigns began, when whites bought it and altered its policy.[2] The black press otherwise backed Hubert H.

3

Humphrey strongly but included supporters of Richard M. Nixon as well.)

2. The publication must be intended for black consumers. (A science magazine presumably is aimed at scientists or persons interested in scientific matters. A paper about music is directed to persons responsive to its contents. Advertising sales depend upon such identification of reader with subject. Similarly, a magazine or newspaper for black citizens deals with their interests and concerns and is not primarily for whites. So long as there is a cultural and ethnic distinction in society between black and white citizens there will be a place for black journalism. These differences still are acute, especially with the possibility that the present trend toward separatism is only temporary.)

3. The paper or magazine must, the report concluded, "serve, speak and fight for the black minority." It also must have the major objective of fighting for "equality for the Negro in the present white society. Equality means the equality of citizenship rights," de Felice said.

Moses Newson, executive editor of the Baltimore *Afro-American,* one of the major black newspapers, noted that the black press of the United States was "founded for the purpose of serving, publicizing, speaking, and fighting for the colored minority." The late E. Washington Rhodes, publisher of the Philadelphia *Tribune,* a leading semi-weekly, although denying the validity of the use of the word *black* or the existence of a black press and accepting *Negro press* as a term, went on to write that the units of this press are intended "to secure for their readers absolute equality of citizenship rights." And from William O. Walker, editor of the Cleveland *Call and Post,* came the clear view that "Black is a color—Negro is a race; so there is a Negro press. It serves the interests and needs of the Negro people."

A parallel can be drawn with another area of communications: theater. Peter Bailey, writing in *Ebony,* insisted that black theater is one that is written, directed, produced, financed by blacks, located in a black community, and uses the community "as its reference point."

Similarly, some black journalists believe that the black press is that owned, produced, and intended for black readers in a black environment. This third proviso, then, makes the black press a special-pleading institution, one with a cause, goal, or purpose going beyond the basic one necessary for survival in the American economy—the making of a profit.

● THE DIFFERENCES DISCERNED

Applying the de Felice specifications to white newspapers and magazines brings out the differences between the black and white presses. Although it usually is owned by whites, the white press need not be. It could be owned by blacks but aimed at whites, for the white press generally hopes to have readers of all hues. The main difference exists in the goals of white publications. Usually they are concerned with the problems of whites, the majority group readers, and only incidentally with those of blacks, Orientals, or other minorities, racial or political. This policy accounts for the complaints against the dominant press which have been made for a century and a half by the black society. During most of the white press' history, in fact, there has been indifference to the black minority's problems, if not downright opposition to that race, giving rise to the black press as a corrective force as well as a weapon with which blacks have been fighting for their rights.

It should be noted, however, that by no means are all black publications dedicated to social causes dear to the country's black citizens. Just as with any other business, there are publications whose goal chiefly is financial profit, sometimes to be used in the interest of the race, other times, as with white entrepreneurs, for the personal benefit of the managers and owners.

● BLACK, NEGRO, OR COLORED?

The black press has existed for almost 150 years, but should it be called a *black* press? This point has become sensitive. A *Playboy* cartoon once showed a white man talking to a black one in an integrated cocktail party scene. Says the white to the black: "I don't want to make any social blunders. What are you people calling yourselves these days?"

Although certain labels have hung on for generations, in the 1960's change came rapidly: *negro* replaced *colored, Negro* came in for *negro, Negro* went to *black, black* then became *Black.* Now the last two are being used interchangeably. All were surrounded by other less widely used terms, although in the black press some at one time were popular: *Afro-American, Aframerican, colored, non-white, race,* and similar variations.

Certain writers and publishers preferred "Negro-oriented" press. *Ebony,* for example, called itself a Negro magazine during its early years, but in its promotion in the later 1960's called itself Negro-oriented. D. Parke Gibson, throughout an entire book, *The $30 Billion Negro,* refers to the "Negro-oriented press," a reflection perhaps of the greater readership of these publications by whites and the desire to direct advertisers' attention to coverage in depth. The term also accommodates the dozens of white-owned radio stations which carry programs for black listeners.

When *Negro Digest,* a companion magazine to *Ebony, Jet,* and *Tan,* underwent a change of name to *Black World* in 1970, the editors explained that "Negro" was in harmony with the times in 1942, when it was founded, but not in 1970. Not only had the magazine's formula changed after its death in 1951 and rebirth in 1961 but its policies also were altered. The editors said that the new name reflected the actual character of the publication.

Although the debate may seem as it did as long ago as 1950 to Roi Ottley, the historian of the Chicago *Daily Defender,* only "a tempest in a teapot," it is worthy of serious discussion because of the semantics of the situation. These terms reflect attitudes. They can indicate the evaluation of a whole race as well as of individual members of the group. For example, a reader sensitive to the various views of this minority would comprehend that someone calling himself editor of a Negro-oriented paper perhaps is conservative socially, certainly at this time nonmilitant, for the militant abhors "Negro," considering it a term applied by whites who feel superior to him. The debate has added importance because it is related to what people of black colored skin call themselves. One needs to know what is acceptable, as the *Playboy* cartoon implies, so as not to offend any group needlessly. Ethnic minorities are particularly tender on this point, as can be seen in the Jewish protests about Fagin and Shylock in theatrical productions and the objections of Chinese, Poles, Italians, Japanese, and the clergy to the various stereotypes of themselves still encountered on cinema and television screens.

As this passage is being written, the press itself and various organizations in this group of Americans have settled down mainly to use of "black," "Black," and "Negro," with the first two seen more and more in print. The Black Academy of Arts and Letters was founded in Boston in 1969, one of dozens of organizations and publications using Black. "Colored" has virtually disappeared except in distinctive and long-used names like that of the National Association for the Advancement of Colored People. "Race" for a time also was widely used by the press, but now is uncommon. "Afro-American" survives more strongly than "colored," since it is in the name of a widely read group of newspapers, and appears as well in some organization titles.

"Negro," although for so long acceptable to both white and black groups (some of the best black magazines have used it for years, *Journal of Negro Education,* for instance), was opposed as long ago as 1896, when Dr. J. C. Embry, a Philadelphia pastor, argued that "Negro" is objectionable because it was derived from color only. He held out for "Afro-American," since Africa is the land of origin of black Americans. More recent objectors say that "Negro" is a word coming from whites and suggests Uncle Tomism. The Congress of Racial Equality barred a Columbus (Ohio) *Dispatch* newsman and a photographer from its 1968 convention because the paper had used "Negro" in reporting its sessions. Dick Gregory, the entertainer, objected to "Negro" because it is related, he once said, to the opprobrious term "nigger," which in turn is derived from the Latin "niger," for black. His view had been voiced many years before by a noted black journalist, T. Thomas Fortune, thought to have originated "Afro-American."

Among the black people there is no uniformity of attitude or practice. But concern over what nonblacks call them is rising as part of the developing consciousness of status and pride in accomplishment.

The term "black" is used in this book because in the author's view it is the choice of many persons actively concerned with the welfare of this ethnic group.

The use of "black" has been defended eloquently by the writer of a letter to *Editor & Publisher*. She discussed a point made by Roy H. Copperud, the magazine's lexicographer-columnist, who expressed surprise that "black," "which might well strike many people as derogatory because of its frequent association in literature and elsewhere with servitude of one kind or another," had been accepted so quickly. That was early 1968.

"It's part of the quest for self-identity, that precious, subtle pride that was so painstakingly crushed in slavery, and has been suppressed all these decades," wrote Elinor Diane Harvin of the public relations staff of the Michigan Bell Telephone Company. "It goes along with the rejection of whitey's insistence that straight hair is better than kinky hair, thin lips are better than thick lips, white skin is better than dark skin.

"It's a way of saying 'Hold on, baby. White is not better than black. We see who we are. Black is on the same level as white. We will define who we are and how much we're worth. You're not going to tell us who we are or who we have to be anymore.' And one doesn't have to be a radical to feel this. . . .

"Whether America's newspapers displace the ever-popular name 'Negro' for black or Afro-American is up to each paper of course. (The black press has already swung overwhelmingly in favor of the 'new' language, still using 'Negro' when they need a nice 'neutral' word)."[3]

● THE NEED FOR A BLACK PRESS

Whatever they may be called, the black newspapers and magazines and their auxiliaries exist. How they developed is related in subsequent chapters. Why they came into being is part of that history.

The aims of the early publications, from *Freedom's Journal* of 1827 to those issued in Reconstruction days, are clear. The exploitation of slaves, their mistreatment and the limitations placed upon them are examined in the historical perspective. But the black citizen of the United States is a free man or woman, education is available (if not always the best), employment can be had at least by some (even if still mainly in the lower echelons), and civil rights slowly are being won. What, then, is the need for a black press still?

It is needed mainly because all the old battles have not yet been won and because there are so many new ones. "Without the black press, the black man would not know who he is nor what is happening to his struggle for the freedom of citizenship," in the words of Valarie Myers, former editor of Syracuse (N.Y.) *Challenger,* one of the many new community papers of recent years. And perhaps less important now than in the past but still vital is the need for facts about themselves, i.e., coverage of the black society, still neglected by the white press which deals mainly in racial conflict, crime, and news of blacks known to whites from the sports and entertainment worlds.

Also, for many years the black people have mistrusted the white press. As Roi Ottley has explained, the white press and news services earned the suspicion of black citizens in the first half of this century because they could not be trusted to tell the truth about blacks. These white agencies were accused of favoring whites against blacks, i.e., tailoring the news to fit the publications' prejudices or at least those of their owners. Both northern and southern papers followed the practice of race identification of blacks only and of ignoring entirely anything but unfavorable black news.

Complaints about the white press treatment of blacks' news today, however, are no less numerous, perhaps more selective because they single out regions, and merely different in nature from those of the early years of black journalism. Representatives of various types of black organizations, for example, met in Washington in 1969 with editors and reporters from the city's three white dailies to discuss "The Minorities and the Press." The session was typical, in the matter of criticisms of the white press, of others held in various parts of the U.S.A. by newsmen's organizations, schools of journalism, and newspaper unions.

The black critics in Washington objected to the papers' practice of displaying civil rights stories next to crime stories involving blacks. They objected also to all news concerning black citizens being handled as civil rights news instead of being put in appropriate departments, such as financial or women's sections. News about blacks, it also was charged, always is negative and the newspapers tend to deal only with conflict stories about what goes on in the ghetto.[4]

As in the early years, blacks still look to their press to fight their battles. A look at almost any black paper and most magazines dramatizes this point. To the middle-class white or other nonblack reader, such as an Oriental, the black world is a separate realm. The use of "world" in black publication titles, such as *Our World, Bronze World, Black World* magazines or Garvey's paper, *The Negro World,* all indicate this separation. The fault is not all that of white publishers. The general white press does not cover the details of life in most industries or professions or other specialized groups of humans, for that would be impossible; that explains the existence of thousands of special publications to compensate for the lack of their news in the consumer or general press.

Blacks can counter, however, that what they do, day by day, is of more importance for whites to know about and to understand than are the doings, say, of the nation's cost accountants or other specialists who have their own publications. The revolt of the black people at mid-century caught many white Americans by surprise; perhaps adequate coverage of the black community and its problems might have helped solve the problems before they became extreme. Yet the continued absence of such coverage of not only the black world but of other minorities as well, the American Indian, for example, is evidence of the lack of perspective of American white-owned journalistic publications, of which there are about 32,000.

● EXTENT OF THE BLACK PRESS

A visitor to the United States from India, whose citizens, being people of color other than white, have a natural interest in and sympathy for the nonwhites anywhere, once remarked to the author that he saw no publications for blacks in his travels around the U.S.A., although he saw many black people. When he was told that at the time the country's black population amounted to 18,870,000, he was astonished.

The experience is a common one for whites as well, although not to be taken too literally. The Indian friend was shown a variety of black periodicals and then recalled having seen several of them on newsstands but of being unaware of their origin. Unless one knows the titles it is not always easy to identify black publications, especially with the greater use by white papers and magazines of black models on covers or the photographs of black celebrities on front as well as inside pages. In general, however, it is true that the black press has little newsstand exposure, for the obvious reasons that only those newsstands where there is substantial black traffic, such as in all-black neighborhoods, would benefit from selling such publications, and that the earning power of almost all blacks has kept down the purchase of publications by single copies. Furthermore, it is too expensive to place publications on newsstands, through distribution companies, unless wide sale is likely. Perhaps one stand on a main street may stock a magazine or two.

Library holdings also have been sparse. Exceptions are private and public institutions patronized by blacks, such as college libraries especially interested in black history and culture, only a recent interest in most instances. It is the unusual public library that receives more than one or two magazines and that number of newspapers aimed at black readers.

Most whites and not a few blacks are unaware of the extent of the black press. College people, except those deeply involved in social movements embracing racial problems, rarely can remember seeing a black publication, a situation the author has become aware of through classroom work during thirty years of teaching journalism courses in which some attention has been given to the black press.

As their circulations attest, most black magazines, aside from a few popular ones, seem to exist in secrecy. White scholars have vague impressions of such capably written and well-edited periodicals as the *Journal of Negro History* and the *Journal of Negro Education.* Several dozen other meritorious publications have functioned for years in quiet, surrounded by white indifference. In their effort to understand the black society, some whites now are beginning to look into these publications.

Preciseness is not possible about the extent of the black press in the eighth decade of this century, with the black population figure at about 23,000,000, any more than it is possible to be exact about its size in earlier years, although not for all the same reasons. Records were not carefully kept and still are not dependable. Today, in addition, the black press is changing in numbers so rapidly that figures on how many publications exist are incorrect the day they are published. The author, for example, assembled the names of more than half a hundred newspapers and magazines, some as much as five years old, never mentioned in any of such listings as the *Ayer Directory,* the *Standard Periodical Directory, Ulrich's International Periodicals Directory,* and other common sources. It is not altogether the list-makers' fault. It is the result of free access to the printing press in the U.S.A., and the quick turnover of publications, for some are born and die without ever getting into anybody's listing.

In the early 1970's black newspapers and magazines appear to have hovered in number between 300 and 325. These figures cover regularly issued publications, not newsletters, bulletins, or other types of borderline journalism. The Department of Journalism at Lincoln University (Missouri), which until 1966 issued an annual report on the number of black newspapers, up to then totaled 140 to 150. Ayer's 1970 *Directory* reported 158 publications, including magazines. *Advertising Age,* in its April 20, 1970, issue, reported "an estimated 225 Negro-oriented newspapers in the nation." The source of that figure, it turned out, was the U.S. Department of Commerce. To that figure for newspapers, which checks with the author's own count, can be added about sixty-five magazines, each accounted for by identification of actual copies by the author. In addition are another thirty newspapers and magazines yet to be verified (see Table 1.1).

While in the numbers game the black press plays a small part, it includes more publications than does any other racial minority group press in the country. Most newspapers are for general consumption; most magazines are specialized, a reflection of the division of the white press.

Brooks divided the black weeklies of the late 1940's into three kinds: six nationally distributed papers with six-figure circulations and several editions—local, regional, or national; about twenty inter-

TABLE 1.1 ● Number of Black Newspapers in the U.S.A.

Year	Non dailies	Dailies
1939	152	3
1958	170	2
1959	149	3
1961	140	2
1962	131	2
1966	170	2
1967	151	2
1968	150	2
1969	158	2

NOTE: This table is useful only to show what the few tabulators have been able to trace, which at best does not approach accuracy. The *Ayer Directory* records mainly papers that handle advertising. It also mixes magazines with newspapers. The Lincoln reports are more discriminating. By actual count the author has records of 199 general circulation newspapers for 1970 and 225 for 1971 (see Table 13.2.)
SOURCES: 1939–66, Armistead S. Pride, Department of Journalism, Lincoln University; 1967–69 *Ayer Directory*.

mediate-size weeklies issued in large cities but not nationally circulated and with sales of from 10,000 to 50,000; the third group, made up of the bulk of the black papers, the unaudited, "minor sheets," published in small cities, and often unstable.[5]

More than two decades later the scene is different. The half-dozen widely distributed papers still are published but their six-figure circulations are no more. The intermediate group circulations also have become smaller. And while the third group still is unstable, it is not the same kind of instability and there is far more hope for survival. In the 1940's and early 1950's these fragile papers were weak because of bad management, lack of capital, too much competition (especially just after television arrived), any one factor or all three. Today there are weak papers because there are more cause or protest sheets, and more attempts at community publications based on the hope of obtaining advertising support, which has come as never before for the smaller, conventional papers and even to some degree for the more militant publications. But the opinion papers of more extreme groups, while they have added to the total numbers, also have a greater mortality. Usually only the subsidized militant papers, like the *Black Panther,* are somewhat independent of the rise and fall of advertising volume.

The most widely read and perhaps influential publications are in the consumer newspaper and magazine groups. One of the three dailies, the Chicago *Daily Defender,* with a circulation of about 35,000 four days a week, extends its influence via a weekly national edition of around the same size. It also is one of the Sengstacke Newspapers and therefore affiliated with several other substantial weeklies, including the *New Pittsburgh Courier* and the Detroit *Michigan Chronicle* as well as a half dozen editions of the *Courier* distributed

TABLE 1.2 ● Black Newspapers with Circulation in Excess of 30,000

Newspaper	Frequency	Circulation	Audit
Muhammad Speaks (Chicago)	weekly	600,000[a]	....
The *Black Panther* (Berkeley)	weekly	100,000[a]	....
New York *Amsterdam News*	weekly	77,708	ABC
Michigan Chronicle (Detroit)	weekly	45,788	ABC
Philadelphia *Tribune*	semi-weekly	38,081	ABC
Baltimore *Afro-American*	semi-weekly	33,687	ABC
Chicago *Daily Defender*	daily	33,320	ABC
Los Angeles *Sentinel*	weekly	38,084	ABC
Atlanta *Daily World*	daily	30,100	....

SOURCES: *Editor & Publisher International Year Book,* 1970; 1970 *Ayer Directory;*
Publishers' statements.
[a] Estimated.

in Ohio, Georgia, Florida, and Pennsylvania. Another black daily,
the Atlanta *Daily World,* a four-day publication, has a circulation of
about 30,000. The third, the Columbus *Times* of Georgia, is a four-
day paper.

Perhaps the best known of the other important commercial papers are the *Afro-Americans,* centered in Baltimore, with editions
also for Richmond, Washington, Philadelphia, New Jersey, and the
nation as a whole. Together they have about 133,000 circulation,
second only to the Sengstacke papers. Other influential southern and
southwestern weeklies are in Louisville, Tampa, Miami, Roanoke,
Jacksonville, Dallas, and Houston.

In the north, aside from the Sengstacke combination, which ex-
ceeds 200,000 in circulation, is the paper with the highest figure for
one newspaper in commercial circles: the New York *Amsterdam
News,* in excess of 70,000.

The most widely circulated paper is the noncommercial weekly
issued by the Nation of Islam, the tabloid *Muhammad Speaks,* with
more than a half-million sales each issue. Also larger than any commercial paper but far below the Muslim paper is the weekly subsidized by the Black Panther Party, the tabloid the *Black Panther,* with
about 100,000 sales an issue (see Tables 1.2 and 1.3).

**TABLE 1.3 ● Circulations of Black News-
paper Groups**

Group	Circulation
Sengstacke[a]	165,740
Afro-American	133,372
Courier	61,548
Scott *(World)*	45,800
Post	50,000
News Leader	46,000
Crusader	30,810

SOURCES: Amalgamated Publishers, Inc., 1970;
1970 *Ayer Directory.*
[a] Includes *Courier* Group.

TABLE 1.4 ● Black Magazines with Circulations of 50,000 or More

Publication	Frequency	Circulation	Audit
*Tuesday*ᵃ	monthly	1,877,375	....
Ebony	monthly	1,176,375	ABC
Jet	weekly	414,555	ABC
*Soul! Illustrated*ᵇ	bi-monthly	250,000	....
*New Lady*ᵇ	monthly	250,000	....
*Essence*ᵇ	monthly	175,000	....
Tan	monthly	113,269	....
The Crisis	monthly	111,641	....
Sepia	monthly	64,992	ABC
Bronze Thrills	monthly	58,265	ABC
Jive	monthly	58,055	ABC
Hep	monthly	56,000	....

SOURCE: 1970 *Ayer Directory;* publishers' statements.
ᵃ Supplement to white newspapers.
ᵇ Estimated.

Circulation data for black magazines are as hard to come by as records of their existence. Those for a few magazines are comparatively large, but the majority, being religious, fraternal, educational, or business, have circulations under 10,000. The bigger periodicals are *Ebony* and *Tuesday,* the only two to pass one million, no other reaching even one-half million. Since *Tuesday* is a monthly supplement inserted in white newspapers distributed in black neighborhoods, it is in a somewhat special category. *Ebony* is the unquestioned leader since it is a separate magazine published and sold in the way consumer periodicals are generally (see Table 1.4).

Direct competition exists between many black newspapers, a situation disappearing speedily in the white press world. Readers in Atlanta, St. Louis, New York, Chicago, Fort Worth, Memphis, Houston and several other cities can patronize second or third papers of entirely different ownership. Some of this competition comes from the local versions of out-of-town-owned papers and by national editions of a few major city weeklies and one of the dailies. The magazine publishing business, as a private enterprise, is dominated by three firms, two with four periodicals each.

● THE SCOPE TODAY

What do these publications tell their readers? What appears in them? The newspapers give their audiences news of the black community as well as of national and international events directly affecting black citizens; a few attempt to offer nonblack news of particular interest. The emphasis is on local or regional news. They also provide entertainment and editorial guidance, although largely the former, as is newspaper habit anywhere in the U.S.A. The magazines also seek to entertain, but more and more are informing and promoting causes. None of this is done with uniform thoroughness or quality. But, along with black radio, the black press is still the main source of the black citizen's information and comment about his life. Through their advertising columns these publications fulfill the commercial function. The segment known as specialized magazines serves as a literary outlet, an opinion forum, or a guidebook for business and professional people. As Henry Lee Moon, director of information for the NAACP and editor of its magazine, *Crisis,* has put it: "colored citizens still look to the Negro press for their side of the story and for an interpretation of the news that affects their vital interests."[6] Or as a perceptive white student expressed it: "A black publication actually is one which helps establish the black identity and serves the black community."[7]

These functions and different kinds of content are, of course, not unique to the black press. The newspapers and magazines of any nation or any minority group have more or less the same purposes if not the same content. The black press differs from the white not so much in kind as in message and in quality. It often reports news not covered by other journalism. It interprets that news differently, from an uncommon standpoint. It ventures opinions about matters not dealt with by other presses and its opinions frequently vary from those of other publications treating the same topics. The reporting and writing, for understandable reasons to be explored in this book, often are superficial; the editing frequently is careless; the printing, especially of the newspapers, is slovenly in many instances.

By and large, the physical patterns of these papers and magazines are like those of others in the U.S.A. The newspapers, at a glance, look like any to be found on the ordinary display. The main news—or news that will sell papers or hold readers—is on the first page; other news stories are scattered throughout the rest of the paper. An editorial page has all the usual characteristics of such pages: two or three essays on local or national affairs down the left; to their right a cartoon on some national topic or event involving black citizens; and columns and letters to the editor in other areas of the page. The columnists frequently are one or two of the nationally syndicated or otherwise regularly available black leaders such as Louis E. Martin, Roy Wilkins, Bayard Rustin, or Benjamin E. Mays. Local columnists abound.

One or two pages may be devoted each to sports, church, society, and entertainment news. A good deal of this often is obvious publicity material. Occasionally columnists appear on sports and society pages. Syndicated copy, obtained from one of the few black feature companies or, more likely, a regular white-oriented one, and news from United Press International (the latter a white agency), or in some instances radical services such as Liberation News Service, appear sparingly, and chiefly in the larger papers. Some of the little weeklies are hardly more than composites of lifted material, with datelines and the symbol showing the source chopped out before the item is pasted for photo-offset reproduction. The rest is advertising, both classified and display. Space is being bought by large corporations as well as by local enterprises seeking to employ blacks but the bulk of the space is filled by the ads of small firms or service-oriented businesses.

Tabloid size is becoming more common among black newspapers, particularly because many of the new community weeklies use that dimension. A national cross-section study of seventy-nine papers made by the author in 1970 revealed that thirty-five were tabloids. Magazines are mainly of two sizes, eight by twelve inches (or newsmagazine) and the six by nine inches used by scholarly journals. But in the numerous variations are the large, flat *Ebony* and *Sepia,* similar to *Life* and *Look,* and the pocket-sized *Black World.* Letterpress remains dominant as a printing method but photo-offset reproduction, especially with new publications, is taking hold rapidly. Of a 1970 sampling that included two dozen new papers, approximately half the total were printed by the newer method.

The magazines are too varied for a single description, the *Negro History Bulletin* having little in common with *Soul! Illustrated.* Just as the newspapers resemble the white counterparts, the magazines, type by type, are much like periodicals for whites serving the same function. *Sepia* is like *Look* or *Life,* superficially. *Phylon* resembles the serious literary and public affairs quarterlies of the *Southern Review* type.

● POINTS OF VIEW

The opinions of these publications, since they descended from a press known for its strong protest function, have in common certain positions. But beyond these particular uniform beliefs there is great variety. It goes without saying that pleas and demands for greater recognition of civil rights can be heard from all except a few dissidents and the highly specialized, technical publications, and even they have their say on the subject now and then.

On racial matters the black press is by and large vigorously outspoken. Although the publications have the same goals, they differ considerably in how they propose to achieve them.

By and large, on most national issues aside from race, the bigger publications are socially and politically conservative or moderate but not reactionary. More liberal viewpoints are to be found in the small community weeklies, the publications of militants, and some of the purely opinion publications than in the big-circulation newspapers and periodicals. Although traditionally loyal to the Republican Party, more and more of the black press members in the past decade turned their support to the Democratic Party, led to that viewpoint by

President John F. Kennedy, Vice-President and then President Lyndon B. Johnson, Vice-President Hubert H. Humphrey, and Senator Robert F. Kennedy. The newspapers have been the principal purveyors of direct editorial opinion. The magazines, since they are issued on a different frequency, with some exceptions either avoid commitment on current issues or find it impractical to have a timely position on any subject outside the publication's realm.   ●

2. THE BEGINNINGS

THE BLACK PRESS in the U.S.A. is approximately half the age of the white press, having begun in 1827, when the white press already had existed 137 years.

Particularly during the early period—1827 to the Civil War—the black press was a leader of protest against injustices to the race; not only that, it was a journalism almost totally committed to a cause. After 1865, however, it began to resemble the white press in its divisions: some publications continuing to crusade for more freedom, others supporting reaction, and still others interesting themselves more in profits than in social progress.

Earl Conrad, a white journalist who worked for the black press in the 1940's, saw that press of the 1830–60 period not merely as a crusader against slavery but also as "the spiritual ancestor of the essentially agitational press of this day [1946] but possibly of the modern labor and radical press," he wrote. It was not a community press in the sense that it did not exist exclusively for the Negro group, he added.[1]

These first publications, despite the African descent of their originators, were modeled after European publications, especially the British, as were all American papers and magazines. No evidence of African influence is apparent; in fact, the first newspaper in West Africa, homeland of many slaves, was founded by Charles L. Force, who went to Monrovia, Liberia, from the U.S.A. He brought with him a hand-run press given him by the Massachusetts Colonization Society of Boston and on it, in 1826, printed a four-page monthly paper, the *Liberia Herald*.[2] He died a few months later and the paper was suspended. But it was revived in 1830 by John B. Russwurm, who was one of the two founders of the first American black paper.

Russwurm had joined with Samuel E. Cornish in bringing out America's first black publication; their *Freedom's Journal* originally was issued in New York City as a means of answering attacks on blacks by another newspaper of that city, the white New York *En-*

quirer. Penn, one of the few historians of black journalism, wrote that the attacking paper was edited by "an Afro-American-hating Jew" who "encouraged slavery and deplored the thought of freedom for the slave" and "made the vilest attacks upon the Afro-Americans."[3] Editor of the *Enquirer* at the time was Mordecai M. Noah.

Although it had newspaper format, the black weekly, whose first issue was dated March 16, 1827, was in content more of a magazine than a newspaper. On the first page of one issue, for example, appear three articles: "Memoirs of Capt. Paul Cuffee," "People of Colour," and "Cure for Drunkenness," none of which can be said to be news. The masthead carried the sentence, "Righteousness Exalteth a Nation." Its columns, as Conrad describes them so well, "were packed with a religious wrath."

The little paper must have been aimed mainly at white readers, since the literacy rate of blacks in the early part of the nineteenth century was low. It is likely that the editors wished to influence the whites, for they were in a position to help free the black man. Doubtless, also, the publishers needed white support, since blacks were not able to help financially.

The two founders and their associates were not experienced journalists. Russwurm, whose name now is borne by both a Harlem public school and a national award given each year by black publishers, was the first black college graduate, receiving a degree from Bowdoin the year before he helped begin *Freedom's Journal.* Later, when he left the paper, he went to Liberia; there are hints that he was dragooned. There he earned his living as a teacher and school administrator but also embarked again on journalism with the *Liberia Herald.* At his death in 1851 he was governor of the Colony of Maryland at Cape Palmas, Liberia.

The two men disagreed over the question of colonizing blacks, Cornish opposing it and Russwurm favoring. As a result, six months after they had launched *Freedom's Journal* Cornish resigned, and Russwurm ran it alone. Within a year, however, Russwurm had left for Liberia, and Cornish returned, changing the paper's name to *Rights of All* in May, 1829. It continued to plead for Afro-American freedom and citizenship. Penn records that it suspended publication in 1830;[4] Pride, a more careful and more recent historian, reports that the last issue extant is dated October 9, 1829.[5]

● **OTHER EARLY PUBLICATIONS**

Cornish, a free black man and Presbyterian clergyman, edited or published other black papers. After he left *Freedom's Journal* to stay, he edited the *Weekly Advocate,* sometimes considered the second black publication because of its tenure. Like its predecessor, it was a New York City paper, and had to rely on the abolitionist movement for support. It, too, went through a change of name. It had many editors in a short time. It first appeared in January, 1837, but in two months became the *Colored American*. As the *Advocate* it was managed by Phillip A. Bell, who was to have something of a career in black journalism, and published by a Canadian, Robert Sears. Financial support, Penn records, came from the anti-slavery movement, including such leaders as Lewis Tappan of the silk merchant family, an organizer of a large abolitionist society. When Cornish left, the editorship went successively to James McCune Smith, an Edinburgh University graduate, and Charles Bennett Ray, a clergyman. There is evidence that it had a Philadelphia edition; if so, it was the first black paper to serve more than one community with separate editions.[6]

The number of publications issued by blacks before the Civil War has been verified as "forty or more."[7] These, the scholar who verified them observes, were journalistic vehicles for views and feelings that, until then, had expression in chants, spoken poems, folk songs, hymns, orations, and sermons, all unprinted forms. Even many of the journalistic publications issued after 1827 were hardly more than pamphlets and were short-lived; thus the career of the *Weekly Advocate-Colored American*, 1837–42, was unusual.

The names of many publications that followed reveal the anti-slavery aims: *Alienated American, Mirror of Liberty*, the *Elevator, Freeman's Advocate, Palladium of Liberty*, the *Genius of Freedom* and *Herald of Freedom*. Most were from New York State. The rest were organized in other northern or western areas. They contained so much opinion rather than news (with their concentration on propaganda for the anti-slavery movement), that they were of far more consequence as persuaders than as news organs.

● **THE *RAM'S HORN***

Although it lasted only a year, the *Ram's Horn* symbolizes the conditions which gave rise to many black publications over the years. Penn relates that in 1846 the New York *Sun* published editorials proposing the curbing of Negro suffrage in that state. A black man, Willis A. Hodges, wrote a reply which was published only when he agreed to pay fifteen dollars and run it as an advertisement. At that, its sentiments were modified. Hodges was told by a staff member, when he protested the changes in his reply, that "The *Sun* shines for all white men, and not for colored men." If he wanted the Afro-American cause advocated, he was told, he would have to publish his own paper.[8] In 1847 Hodges established the *Ram's Horn*.

His partner in the venture was Thomas Van Rensselaer; neither had capital with which to work, so Hodges agreed to raise money and write for the paper. He spent two months earning what was needed by doing whitewashing. He paid for the first issue and wrote its first article. January 1, 1847, saw publication of 3,000 copies, with the motto, "We are men, and therefore interested in whatever concerns men." A weekly, it had as contributors a distinguished black journalist, Frederick Douglass, and a noted white fighter for blacks, John Brown, although Penn wrote that Douglass did little writing but mainly lent his prestige to the paper as editor in name if not in fact.

Penn reports that it reached 2,500 subscribers and survived until 1848, Hodges having withdrawn in a dispute and Rensselaer remaining as editor and owner for its last few issues. Penn called it a strong anti-slavery paper that "had done good work for the race, in whose special interest it was run."

● DOUGLASS AND THE *NORTH STAR*

In its forty-third issue the *Ram's Horn* carried a prospectus for a new anti-slavery paper, to be called the *North Star*. A weekly to come from Rochester, New York, it was to sell for two dollars a year (if paid in advance, fifty cents more if not within six months) and to be published by Frederick Douglass.

The *Ram's Horn* was the first of a series of newspapers and magazines edited or published by Douglass, the great journalistic and oratorical hero of American blacks and one of the outstanding leaders in their struggle for freedom. He set forth the platform for his new paper thus:

"The object of the *North Star* will be to attack slavery in all its forms and aspects, advocate Universal Emancipation; exact the standard of public morality; promote the moral and intellectual improvement of the colored people; and to hasten the day of freedom to our three million enslaved fellow countrymen."[9]

November 1, 1847, saw the paper born. It was the *North Star* until 1851 when it was merged with the *Liberty Party Paper* and renamed *Frederick Douglass' Paper*. Doubtless that is what everyone actually called it, for he was by then a widely known and admired lecturer. Douglass said he did it to distinguish it from the many other papers with *Star* in their names.

The $2,175 with which the paper was established came from English friends. It cost two dollars an issue to produce and had an average circulation of 3,000. Assisting at first as an editor was Martin R. Delaney, who had edited and published the Pittsburgh *Mystery* and was the first black graduate of Harvard. Delaney, sometimes considered the original black nationalist, began the *Mystery* when he was thirty-one and edited it from 1843 to 1847. He met Douglass when the orator visited Pittsburgh in 1847. After six months he parted with Douglass, leaving journalism to study medicine, and went on to a career of importance in that field. He wrote books also, including at least one novel.[10]

Douglass not only met local opposition in Rochester from anti-black elements but also after a time the plague that besets black journalism even today set in upon him, lack of both money and staff help. With the aid of his sons and many friends, however, he kept the paper alive until 1860, pouring into it what money he could make in public speaking, at which he excelled, and writing.

Several inches larger overall than the regular eight-column standard newspaper of today, *Frederick Douglass' Paper* would not be considered particularly readable. Each of its four pages contained six wide columns packed solid with type; its front page usually carrying no breaks except spaces between its small headlines. It consisted largely of abolitionist material, looking and sounding much like the *Liberator*. But that was the journalistic vogue. The vigor of Douglass' writing and the excitement of the times compensated to some extent for the lack of typographic attractiveness.

● FREDERICK DOUGLASS

The words and works of Frederick Douglass appeared for many decades chiefly in biographies written by blacks and anthologies of black writing edited by black scholars and literary people. White authors and scholars usually relegated him to the footnotes. But in recent years children's books about him have been issued, his autobiography has been republished, estimates of his importance and contribution have appeared, as have new biographies and collections of his writings. Two motion pictures based on his life are reported to be in preparation; the U.S. government has issued a postage stamp carrying his portrait. The emphasis today has not been upon his journalism as much as upon his leadership of his race, which is as it should be, for he was only secondarily a journalist, although an extremely active one. Whatever the emphasis, his story is extraordinary.

Originally his name was not Douglass but Lloyd. He was born in Maryland in 1817 or 1818 (he was unsure of the year, as slaves' children often were) of a slave owned by a wealthy planter, one Colonel Edward Lloyd. His mother was Harriet Bailey. As was the custom, he bore his master's name. The boy knew nothing about his father, as slave children often did not. But Colonel Lloyd was gossiped as the father; in his autobiography Douglass allows the reader to think that the colonel might indeed have been his parent.[11]

Until he was seven he was reared by his grandmother, and then taken to the plantation home. There for three years he saw the cruelty with which slaves were treated, sights that never left his memory. When he turned ten he was sent to Baltimore to live with a relative of the Lloyd family. There he learned to read and write a little, taught secretly by the mistress of the house. But when the white master found out he prohibited his wife from continuing the lessons to the slave boy.

Douglass soon was allowed to hire himself out. He earned three dollars a week as a shipbuilder's employe. While doing such work he tried many times to escape slavery, succeeding finally in 1838 and fleeing to Philadelphia. From there he went to New York and New England, taking laboring jobs. He used the name Lloyd, but after several years took the name Bailey, was married, and continued work as a laborer. He shortly assumed the name he retained for life: Douglass. At about the same time he came to know a man who was to influence his life sharply: William Lloyd Garrison, the abolitionist-journalist. Garrison helped educate him and encouraged him to become a writer and author, Douglass having improved his reading and writing ability while working.

Douglass' first public writing was letters to newspapers, in which he attacked slavery. As Quarles and some of his earlier biographers point out, his experiences on the plantation provided him with graphic examples of the effect of the system. He also attended anti-slavery meetings; at these he had opportunities to demonstrate his oratorical ability, beginning a public speaking career which was to bring him to international fame. In 1845 he went to Europe to lecture there, stirring opposition to the evil he was fighting. Still a slave, he was in constant danger of recapture by Colonel Lloyd. Realizing this, English Quaker friends collected $750 and in 1846 bought his freedom.

Upon his return to the U.S.A. the next year, Douglass went to Rochester, beginning the venture which most entitled him to a place in American journalistic history but which is scarcely mentioned in the volumes on that history. His editorship of the *North Star–Frederick Douglass' Paper* was interrupted in 1859 when he was rumored to have been involved in the John Brown raid and threatened with arrest. Friends spirited him to Canada; from there he went to England. After the threat died down he returned and resurrected the paper. In it he urged Lincoln to use black troops and to issue a proclamation of emancipation. By now he had come to oppose the Garrisonites, many of whom had failed to support his publications because of disagreement over policies in combatting slavery. He refused to believe, as did most abolitionists, that the Constitution was pro-slavery per se. He also had no confidence in the view that politics was unavailing in fighting slavery. He wanted to use the Constitution and the democratic right to vote as weapons against evil.[12]

Douglass again gave his name to a publication when in mid-1860 he issued *Douglass' Monthly*, a magazine aimed mainly at British readers and devoted largely to abolitionist material. It came to an end three years later. As the magazine began the newspaper ceased, deeply in debt and almost devoid of support. Little sustenance was coming from whites and virtually none from blacks—who were in no economic condition to provide it in any case.

For the next decade Douglass devoted his time largely to lecturing and working with labor and political groups, at which he was impressively successful. A big man, with a powerful voice, he was an eloquent speaker invited everywhere in the fight of the black man for justice. In his prime he resembled Mark Twain or Walt Whitman, for he had a striking head and beard of white hair.

Douglass returned to journalism in 1870. A new weekly, the *New Era,* appeared in Washington, with Douglass as corresponding editor. It was devoted to righting the wrongs against black people. But it soon, despite Douglass' warnings, went into debt deeply. Douglass rescued it by buying a half interest, changing its name to *New National Era* and assuming its editorship.

Its policies, he wrote, were: "Free men, free soil, free speech, a free press, everywhere in the land. The ballot for all, education for all, fair wages for all." He published many of his own articles on issues confronting the black citizens in the 1870's. But by late 1874 it failed again; it had absorbed another paper, *New Citizen,* but the financial panic of 1873 was too much and Douglass' two sons, who had bought it, could not save it, even by making it anti-union and a Republican Party voice. It ceased in 1875,[13] Douglass saying later "This misadventure"—it had cost him $10,000—had been a useful investment, for from the experience he had learned to stay out of newspaper work, which he did thereafter. His main interest became his activities in government appointments.

Douglass died in Anacostia Heights, D.C., in 1895, aged seventy-eight. His Washington home has become a shrine; in 1969 the House of Representatives passed a bill appropriating $338,000 to rehabilitate it.

What was his contribution to journalism? He had a clear idea of what it might be, as he explained it in one of his several autobiographies in a passage written just before he launched his major publication:

> The grand thing to be done, therefore, was to change the estimation in which the colored people of the U.St. were held; to remove the prejudice which depreciated and depressed them; to prove them worthy of a higher consideration; to disprove their alleged inferiority, and demonstrate their capacity for a more exalted civilization than salary and prejudice had assigned to them. I further stated that, in my judgment, a tolerably well conducted press, by calling out the mental energies of the race itself; by making them acquainted with their own latent powers; by enkindling among them the hope that for them there is a future; by developing their moral power, by combining and reflecting their talents would prove a most powerful means of removing prejudice, and of awakening an interest in them. I further informed them—and at that time the statement was true—that there was not, in the United States, a single newspaper regularly published by the colored people; that many attempts had been made to establish such papers; but that, up to that time, they had all failed. These views I laid before my friends. The result was, nearly 2,500 dollars were speedily raised toward starting my paper.[14]

In spite of his difficulties, he was to persist, and in the long run be successful. For it was not a small accomplishment, in those pre-Civil War years, to keep a black paper which we now would call an example of advocacy (or militant) journalism alive for more than a dozen years. It was an encouragement to other black publishers; it went on to be a source of inspiration for dozens of others to follow, even today.

Clearly the positions Douglass took in his papers provided leadership against the slavery system. And, although he differed later with other abolitionist leaders, his editorials and articles helped clarify the direction in which the movement was going.

Thus Frederick Douglass fulfilled several of the traditional functions of the newspaper publisher: he provided information as well as guidance and encouraged others to continue with their efforts.

● THE EARLY MAGAZINES

Although little news appeared in these early papers and much of the material that did appear was of the kind now usually bound into magazines of opinion, they are classified generally as newspapers rather than periodicals because of their appearance, frequency of issue, and their habit of calling themselves news organs. Charles S. Johnson, a black scholar and editor, has observed that the first black publications were like magazines. But there were orthodox periodicals of a type other than *Douglass' Monthly*. Conflicting claims exist about which was first, largely revolving around whether it was one of broad or specialized appeal. Johnson notes that the first with a black editor was the *National Reformer*, the monthly issued by the American Moral Reform Society of Philadelphia.[15] Because it had more white readers than black and was intended for abolitionist readers and had integrated ownership and management, it is not by definition a black magazine. Penn records 1833 as its year of first issue; Johnson gives 1838.

A general magazine edited and owned by blacks and aimed at black readers was the *Mirror of Liberty*, a quarterly issued in New York City, edited by David Ruggles. It lasted from 1847 to 1849. It was not the first magazine, however, for from the black church denominations came several, including the *African Methodist Episcopal Church Magazine*, a short-lived quarterly started in September, 1841, but halted in the following December, and published from Brooklyn.

Another early one was the *Christian Herald*, later called the *Christian Recorder*. It grew, as did so many church periodicals and newspapers, out of the common goals of the black church and the black press. Like white church publications of the time, some of this religious journalism for blacks ventured into social problems. The *Herald*, a Pittsburgh publication sponsored by the African Methodist

Episcopal Church, had grown out of *Mystery*, the Pittsburgh paper edited by Douglass' aide, Delaney. Founded in 1848 as a quarterly, after four years it was moved to Philadelphia, where the name change occurred and it was issued each week.[16] As the *Recorder* it was to continue into the twentieth century and rank among the longest-lived of black publications. Penn called it a bishop-maker among church periodicals, for Jabez Campbell, its first editor according to Penn, later rose to the episcopacy, as did his successor, John M. Brown.[17] It was being published in newspaper format in Nashville, Tennessee, in 1970, and claiming seniority among black church weeklies.

Subsidy, as with many religious publications still, was the only practical means of financing magazines like the *Recorder*. That circumstance accounts for the existence, over the years, of numerous church, lodge, club, educational, and college publications. Detweiler records that in some states even these relatively innocuous publications suffered from the fact that blacks were not allowed to go to school or read papers, magazines, and books.[18] It was one reason for the scarcity of publications before Emancipation.

During the Civil War establishment of new publications naturally fell off. Penn and other early writers were able to discover only one black paper founded between 1860 and 1865, the *Colored Citizen* of Cincinnati; it died once the conflict ended. But there were others. An important one, significant because it was the first to be established in the South, was *L'Union* of New Orleans, a French-English weekly started in 1862. The next year it became a tri-weekly, but could not survive past 1864.[19]

● AFTER THE CIVIL WAR

When the Civil War ended there was a rush to establish new black publications. Pride's study shows that a dozen were begun just from April, 1865, to January, 1866; half were in the South, the first real breakthrough for that area.[20]

During the decade after 1865, black newspapers sprang up in eight states that had had none and in four others that already had papers. From 1875 to 1895, more were founded, for this was a period of migration to the north. In 1887 alone 68 papers were begun. And by 1890, according to Pride, 575 had been established. Many of these were intended to be regular newspapers, but various other types of black publications were born as well, some as political organs, others to serve churches or other special groups. One of the religious papers survives. The *Star of Zion* of the African Methodist Episcopal Zion Church, begun in 1867, today is a tabloid newspaper published for the denomination in Charlotte, North Carolina.

Another paper that reached into the next century, although unlike the *Star of Zion* it lacked subsidy and so did not live, was the Wash-

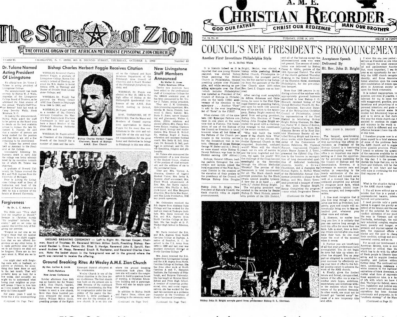

FIG. 2.1. Newspapers issued by two of the long-established black church denominations.

ington *Bee* which was published from 1882 to 1926. Founded by William Calvin Chase, who had edited the Washington *Plaindealer* from 1879 to 1881, and the *Argus* from 1880 to 1883, the *Bee* left "a record for endurance, forthrightness, and racial appeal," Pride observes.[21] And Penn wrote that "Nothing stings Washington City, and in fact, the Bourbons of the South, as the *Bee*." A weekly, during its forty-four years Chase made it an exciting if bitter paper. He was fond of exposés. He took sides on many subjects; his position always was clear if not consistent.

The war's end meant not only more publications but also a change in their content. The dominating subject of slavery was replaced with material of great variety. Immediately at the end of the war, for example, a Friday publication, using the name of an earlier, Albany, New York, paper, the *Elevator,* was launched in San Francisco by Phillip A. Bell, who had managed the *Colored American* some years before. It contained material on science, art, literature, and drama.

Another new element was illustrated by a paper issued later in 1865 by Republican party members in Augusta, Georgia. The *Colored American* again was to serve as the flag of a newspaper "designed," as its prospectus put it, "to be a vehicle for the diffusion of Religious, Political, and General Intelligence." The new element in this publication's formula was the plan to devote it "to the promotion of harmony and good-will between the white and colored people of the South. . . ." It was to cost four dollars a year, a reflection of the rise in expenses. Its publisher, however, had bad luck with his share-holders and the paper was sold in 1886 and its name changed to the *Loyal Georgian*. After two years it was merged with the *Georgia Republican*.

In certain other states postwar papers came into being quickly and were serving black readers of different sections. Among the earlier ones noted by Penn were the *Colored Tennessean* and the *True Communicator,* the latter of Baltimore. Neither survived for long nor, for that matter, did many of those in the rush to the presses. Among the more important new black papers was the *New Orleans Louisianian,* the first to be issued twice a week; *Our National Progress,* of Wilmington, Delaware; the *Progressive American,* of New York; the *Argus* of Washington, and the *Western Sentinel* of Kansas City, Missouri.

Penn included in his account a table showing the growth in the number of papers by states from 1880 to 1890. Texas began with one and a decade later had fifteen, according to the tabulation. Georgia went from none to ten; Pennsylvania, Virginia, and Alabama each added nine to their original one publication. In 1880, Penn calculated, there were thirty-one publications; at the end of the following decade 123 had been added, for a total of 154.[22] Years later Pride was to prove that many more were founded but that most did not survive to 1890.

Six reasons for the upsurge of black papers after the Civil War have been given by Pride.[23] The black populace was becoming better educated; freedmen were able to earn a little more; social service and other groups gave financial support to the press; religious organizations entered journalism to advance their views; the blacks able to vote provided an audience for politically sponsored publications; the last, suggested to Pride by Rashey B. Moten Jr.'s thesis at the University of Kentucky, was that it was realized that the editor of a paper is a person of wider influence than some other professionals.

To these reasons can be added the fact that social changes other than the end of slavery and war were affecting the black citizens at this time as well. During the Reconstruction years blacks were pushed into ghettos in the larger cities of both North and South. Segregation became the enforced way of life for them. Conrad, commenting on this change, observes that it led to a community-conscious press devoted to protest against discrimination as well as to reporting the minutae of black life.[24]

Such protest kept the papers alive when other content failed, as in the instance of the Chicago *Defender* (see Chapters 3 and 4), which lived on scandal and crime stories for a time but did not thrive until it became the champion of the black people.

● WOMEN JOURNALISTS OF THE PERIOD

The women journalists of the black race in America who have achieved distinction through their accomplishments on newspapers are largely those of the present century. Perhaps "attention" is a more nearly fair word than "distinction," for the women editors and writers of the nineteenth century have been ignored, as journalists, by almost all who have written on black journalism. An exception is I. Garland Penn. His writing is so gushy, however, that it is impossible for one reading his history today to depend upon his judgments. At least he exhibited a sensitivity about a minority within a minority. A sixty-page chapter in his *Afro-American Press and Its Editors* tells the stories, in his usual somewhat florid style, of nineteen women engaged in black journalism in this period. An example of his style is this portion on Professor Mary V. Cook, chiefly a teacher who in the 1880's and 1890's wrote columns for the *American Baptist* and the *South Carolina Tribune* and edited a magazine, *Our Women and Children:* "There is a divine poetry in a life garlanded by the fragrant roses of triumph."[25]

Far more active than Professor Cook was Mrs. W. E. Mathews, who during the same years wrote under the name of Victoria Earle. She freelanced to the New York *Times,* New York *Herald,* New York *Sunday Mercury* and several lesser known papers; she was New York correspondent for the Detroit *Plaindealer, National Leader,* and *Southern Christian Recorder* as well as contributor to others. Among the better-known black papers in which her work appeared were the Washington *Bee,* New York *Globe,* Boston *Advocate,* New York *Enterprise,* and Cleveland *Gazette.* The Associated Press used her copy and several magazines bought her fiction.

Possibly the one woman journalist of the nineteenth century remembered in this century was Mrs. Ida B. Wells-Barnett. Penn compares her to the once internationally known Mrs. Frank Leslie, widow of the English editor whose name was on various versions of a once highly popular illustrated magazine during and after the Civil War. Bontemps and Conroy, writing many years after both Penn and Mrs. Barnett had died, have provided a little sketch of her career. A Mississippian born about 1869, she was left by her parents' death to support four (Penn says five) younger brothers and sisters when she was 14. She worked but also studied. After a time, at Fisk University, her interest in journalism cropped out when she wrote for the student paper. She then became a Memphis teacher but continued her journalism by writing for a local black paper, the *Living Way.* She was Ida B. Wells but used only Iola in her by-line. In the ensuing years she wrote for many other black publications and also entered publishing by becoming half-owner as well as editor of the Memphis *Free Speech,* a black paper that campaigned against racial injustice.

In 1892, however, her paper's plant was sacked because it had carried accusations that white competitors had inspired the murder of three black business men. The hoodlums, Bontemps and Conroy relate, demolished the press and the paper's offices. Miss Wells had to move from the city to save her life. Because she had been free-lancing to the New York *Age* she went to that paper, then published by T. T. Fortune. She worked also with Douglass and William Monroe Trotter in their anti-slavery enterprises. Like Douglass she made a strong impression when she lectured against lynching in the British Isles. In the mid-1890's she settled in Chicago, organizing various women's clubs and kindergartens. Anti-lynching leagues were formed after her lectures in both Britain and the U.S.A. She continued to write for both the black and white press, particularly the Chicago *Inter-Ocean*. In 1895 she married Ferdinand L. Barnett, a lawyer and part-owner of the first black newspaper in Illinois, the *Conservator*. After their wedding they continued to fight racial injustice and Mrs. Barnett began planning an ambitious political and teaching career, but in 1931, aged 62, she died suddenly. Nine years later a large low-rent housing project in Chicago was named for her; certain women's groups carry her name today.[26]

3. BLACK JOURNALISM ENTERS THE TWENTIETH CENTURY

SOME OF THE most important papers extant were launched just before or after the turn of the century, as the American black press became better established. More newspapers were founded as commercial ventures and to serve as news rather than propaganda organs, but cause papers continued to appear as well. Some weeklies were to become leading papers in later years. The magazines, however, were by and large still organs of opinion or of organizations rather than vehicles of entertainment.

The turn of the century saw the rise of several important black leaders in American history—men able and skillful enough to use journalism as a tool to support their causes and views.

● THE PHILADELPHIA *TRIBUNE*

The Philadelphia *Tribune,* which considers itself the oldest continuously published black newspaper in the country, was organized in 1884 by Chris J. Perry, Sr. One of the most substantial of the black papers, it owns its own plant and engages in various public enterprises, such as charities and scholarship programs (see Chapter 14). After Perry died in 1921, the paper was published by his widow and two of his daughters. The husband of one, E. Washington Rhodes, a lawyer, was publisher and editor until his death in 1970. Rhodes had taken a decided position about the black race, singling out what he called "affluent middle-class Negroes" because they did not in his opinion do enough to help the poor.

● THE *AFRO-AMERICAN*

The *Afro-American* is the name for a Baltimore paper with five editions, four regional and one national, which have made it one of the oldest and most powerful black journalistic institutions in the United

States.[1] Like so many other black papers, the *Afro,* as it is called by most readers, had its origin in religious circles. Three Baltimore church people figured in its first few years. The first was the Rev. William M. Alexander, who had started a provisions store in the city. Wanting to advertise Sharon Baptist Church and community enterprises, he published on August 13, 1892 a four-page paper to which he gave the name, *Afro-American.*

Another churchman, a layman who was superintendent of the Sunday School in St. John African Methodist Episcopal Church in the same city, wanted all such black church schools to organize statewide, as did the white groups called the Epworth League and the Christian Endeavor Society. This man was John H. Murphy, Sr., a whitewasher by trade. He, too, thought a publication would be a force for achieving his aim. He bought type fonts and a press; from the cellar of his home in Baltimore he printed *Sunday School Helper,* a small paper.

A third man printed a paper with the same purposes as the Rev. Mr. Alexander's, calling it the *Ledger.* This editor was the Rev. George F. Bragg, pastor of St. James Episcopal Church.

Murphy acquired the *Afro* by borrowing $200 from his wife and buying it at auction; it had a circulation of 250. When in 1907 the *Afro* was merged with the *Ledger* it was called the *Afro-American Ledger.* Murphy was publisher and Bragg wrote the editorials. For the publisher it became a lifetime occupation, for he owned the paper until his death in 1922; his family continues it still.[2] It went first into the hands of a son, Carl Murphy; by then it had gained recognition as a national publication. D. Arnett Murphy, still another of John Murphy's sons, served as vice-president and advertising manager. A grandson, Howard E. Murphy, was business manager. Mrs. Elizabeth Murphy Moss, a granddaughter, was at one time assistant managing editor and a war correspondent, and today is a vice-president and the treasurer of the firm as well as general editorial supervisor. John H. Murphy III now is president, succeeding Carl Murphy at his death in 1967.

The *Afro* has during its history followed a policy of moderation in direct editorial opinions and an emphasis on news coverage as a tool with which to inform and mold public opinion. A credo formulated in 1920 by John H. Murphy, Sr., and published regularly since on its editorial pages sets its tone (see Chapter 8).

● **IN NEW YORK AND CALIFORNIA**

Booker T. Washington frequently is linked with the *New York Age,* a prominent weekly that stemmed from a downtown New York tabloid, the *Rumor,* begun in 1890. In 1903, Washington said he believed that a strong national Negro paper was needed. Remaining behind the scenes, he began to subsidize the *Age* and by 1907 had completed purchase of the weekly. "His influence over the Negro press was achieved by loans, advertising, printing orders and political subsidies," wrote one of Washington's critics. "He saw to it that critical papers received editorial material favorable to his cause and at times was even able to disrupt the distribution of such publications."[3]

Because of Washington's connection with the paper it was severely criticized by W. E. B. Du Bois and other black leaders who disagreed with a philosophy that they believed condemned the black man to segregation and subservience to whites.

In its earlier, less controversial days the paper, as *Rumor,* called itself "A Representative Colored American Newspaper" and was published by George Parker, who changed it from a twelve-page tabloid to standard size and renamed it the New York *Globe.* As *Rumor* it carried news, verse, short stories, and articles; its first page usually was a woodcut of some black leader; on one occasion it was Douglass. Parker took on two partners, W. Walter Sampson and T. Thomas Fortune, who was to become a leading figure in black journalism.[4] In a few years Parker sold his interest to Bishop William B. Derrick. But the bishop could not pay his share so the paper went into the hands of the marshal. Fortune took over as sole owner in 1884 and changed the name once more, to the *Freeman.* After also withdrawing for a time he returned in 1888; by now it had become the *New York Age.* On rejoining it, Fortune became co-owner with Fred R. Moore, as well as editor. Moore bought Fortune's share in 1907, continuing to publish it until 1943, and it remained in the Moore family after his death that year. During Moore's regime the paper exposed the Ku Klux Klan before white papers brought that organization's actions into the open. Moore, however, was better known for his business and political activities than his journalism. He worked in New York banks, in 1893 organized the Afro-American Building and Loan Company, and in 1903 was elected national organizer of the National Negro Business League, four years before joining the *Age* staff. He once was U.S. minister to Liberia.[5] A later editor who became even more widely known was James Weldon Johnson, the poet.

A white couple, Mr. and Mrs. V. P. Bourne-Vanneck, of England, bought the *Age* in 1949; the Chicago *Defender* took it over from them in 1952 and merged with it; for a time the *Defender*'s New York edition was called the *Age-Defender,* but within a few years the *Age* name no longer appeared in the flag.

Another paper which made some, if less, impression, and which did not survive was the *California Eagle,* founded in 1879 in Los Angeles. Of standard size, it became the property in recent years of a leader of the NAACP, Loren Miller, but he sold it in 1964 when he was appointed a municipal judge. It ceased in 1967.[6]

● T. THOMAS FORTUNE

In any occupation there always is someone who, during the latter part of his life is called "the dean" of whatever it may be. T. Thomas Fortune was one of those so dubbed. Ottley, the biographer of Robert S. Abbott and author of several essays on the black press, wrote that Fortune was in his time considered the dean of black journalism in America. Fortune, along with Frederick Douglass and William Monroe Trotter, is recalled almost a century later, unlike most black journalists of the past. He deserved Ottley's title because he had a far greater background of professional experience than most of his contemporaries and was treated as a spokesman for the black press. He came of slave parents, and was a boy of all errands in a southern white newspaper office. After working as a mail agent and then a special inspector of customs in Delaware, he went to work in a composing room, and then joined *Rumor*. Meanwhile he was an assistant to Amos Cummings on the New York *Evening Sun* and later wrote for the companion daily, the New York *Sun,* when the noted Charles Anderson Dana was its editor.[7]

Many years later, in a magazine article, Fortune recalled his early journalism.

> When I entered upon the active work of journalism, in New York City in 1879, my partner and I were the first to set the type of the *Globe*. At night we prepared the forms for the press, and in the day we worked as compositors. Mr. William Walter Sampson and I had worked together as compositors on a daily newspaper, now the *Daily Times-Union,* at Jacksonville, Florida. Through him I secured a position on the *Daily Witness* in New York. Here I found my previous experience of great value, for it had been my good fortune to have met and collaborated with such men as John W. Cromwell, Charles N. Otey, and Robert Peel Brooks, among the most brilliant men that the race has ever produced. My acquaintance also included the great Frederick Douglass, the lion of them all. . . .[8]

While editor of the *Age,* Fortune attracted notice in the white press with his editorials. Ottley quotes Theodore Roosevelt as saying: "Tom Fortune, for God's sake, keep that pen of yours off me." Fortune helped Booker T. Washington with the writing of his autobiography. Late in his life he came to believe in the back-to-Africa movement of Marcus Garvey, discussed later in this chapter

● TROTTER AND THE *GUARDIAN*

The first important paper born after the turn of the century was the weekly Boston *Guardian,* founded in 1901 by William Monroe

Trotter and George Forbes. Both were 1895 college graduates, Trotter from Harvard and Forbes from Amherst. A provocative paper, it would now be considered militant. W. E. B. Du Bois, himself a perceptive journalist, described the *Guardian* as "bitter, satirical, and personal . . . well edited . . . earnest, and it publishes facts." He reported also that "it attracted wide attention among colored people; it circulated among them all over the country; it was quoted and discussed." Few blacks agreed with it wholly, he believed.[9]

Of greatest significance was the fact that it was the start of organized opposition to Booker T. Washington. When he came to Boston in 1905 to speak, Trotter and Forbes raised questions with him about his views on black education and voting. The result was "a disturbance," as Du Bois described it, and "a riot" in the view of Boston's white dailies. Trotter was arrested and served a jail term. The whole incident led to a major event in black history in America. Du Bois' resentment of the treatment of Trotter led to forming of what in 1906 became incorporated as the Niagara Movement, so named because its founders originally met near Buffalo, New York. Among its principles were promotion of freedom of speech and criticism and "an unfettered and unsubsidized press." More will be heard of this movement when Du Bois' own career as a journalist is examined.

Trotter also worked for improvement of the lot of the black people through the New England Suffrage League and the National Equal Rights League. Because he had experienced race prejudice he dedicated himself to its defeat through journalism. On one occasion he led a delegation to a personal interview with President Woodrow Wilson to protest prejudice against blacks. This editor's place in black journalism can be gauged from a statement by Lerone Bennett, Jr., a specialist in black history, who credits Trotter with having "laid the first stone of the modern protest movements" and "mobilized the forces that checked the triumphant advance of Booker T. Washington's program of accommodation and submission." Washington replied to the assault on his views by subsidizing another paper to compete with the *Guardian,* Bennett reported.[10]

Unlike many other black journalists who came to positions of power, Trotter was reared in a comparatively luxurious home in a predominantly white Boston suburb, Hyde Park. He was born in 1872, in Chillicothe, Ohio, a son of a white merchant and a former slave. His family moved to Boston when he was a baby. At Harvard he was a cum laude graduate and elected to Phi Beta Kappa, the first black to be accepted by that elite group of scholars. He then completed a two-year master's program in one year. From his father he learned to fight for equality. James Monroe Trotter, while a Union Army lieutenant, led a successful campaign to equalize the pay scales for black and white soldiers. After graduation William Trotter began a real estate business; in 1901 he started his paper. Judging by a 1902 issue, it was one of six columns, with cartoons and halftones and the familiar unbroken columns of type so common in all U.S.A. newspapers in those days.

When the offices were moved into a Boston building where Garrison's *Liberator* once was published, Trotter, an admirer of the abolitionist leader, found this fitting. He spoke out against segregation in federal employment and protested "The Birth of a Nation" film as racist; it then was banned. Bennett calls him the "Boston Cato."

But all was not well with his paper. For a time Trotter had been well off, but in the second decade of the century he and his wife lost their home and lived in poverty; the paper was too great a drain on their resources. He held on through the depression years of the early 1930's but died in 1934, in what was either an accidental fall or suicide. The paper was continued by his sister, Maude, until her death in 1957. An indication of new appreciation of his fight for his people was the naming of a high school for him in 1969 in Roxbury, Massachusetts.[11]

● **ABBOTT AND THE *DEFENDER***

Trotter may have laid the first stones for the modern protest movements but Robert S. Abbott, after a somewhat slow start, built the foundation, using his Chicago *Defender,* now the anchor newspaper in the largest group or chain of black publications in the country and itself one of the only three dailies in black journalism.

Roi Ottley, his biographer, ranks Abbott with "the giants of his time: Booker T. Washington and W. E. B. Du Bois." Abbott's activities and personality were far different from those of the other two men, who were more personally conservative and more politically distinctive. Ottley notes that Abbott was "almost inarticulate" and humble, whereas Du Bois was clearly an intellectual and a considerable egotist. The greatest praise of Abbott came from an influential white scholar, a keen analyst of American life, the Swedish economist Gunnar Myrdal, who considered him, as Ottley summarized it, "the greatest single force in Negro journalism, and indeed the founder of the modern Negro press."[12]

Abbott's background was complex. A Georgian, he was born in 1868 on St. Simons Island. His father, Thomas Abbott, had been head butler in an aristocratic household. His mother was a hairdresser in a Savannah theater. Various relatives worked as servants in Thomas Abbott's employer's household. His family, apparently of Ibo stock, was literate. After the Civil War his parents ran a small grocery store on the island. Thomas, despite his record of service, is reported by Ottley to have neglected his wife, and was not even on the island when Robert was born.

Robert's mother, Flora Butler Abbott, was snubbed by the other

Abbotts. She had learned to speak German, going for a time to a secret slave school; learning that language was to change her and her son's lives. When Thomas Abbott died the family brought legal proceedings against Flora because she refused to surrender her son. John H. H. Sengstacke helped her fight the case and won it for her. Sengstacke was the son of a well-to-do German merchant, Herman Sengstacke, who had married a slave girl in 1847. John was their first child. He was taken to Germany by his father, who did not want his children reared as slaves. When the elder Sengstacke returned to Savannah, he was defrauded of his inheritance and John came to the U.S. to find out why. It was then that he met Flora Abbott and became Robert's stepfather.

As a youth Robert and his seven brothers and sisters (Flora and John's children) lived in a black settlement in Savannah. Robert's first exposure to journalistic work may have come when his step-father became a translator for the city paper, the *Morning News*. His own first newspaper job was in the print shop of the Savannah *Echo*, but he botched it by damaging an imposing stone. After periods at several colleges he went to Hampton Institute, but left in 1888 to resume work at the *Echo*. About this time his stepfather decided to enter the publishing business by founding a paper, the Woodville *Times*. Alexander, a brother of Robert, was editor when the elder Sengstacke died.

At Hampton the future founder of the Chicago *Defender* had studied printing as well as an academic program, which he completed in 1896. During this period he was influenced by Frederick Douglass and Ida B. Wells, two noted black journalists whom he had heard speak. After graduation he became a printer in Woodville and helped get out the *Times*. Printing jobs being hard to get and ill-paid at that, and lack of money having thwarted him in a romance, Robert decided to study law. He took his own father's name, changing from Sengstacke to Abbott. The only black in a class of seventy getting law degrees, he was not admitted to the bar. His search for work in several midwestern cities was no better as lawyer than as printer until 1904, when a political friend pried him into a printing house job despite his color. After his stepfather died Robert resolved to be a teacher, and began in a Woodville school. Journalism continued to beckon, however, so after a time he decided to start his own newspaper.

Founding of the Defender. Abbott selected Chicago because it had a large black population, about 40,000 then. Before the paper was launched in 1905 he had attempted a daily; apparently the two or three numbers issued were scrapped and none has been found. He ignored the fact that the black press field was crowded: Chicago had three already: the *Broad Ax, Illinois Idea,* and the *Conservator.* The black citizens also had access to two important out-of-town papers, the *Indiana Freeman* and the *New York Age.* The goal Abbott had for his paper was to fight for the black race, so he called it the *Defender*. In rented space on State Street he put a card table and a borrowed chair; he arranged for the paper to be printed on credit, since his total capital was twenty-five cents—needed for paper and pencils. His staff was himself, helped by his landlady's teen-age daughter. One early issue of the weekly, now on display at the Chicago *Defender* building, is impressive for so feeble a foundation. The first was dated May 5, 1905, but all copies now are lost. It was, in contrast to its rivals, an offering of news, much of it in the form of personals. Politics and black problems at first were avoided. Paid advertising was there, but not enough. In fact, the paper would have died if Mrs. Lee, Abbott's landlady, had not let him use her dining room as an office, provided his meals, given him money for small expenses, mended his clothes, and let him use her telephone. It remained the paper's address until 1920. These good deeds not only saved the paper but also saw it to prosperity. In time Abbott showed Mrs. Lee his gratitude by giving her the deed to an eight-room house.

With the paper beginning to catch on, Abbott began a policy of muckraking, running campaigns against prostitution in the black community and for black causes. Accompanying the muckraking was a policy of sensationalism, but the use of so many crime and scandal stories brought the paper heavy criticism. During World War I he combined support of the war with the battle for black rights.

The campaign for which Abbott and the *Defender* are best remembered came during and after World War I. When the black soldiers returned it still was obvious that blacks would not be granted first class citizenship, even though many had lost their lives or been wounded. By 1916 the Ku Klux Klan had gained new strength, boasting of its five million members. They and their sympathizers were tarring and feathering, branding, hanging, and burning the black people; in one period in 1919 as many as seventy were lynched.

Abbott had suggested through the paper in 1917 that the blacks come north, pointing out that conditions were better. The paper led in formation of clubs that could get group railroad rates. And north they came. Ottley reported that 110,000 moved to Chicago alone, almost tripling the black population.

One result Abbott had not counted on, however, was the race riots in Chicago after the great migration. He tried to calm the rioters but was not heeded. The *Defender* did not come off well in a report of a commission on race relations, being accused of irresponsible journalism, although complimented for running balanced editorials

The *Defender* nevertheless went on to prosperity, its own presses, and another, larger building. Abbott's personal characteristics now became more evident in his paper's tone: Ottley notes a tendency toward penuriousness, but self-indulgence about automobiles. His policy about black progress, at first militant, gradually changed to one of moderation, in his biographer's opinion. He saw to it that the paper emphasized black accomplishments and abandoned an earlier abrasive tone. It continued, however, to sensationalize crime for the sake of sales. When he was fifty Abbott married and began to travel. He went to Brazil, where he learned of the low status of blacks, which prompted demands for more reforms in the U.S.A., including integration, a stand that lost him supporters. A European trip, in which he met discrimination, moved him to write a series of articles for his paper. Ottley writes that Abbott came to fear personal attack and was cautious when traveling, sometimes disguising himself or using another name.

The Defender Goes On. The *Defender*'s history illustrates the use of sensational treatment of news in order to sell papers. After it no longer was necessary for Pullman porters to bring newspapers from other cities so that Abbott could rely on them for news of the black people, the paper stayed in a leading position primarily because of what then was called race-angling the news. Ottley notes such headlines as "White Gentleman Rapes Colored Girl" and "100 Negroes Murdered Weekly in United States by White Americans," those lines being in red ink. The stories, he discovered, at times were from the imagination of a staff member.

By 1915 the paper was enlarged; branch offices were opened, including one in London. Several thousand agent-correspondents worked to increase sales and gather local news. By that year circulation reached the astonishing figure of at least 230,000, a total found by Ottley's own investigation. Along with this prosperity came evidence of influence, for whites began attacking it as divisive of the races and subversive because it challenged racial traditions. Ottley reported that several cities tried to prevent distribution by confiscation. Ku Klux Klan members threatened owners of copies. Two distributors were killed. A riot broke out in Texas that resulted in whites burning blacks' homes and the public flogging of a black school principal because a black teacher covered a lynching for the paper.

But after World War I circulation dropped gradually to 180,000. By now readers were getting much for their dimes: thirty-two pages, although a few years before it had been four to eight. The circulation decline was to be expected; no war or riot news was there to whip up sales. Also, competition had appeared in the Chicago *Whip*, which sold for a nickel.

The *Defender* was the first unionized black paper as well as the first integrated one. Technically trained black men were scarce, so a white foreman and printers were hired, as were advertising salesmen, not without bringing criticism and a fall of support. After the early 1930's the paper settled down to a modified news policy on racial events, a social philosophy asking patience, and moderation in matters of racial change and conflict. The *Defender* had suffered during the depression, like all other businesses, and by 1935 was down to

73,000 circulation. It also was showing the effects of absentee owner-ship, for Abbott was away much of the time. Slashes in personnel and salaries were ordered; Abbott cut his own earnings to $200 a week and subsidized the paper to the tune of more than a quarter of a million dollars, Ottley discovered. Misdealings with the paper's funds also occurred at this time.

The paper continued the fight for fairer treatment of black citizens at the same time that it added features such as cartoons and personal columns. Much space was devoted to society, cultural, and fashion copy, a practice that later moved Frazier, the sociologist, to write: "Since the Negro newspaper makes its appeal to the awakened imagination of Negroes in urban communities, it provides a ro-mantic escape for Negro city-dwellers."[13]

Advertising was slim still; circulation revenue remained, as with the black press in general, the main income source. Ads often were the kind long ridiculed by adverse critics—hair straighteners, magic symbols, sex books, and skin color potions.

Politically the paper up to the 1920's had been independent but leaned toward the Republicans, the traditional stand of the black press. In 1928, however, Abbott opposed Herbert Hoover and sup-ported Alfred E. Smith. When much of the responsibility for the *Defender* was turned over to John H. Sengstacke, the weekly not only regained its secure foundation financially but also took different political stances than in the early days.

Abbott's Decline. When the depression struck the nation, Abbott tried to discourage a new migration of blacks from south to north, but this time was as ignored as he had been heeded earlier. This failure, plus the loss of his mother in 1932, affected his health, and Ottley says he often was away from the office. Meantime, he also had begun a magazine, *Abbott's Monthly,* the attention to which did not help his health, for by now both the magazine and the paper were in financial trouble. The magazine died in the depression and bank failures affected his personal fortune. The next calamity was a suit for divorce, which was costly.

The year Abbott was seventy-one he decided that his nephew, John H. Sengstacke, son of his brother Alexander, should carry on the paper. In 1939 he willed two-thirds of the estate to the young man and a third to his second wife, whom he had married in 1934. Most of his time was spent in bed, for he was becoming weaker daily. He began to dictate an autobiography; it never was completed. Death came in February, 1940.

Lochard and Harper. A characteristic of newspaper and magazine publishing is that certain publications attract talented writers and editors. They are not always large publications; *The New Yorker* is an example. The black press has had a similar experience. *Ebony* magazine, the Atlanta *Daily World,* the Chicago *Defender,* and the Pittsburgh *Courier* among them have had as staffers most of the more capable craftsmen (see Chapter 10). Few of these stars are known as stars in the world of journalism in general; only a few, in fact, have received recognition within the black press itself. Glances at only two will be found here; a dozen more could be listed, some tragic, some amusing. Metz Lochard and Lucius Harper were selected because they represent different types.

Metz P. T. Lochard appears to have been one of the best educated of the *Defender's* staffers. Although Ottley, historian of the *Defender* and its publisher, thought Lochard was "the first foreign editor in the Negro press," this distinction, if correct (as it probably was), was not Lochard's major contribution. A Frenchman educated at Oxford University as well as at the University of Paris, he had been an interpreter for Marshal Foch and then a language teacher at two noted black universities, Fisk and Howard. His French background and linguistic ability attracted Abbott. After the publisher's death Lochard became editor-in-chief of the paper.

Lucius C. Harper is remembered around the *Defender* office, at least among those who recall any of the oldtimers, as the staff member who once headed two of Robert Abbott's major enterprises, for he served as editor both of the paper and of *Abbott's Monthly,* the short-lived venture into periodical publishing. Outside the office, however, he was known because of his "Dustin' Off the News" column, a lively and popular feature that appeared in the 1940's and 1950's.

Harper's first connection with the Abbott enterprises came through a fluke. Somehow his letter of application in 1916 to *Overton's,* a black magazine, was delivered to the *Defender* offices in error. Harper had a typewriter and could use it—few black people were interested in journalism in those days and the few scarcely ever were thus equipped. He was hired. Harper had learned barbering, but had come to the paper with more than that skill and a typewriter. A graduate of Oberlin College, like Abbott he began as a printer's devil, working for the *Georgia Baptist.* He wrote articles for the Indianapolis *Freeman,* the Cleveland *Gazette,* and the *New York Age.* His interest in being a journalist arose, Ottley writes, from knowing newsmen at the Chicago Press Club, where he once worked as a bellboy. When Abbott hired Harper in 1916 he began a term of service that lasted thirty-six years.

● W. E. B. DU BOIS THE JOURNALIST

So controversial was William Edward Burghardt Du Bois' life—he was the center of disagreements as a teacher, as an NAACP executive, and as a political partisan—that his close association with black journalism is submerged. He founded five magazines, two of which still are published; he was a correspondent for four newspapers, columnist for numerous both black and white papers, and contributor of articles to many general as well as scholarly periodicals, black and white.

Journalism to Du Bois, it is true, was only a tool to advance his sociological studies of the black race or to aid him in his plans to help the race. But he used it effectively and far more than some others who considered themselves journalists but engaged in that profession as entrée to another: politics.

A New Englander, he was born in the same year, 1868, as Abbott. He was of partly slave and white ancestry, for his parents both had white blood in their backgrounds. He barely knew his father who had left to make a home for his wife elsewhere in the country but Du Bois' mother was too timid to follow. She and the boy lived in near poverty, aided by family and friends. He attended public school in Great Barrington, Massachusetts, and also was active in church there. He was a booklover.[14]

Yet in none of his town life did he personally encounter racial discrimination or segregation. He learned of it by being told by others.

Du Bois' first journalism was the editorship, with a white classmate, of a short-lived, hand-produced high school paper called *Howler.* A local bookshop operator got him his first professional news job—as correspondent for the Springfield *Republican,* a famous white daily. He also wrote for the notable black weeklies, the *New York Age,* the *Freeman,* and the New York *Globe.* When he went to Fisk University in 1886, his first venture into the South, he edited the *Fisk Herald.* Many years later, in 1924, he helped bring out what might be called an off-campus version of it in New York in support of a student rebellion at his alma mater.

From Fisk he went to Harvard, but did no journalistic work there, nor again until his return late in the century from graduate study in Germany. He began contributing sociological articles to the *Atlantic Monthly* and *World's Work,* two of the most important white periodicals then being published. A clue to his developing concept of journalistic responsibility appeared when a committee made up of several dignitaries, including Walter Hines Page, editor of the *Atlantic,* approached him about editing a magazine to be published at Hampton Institute. When he said, in submitting his plans, that he would expect all editorial decisions to be his own only, the project was dropped. This position was to disturb his journalistic life ever after but also may account for the effectiveness of several of the publications he edited.

By 1905 Du Bois had become fully aware of the power of the press. He wrote to a wealthy man he had met two years before, he relates in the autobiography, the need for "a high class journal to circulate among the Intelligent Negroes. . . ." In his letter he characterized the black press of the time thus: "Now we have many small weekly papers and one or two monthlies, and none of them fill the great need I have outlined." He thus described that need:

"The Negro race in America today is in a critical condition. Only united, concentrated effort will keep us from being crushed. This union must come as a matter of education and long continued effort."

The publication he had in mind would tell black readers of their own and their neighbors' needs, "interpret the news of the world to them, and inspire them toward definite ideas." And it would be a monthly. But the wealthy men he approached expressed sympathy and nothing more. There it ended until a few years later.

Du Bois' proposal of a magazine reflected his social views. They put him into conflict with Booker T. Washington. Du Bois himself "believed in the higher education of a talented tenth who through their knowledge of modern culture could guide the American Negro into a higher civilization." Washington believed that blacks would gain their best place by being skilled workers and businessmen and finally capitalists.

Du Bois saw his plans for a publication born at last in 1906. With the help of two Atlanta University graduates he had started in Memphis a small printing establishment. It now produced the *Moon Illustrated Weekly,* and may have given the editor the formula for the magazine he edited later, the *Crisis.* The *Moon* soon ranged itself against Washington. It contained miscellany, much of it reprinted from other black publications but also original editorials and biographical articles. After a year it was discontinued and in 1907 replaced by *Horizon,* which its founder dismissed by merely calling it "a miniature monthly." Rudwick, one of Du Bois' biographers, reported that *Horizon* was begun as a voice for the Niagara Movement. It failed, he believed, because the black people of the period were not ready for the Niagara philosophy. But producing this periodical laid more of the foundation for Du Bois' later editorial work. *Horizon,* in turn, gave way in his affections to the *Crisis.*

That magazine came from Du Bois' decision to resign his faculty post at Atlanta University and become director of publications and research for the NAACP, of which he had been an incorporator. His work brought him into association with Oswald Garrison Villard, publisher of the *Nation* and editor of the New York *Evening Post* as well as a grandson of William Lloyd Garrison. Ever the egotist, Du Bois was critical of Villard because the far more experienced white journalist gave him advice on editorial matters.

He began the *Crisis* on his own and despite, as he put it, "the protests of many of my associates." He saw in the magazine a chance to interpret to the world "the hindrances and aspirations of American Negroes." His work with it was a deep interest for nearly a quarter of a century: 1910 to 1934. During those years he made the magazine a vigorous critic of any national policy or event which resulted in harm to the black people—whether it was discrimination in the military services or the wartime lynchings of the 1914–19 conflict.

"As *Crisis* editor," Bennett has written, "Du Bois set the tone for the organization and educated a whole generation of black people in the art of protest."[15] But he was so possessive of the magazine and so prone to use it to comment on the NAACP itself (of which, it should be remembered, it was the official organ) that there was dissension within the organization. Through the magazine he advocated a program which certain other NAACP leaders could not accept.

Another Du Bois journalistic idea was founding a magazine for all children but written from a black standpoint. Launched in 1920, it was called the *Brownies' Book* and was intended to "help foster a proper self-respect," as its editor put it years later. It lasted two years, becoming one of the few black juvenile publications.

When he became sixty-five, Du Bois resigned from the NAACP and the editorship of the *Crisis,* returning to Atlanta University in 1934 as sociology department head. One of his purposes, he said, was "to establish . . . a scholarly journal of comment and research on world race problems." It took six years for this goal to be reached. The result was *Phylon,* being published still at the university as a scholarly and literary quarterly. He was editor for four years. It was to be his last major editorial work. Thereafter he wrote articles for black as well as white publications: *New York Times Magazine, New Masses, Nation, Journal of Negro Education, Negro Digest, Freedomways, Masses,* and *Mainstream,* among others. He was the author, from 1896 to 1963, of a score of books, editor of a dozen more, author of countless articles, and regularly contributed newspaper columns.

Because he placed his confidence in college-educated blacks to "save the race," as Rudwick puts it, Du Bois naturally believed in the use of books, magazines, and newspapers as vehicles of communication.

In the 1960's, as attempts were made to catch up with black history, it was popular to name schools for noted black people. Du Bois was not overlooked. The Chicago board of education in 1969 renamed a South Side elementary school for him, not without a debate, however. For toward the end of his life he joined the Communist Party, moved to Ghana, and became a citizen of that African nation. He died there in 1963, aged ninety-five. His new publishing project he was not to live to see realized—the *Encyclopaedia Africana* he had been commissioned to direct. His views were recalled in 1970 when his widow, Shirley Graham, also a writer and a New Yorker living as a Ghanian citizen in the United Arab Republic, for a time was denied a visa to enter the U.S.A. The reason given by the Department of Justice was based on a section of the McCarran-Walter Act that forbids entry into the country of persons associated with subversive activities, as a New York *Times* dispatch put it.

A memorial park was dedicated to Du Bois on October 18, 1969, at Great Barrington, on the site of the farmhouse where he spent his childhood. It was opposed by the John Birch Society and a white weekly, the Berkshire *Courier,* but supported by many other cities and the white daily, the Berkshire *Eagle.*

● **OTHER MAGAZINES OF THE PERIOD**

Du Bois' magazines were not the only important ones of the first few decades of the century. One group now remembered because of the social climate then and today was what might be called mildly leftist in sympathies. These included *Opportunity, Crusader, Promoter, Triangle, Messenger, Black Man* and *Negro World,* most issued from New York City. Like so much of the black press, several of these were organs of protest, some asking for a black state, others espousing a vague radicalism that avoided both socialism and communism of the brands then current, a radicalism centered on battling for the rights of blacks or for blacks to be in all government departments. But others supported some brand of socialism as a social order, with stronger labor and farmers' unions and cooperatively owned businesses.[16]

Black Man was among the more than half-dozen publications of Marcus Garvey, whose journalism will be noted in more detail. Intended as a monthly and published from Jamaica, the periodical, according to Cronon, a Garvey biographer, was irregularly published. It first appeared in 1933, carrying organization news and much of Garvey's own writing, such as poetry, editorials, and other communications from the messianic editor. It had many financial problems but managed to maintain an international circulation and continue for five or six years to help unite members of Garvey's Universal Negro Improvement Association. In one of its final issues was an appeal for support of a bill asking repatriation of U.S. blacks to Africa. It had been introduced by a notorious racist, U.S. Senator Theodore G. Bilbo. But it tied in with the magazine's and Garvey's program for American blacks.

An earlier Garvey magazine was *Negro Churchman,* launched as an organ of the denomination which the Black Moses, as Cronon calls him, had stimulated, the African Orthodox Church. A monthly, it supported Garvey's belief in an all-black religion, to which much of the rest of the black press gave no encouragement. The bulk of the other religious groups rejected it, evidently thinking the new denomination and its organ were merely political tools for Garvey.

Probably as much condemned and feared in its day—toward the end of World War I—as the *Black Panther* is at the other end of

the century, the *Messenger* today seems placid. At first it was edited
jointly by Chandler Owen and A. Philip Randolph, the latter now
a revered black leader long identified with the labor movement.
Openly Marxist, a dangerous position for those days of government interference with the press, it opposed Du Bois as much as Washington,
although they were in sharp disagreement. Representative James
Byrnes, of South Carolina, attacked the *Messenger* (as well as the
Crisis) in the House and blamed black journalists for the post-war
race riots. Consequently it was investigated by the Department of
Justice. Its report named the *Messenger* as "the most dangerous."[17]

Detweiler illustrated the tone of the *Messenger* when he noted
that a poem by Archibald H. Grimke, "Her Thirteen Black Soldiers,"
had been rejected by the white *Atlantic Monthly* and the black *Crisis*
but accepted and published by the *Messenger*. He describes the verse
as "a sombre invective against the nation, which is held guilty
for the fate of the Negro soldiers who rioted at Houston in the summer of 1917."[18] Another issue of the *Messenger* carried a cartoon
showing a black riding in an armored car and shooting down his
white opponents in race riots. Claude McKay, one of the best of the
black poets, published in this magazine one of the poems for which
he is best remembered, beginning: "If we must die, let it not be
like hogs." And the magazine devoted itself to urging blacks to form
and join labor organizations of their own. George S. Schuyler notes
in an autobiography that the magazine began as the *Hotel Messenger*.

Like Henry R. Luce, founder of the Time Inc. empire, Robert
S. Abbott started a magazine during an economic depression, one
sharply in contrast to the radical *Messenger*. Luce's *Fortune* went
on to thrive, but *Abbott's Monthly*, as already noted, did not last.
Roi Ottley assigned it the distinction of being "the first popular-style
periodical published for Negroes," perhaps a challengable assertion
in 1919, when it first was issued. Ottley also called it a forerunner of
Ebony, although that picture magazine owes as much to *Life* and
Look as to any other, and *Abbott's* little resembled either.[19] It was
a melange of articles on many different topics, international and
national, of special interest to black readers. Much of it was race-
angled. Poetry and photographs were included. It was going well
until the depression caught up with it. Unlike *Fortune*'s readers,
its clientele were persons to whom the cost of a magazine was a
personal sacrifice from an always low income. Its diffuse content
and absence of any discernible formula may have undone it also. In
any case, it was no more after 1933.

Perhaps far more to be lamented was the death of a periodical
begun in 1923 which outlasted Abbott's magazine. This one was
Opportunity, often confused with a still-published salesman's journal but actually the voice until 1949 of the National Urban League.
Charles S. Johnson, one of the few scholars interested in black periodicals, not only wrote about them but also began and edited *Oppor-*

tunity, making it one of the best in its day. He saw the need to give
the magazine an auxiliary activity by sponsoring the Harlem Writers'
Guild and set up literary competitions. As Frank W. Miles, a writer
on black periodical journalism, noted of it, "thus living up to the
Urban League's motto—not alms but Opportunity."[20] Bearing the
subtitle, "Journal of Negro Life," it was a quarterly of about fifty
pages an issue, carried serious articles on black problems, reviewed
books, and reported on business and professional opportunities. Personality sketches and literary work were staples, as was League news.
When it ceased it had a circulation of 10,000. The League explained
that it was discontinued because "Many other outlets are now available
for the creative work of Negro writers and for serious articles on
Negro life" and because increased costs of production made the
deficit too great. In those words rests the explanation for many subsequent publication failures.

During the 1920's new magazines of a more specialized type than
Opportunity appeared quickly: *American Musician, Master Musician,
Music and Poetry, Encore,* and *Negro Musician* were those particularly
devoted to music. In another decade, a dozen and a half more were
begun, including *Brown American* and *Challenge,* but did not live
to see the last of the 1930's. But in the 1940's, as to be seen later,
came the surge that produced several highly successful consumer magazines and the rise of various more specialized periodicals, these dealing with the trades, education, travel, and other topics. *Pulse, Negro,
Spotlighter,* and *Headlines,* among the general ones, did not survive;
Negro Digest did so, although it was buried for a decade and in 1970
became *Black World.*

● WASHINGTON AND GARVEY

The newspapers during this period had just as unsteady a history.
Prominent in the first quarter of the century were two figures, one
that of an educator, the other of a politician-editor-churchman, both
interested in newspapers rather than periodicals as tools for their
purposes. These men were Booker T. Washington and Marcus Garvey.

Washington's vague connections with black newspapers already
have been noted. He was thought, according to Rudwick, to have
provided some with financial assistance; it may or may not be significant that his articles appeared in those particular papers. Du Bois
accused him, as early as 1905, of having provided several with $3,000
in hush money the year before. In time Du Bois even named them:
the *New York Age,* Chicago *Conservator,* Boston *Citizen,* Washington
Colored American, Indianapolis *Freeman,* and *Colored American*
magazine, all now defunct. Rudwick asserts that Washington secretly
invested that sum in the magazine and assumed its operations.[21]

Rudwick also goes on to say that advertisements were bought in papers which supported him, such support including publication of editorials sent to the editors. Among the papers so favored, he declares, were the Charleston *Advocate* and the Atlanta *Independent.* These editorials appeared in several papers simultaneously, a situation to be expected in chain or group papers but not in those independently owned and separate. To these assertions Ottley adds the view that Washington gained press support by persuading supporters to buy financially weak papers; at one time as many as thirty-five were available to publicize his work or that of supporters. Among them were the Chicago *Broad Ax* and Chicago *Conservator.*[22]

Washington did more than operate behind the scenes, however. After publication of his classic of black literature, *Up From Slavery,* he was asked to write magazine articles. Ever his opponent, Du Bois declared in one of his autobiographies that these were prepared by black and white ghost writers, with their headquarters at Tuskegee, of which Washington was president.[23] Perhaps, like many a presidential and gubernatorial speech and article, his were composed with the help of others. Nevertheless, they were important in advancing Washington's views, especially that the black man was best able to improve his lot by using the worlds of labor and business as the paths to power.

If Washington was largely on the fringe of black journalism, Marcus Garvey, at least in the early part of his life, was steeped in it. Unlike other prominent editors and publishers such as Du Bois, White, Abbott, and Trotter, Garvey was racially pure, for he was entirely of black ancestry. Born in 1887 in Jamaica, his story differs from most of theirs also in that he was prone to demagoguery and had a most unhappy end to his career.

One of his first jobs was as a printer, at which he worked from his fourteenth to his twentieth year in Kingston. In 1907 he became a master printer and a foreman. When he took part in a printers' strike that year he lost his job, an experience that led him to begin what was to be a lifelong career as an organizer for members of his race to improve their social, political, and economic condition. His plans were not limited to the West Indian or U.S.A. black, but were international. The organization for which he is most remembered, the Universal Negro Improvement Association, he formed and headed in 1914. It was his platform. Garvey had a sense of the dramatic that made his own and his followers' activities newsworthy. In appearance they were attention-getting. The men were part of what he called the African Legion; they wore blue uniforms and red trousers. The women belonged to a Black Cross Nurse Society.[24]

His following was large among the working class blacks but not among the middle class or its leaders, many of whom were disaffected by such bombast as calling himself the Provisional Ruler of Africa in Exile. His plans were far too big, involving establishment of a Black Star Line, a steamship company with small vessels in poor condition.

American blacks invested $750,000 in the firm, which could not carry out his glowing plans. Garvey was indicted on fraud charges, accused of making rosy promises which were not kept. He received a five-year sentence and later was deported to Jamaica. The account in his paper, the *Negro World,* on August 11, 1926, carried the headline: "150,000 Honor Garvey" and the story began: "Harlem, the largest Negro community in the world, paid a tribute today to the greatest Negro in the world."

Black journalism had played an important part in Garvey's life. His first venture into publishing began while he was on a government printing office job in 1910 in Jamaica. He started a magazine, *Garvey's Watchman,* the first of a series of short-lived publications he was to sponsor. Next came a fortnightly, *Our Own,* a political organ.

By now he had concluded that organization was needed if he was to help improve the conditions of his people. He quit his job, went to Costa Rica and while there started *Nacionale,* but it too failed through lack of response. Then came another Spanish-language paper, *La Prensa,* likewise short of life. He traveled through South America, where he saw more exploitation of black workers. Eventually he reached England, where he saw a copy of Washington's *Up From Slavery.* It inspired him to more efforts to lead his race; it was then that he returned to Jamaica to form the Improvement Association. In two years he went to the U.S.A., in another two he started the New York paper which was his most important journalistic contribution: the *Negro World,* the Association organ.

A weekly, the *World* rapidly became popular and went to a circulation of about 200,000 at its best, perhaps 50,000 in an average week, with a wide distribution. Garvey was responsible for the paper, writing editorials and at times longer articles, but the bulk of the writing was done by others.[25] It was more an opinion organ than a newspaper, hitting hard for the nationalistic aims of Garvey's group, harking frequently back to Africa. Among the several capable journalists who wrote for it were T. Thomas Fortune and John E. Bruce. The *Negro World,* in fact, for a time was a rival for the Chicago *Defender* as a leading black paper. Garvey's strong personality and the actions of some followers put the *Defender* in the opposite camp. The *Negro World* naturally espoused Garvey's major campaigns for his shipping company, a Black House to match the White House, black generals, black congressmen, and even a Black God.

When Garvey was not relating his accomplishments, he wrote forcefully and convincingly. An example of his writing is this portion of an article in the *Negro World* in 1921:

> Some people ask, "Why hasn't the Universal Negro Improvement Association protested against so-and-so, and why hasn't it sent a telegram to the President denouncing lynching? Why hasn't it asked for interviews from Congressmen and Senators over the question of injus-

tice to the Negro?" Why should you want to do this when other organizations have been doing this for the last twenty years without any result?[26]

The *Negro World* was suspended in 1933, a depression year, outliving several other short-lived Garvey ventures, such as *Negro Times,* a daily; *Black Man,* a monthly magazine; *African World,* a paper distributed in South Africa; the monthly *Negro Churchman,* and the *Negro Peace Echo.* When Garvey died in 1940 a follower revived the *World* in Cleveland as the *New Negro World,* in magazine form, but it soon ceased. Garvey himself has not been forgotten, however. On the contrary. His nationalism appealed to the new separatist movement of the 1960's and 1970's. The black press reported various Garvey Day ceremonies in August during recent years, with proclamations, parades, and entertainment in his memory. A Garvey housing project was launched and a New York park was given his name.

● THE RISE OF THE *COURIER*

Today it calls itself the *New Pittsburgh Courier,* but it is one of the oldest black newspapers of general distribution. Founded in 1910, the *Courier* at one time had the largest circulation of any black paper in the country, close to 300,000. Credited with developing the paper was Robert L. Vann, whose manner of directing it was continued after his death by his widow, who became publisher in 1940. Until recently the *Courier* has been one of the top papers in circulation, and still is influential because of its traditions.

Vann was brought in by the four Pittsburgh Methodist church people who founded the paper but who could not make a go of it financially. He was a lawyer with journalistic experience on two other black papers in the same city. His formula was to launch the paper on numerous crusades in behalf of the black community and black citizens generally. These campaigns were against jim-crowism and discrimination against blacks in major league baseball, two of the classic targets of papers out to fight for black rights. He put the *Courier* behind nationally known black figures, such as Jackie Robinson and Joe Louis, early in their careers. Vann did something even more difficult: he saw to it that the paper was taken into the South, for in some localities black citizens were prohibited from reading black publications.

The story of the *Courier* follows what now is a familiar pattern: printing sensational news for the sake of sales, running campaigns in the news columns, printing editorials in behalf of readers, and struggling for advertising. But it went a step further: it attracted to its staff some of the major black journalists of the first half of this century, such as George S. Schuyler, P. L. Prattis, William G. Nunn, and a good many young writers who later became important on other papers.

● OTHER JOURNALISTS AND PAPERS

Douglass, Du Bois, Abbott, Garvey, Trotter, Fortune, Vann—these were among the effective men in black journalism by the end of the first century of its existence. Until another two decades had passed there would be none who made the same national impact. But there were other important black publications and publishers in the early 1900's. Among the papers are the St. Louis *Argus,* the *Informer* papers of the Southwest, the Kansas City (Mo.) *Call,* the Buffalo *Star* and the Norfolk *Journal and Guide.* And the New York *Amsterdam News,* among other papers begun before the turn of the century, went into the forefront by the 1940's.

Among the publishers of that time who carried on their work into the 1960's was the late Carter W. Wesley, of the *Informer* group. When Lincoln University gave two of its citations of merit in 1960, one went to Wesley for his work as head of black papers in two Texas cities: the Houston *Informer* and the Dallas *Express.* Born in 1892, Wesley was both a lawyer and publisher and a founder of the National Newspaper Publishers Association. In law he specialized in civil rights cases, one leading to the Supreme Court decision permitting blacks to vote in primaries.

About ten years his senior was Chester Arthur Franklin, identified with the black press for fifty-seven years. He founded the Kansas City *Call* when he was thirty-eight, but he already had been in publishing for twenty-one years. When he was seventeen he began by running the Denver *Star,* earlier called the *Statesman.* At his death in 1955 the *Call* was one of the larger papers and still is a leading weekly. A distinguishing feature of the *Call* under Franklin was its avoidance of sensationalism; frequently its front page had no crime stories.

Another lawyer-publisher was Andrew J. Smitherman, but unlike Wesley he has received little attention. He was a versatile publisher in the Southwest and East. His specialty in law was criminal trials. His first papers were published in Tulsa, Oklahoma, a daily as well as a weekly. Both, as well as his home, were lost in race riots in 1921. Smitherman began another paper in Springfield, Massachusetts. Then in 1925 he moved to Buffalo, New York, at first working for other black papers, but the satisfaction of ownership was missed, so he borrowed $100 and in 1932 founded the Buffalo *Star,* later called the *Empire Star,* and remained its editor and publisher for twenty-nine years. At his death in 1961 the white press in Buffalo credited him with having founded the nation's first black daily, but several such papers of that frequency had been published before Smitherman was born in 1885.[27] The *Star* ceased soon after his death.

● **THE** *AMSTERDAM NEWS*

With certain individuals, publishing was only one of their activities; we already have encountered several lawyers. Others ran
real estate firms, were doctors, bankers, or politicians; a few were
diplomats. These connections indicate that especially in the early
years of this century publishing was not lucrative, newspapers and
magazines receiving neither enough advertising nor circulation revenue. But it also may indicate that successful businessmen were not
putting their primary effort into publishing or perhaps were unaware
that it takes certain talents and abilities different from those of the
more widely followed occupations, such as real estate and banking.

Medical men were involved, as one still is, in the publishing of
the New York *Amsterdam News.* James H. Anderson, who began the
paper in 1909, was not a physician. He wanted to start a weekly and
evidently used the name of the street on which he lived for its title.
James Booker, author of a brief history of the paper, wrote that Anderson had "a dream in mind, $10 in his pocket, six sheets of paper
and two pencils" when he put out the first copy. Despite its owner's
weak finances, it continued. It has had several owners since, including
two physicians who purchased it in 1936. They were Dr. Philip M. H.
Savory and Dr. Clelan Bethany Powell. Dr. Powell diversified his business activities by running as well the Victory Mutual Life Insurance
Company, a photoengraving firm called Rapid Reproduction, and
other enterprises. Dr. Powell's partner died in 1965; today he is owner
and publisher, owning several other businesses in addition to the
paper.[28]

For a time the paper was a semi-weekly, tabloid on one day a
week, a standard-size sheet on the other. That policy was followed in
1945, when it was meeting competition from Adam Clayton Powell's
People's Voice and the *New York Age*. It was moved by this strong
competition as well to sensationalize the black community's news, but
ran what have been called sedate editorials in the midst of accounts
of brutal murders, stabbings, and sex crimes. Significantly, perhaps, it
outlasted both rivals and today is one of the leading weeklies (see
Chapter 5).

● **THE YOUNGS IN NORFOLK**

The story is that when P. Bernard Young went to work in 1907
for what now is known as the Norfolk *Journal and Guide,* it was the
fraternal organ of the Knights of Gideon. Its circulation was 500, it
was six years old, and called the *Lodge Journal and Guide.* He got
the job because one day the editor did not appear, and Young wrote
an editorial. As a result he was made associate editor, and in 1910
bought it and converted it into a general black newspaper.[29]

The Young family has been running it ever since and has served the black press by holding office in the national organization of publishers and by placing the *Journal and Guide* on a par with the large national newspapers.

Plummer Bernard Young, the founder, who preferred simply to sign himself P. B. Young, was a North Carolinian. He ran the paper from 1910, when he was twenty-six, until his death in 1962. A son, Thomas White Young, holder of law and bachelor's degrees from Ohio State University, succeeded his father, after working two years as a war correspondent. But in 1967, after having served as editor and publisher only five years, he died. His widow now is vice president of the publishing firm. Like many other publishers, he had interests as well in banking and insurance.

The weekly, although until recent years somewhat more conservative in its policies than other national papers, was never silent about the black citizen's place in wartime, but at the same time supported the wars without pretending that blacks were faring better at home. The *Journal and Guide* also has the reputation of avoiding ultrasensationalism more than most of the medium-sized or large black papers.

● **IMPACT OF WORLD WAR I**

Several more papers and entrepreneurs must be noted, especially since they are influential. One is the Oklahoma City *Black Dispatch,* a weekly begun in 1915. It got its unusual name, according to its editor, and publisher, Roscoe Dunjee, ". . . as a result of an effort to dignify a slur." There was an Oklahoma expression, "That's black despatch gossip." But, he went on to say to his interviewer, "the influence of this statement is very damaging to the integrity and self-respect of the race. All of this has developed a psychology among Negroes that their color is a curse and that there is something evil in their peculiar pigmentation. It is my contention that Negroes should be proud to say, 'I am a black man.'" In saying this Dunjee anticipated the popular expression, "Black is beautiful."[30]

Four years later another paper important today was founded, the Kansas City *Call* and in 1934, one more major weekly, the Los Angeles *Sentinel* (see Chapter 4).

Many editors and publishers were confronted with a dilemma when the U.S.A. entered World War I. American black citizens had little enthusiasm for the conflict, an attitude reflected in the leading publications. Too much for some editors was the contradiction of expecting blacks to fight to save a democracy they did not experience. Most cynical were the socialist and other left-of-center magazines. The Chicago *Defender,* the *New York Age,* the Washington *Bee,* the Baltimore *Afro-American,* and the Norfolk *Journal and Guide* pointed up the irony of the situation in editorials and cartoons. But they concluded that at the same time that the American black should be treated more fairly by the military it was essential that the U.S.A. and its allies overcome the enemy, for if they did not the black as well as the white on the American continent would suffer. The *Bee* said editorially:

> But the Negro is willing today to take up arms and defend the American flag; he stands ready to uphold the hands of the President; he stands ready to defend the country and his President against this cruel and unjust oppression. His mother, sister, brother and children are being burned at the stake and yet the American flag is his emblem and which he stands ready to defend. In all the battles the Negro soldier has proved his loyalty and today he is the only true American at whom the finger of scorn cannot be pointed.[31]

Such attitudes naturally led to charges of sedition by the super-patriots. The Department of Justice placed charges of disloyalty particularly upon the leftist magazines. The effect upon the publications was to stimulate interest in their content and to win the loyalty of readers, who realized that the publications were fighting the battle for them.

● A NOTE ON DISCRIMINATION

The black press, serving a people with a long history of being the butt of racial discrimination, has been the victim of discrimination as well. During the nineteenth century, especially in the years before the Civil War, it faced the problem of interference with distribution and the right of blacks to read their own publications. In the twentieth century, the discrimination sometimes has been more subtle, depriving publications of advertisers, interfering with their distribution, and ignoring their existence as a force in society.

In the first quarter of the century publishers encountered the problem of suppression. Detweiler records not only the raids on publication offices by the Ku Klux Klan and other hooded hoodlums and the cancellation of advertising by white merchants but also the passage of laws forbidding dissemination of the publications. The Mississippi legislature in 1920 passed "An act to make it a misdemeanor to print or publish or circulate printed or published appeals or presentations of arguments or suggestions favoring social equality or marriage between the white and Negro races."[32] The year before, the Chicago *Defender* had printed this dispatch; from Yazoo City, Mississippi: "Threatening her with death unless she stopped acting as agent for newspapers published by people of her Race, Miss Pauline Willis was compelled to leave town."[33] And in 1920, a black minister who distributed copies of *Crisis,* the NAACP magazine, on a train

in the same state, was mobbed, put in jail, and then on a chain gang
when he asked for police protection. The lieutenant governor and
the governor both refused to intervene.[34]

Mississippi was not alone. A Somerville, Tennessee, paper
printed, on February 7, 1919, this account: "White people of this
city have been issued an order that no 'colored newspapers' must be
circulated in this town, but that every 'darkey,' the petition read,
must read The Falcon, a local white paper edited by a confederate
veteran. The whites stated this step was being taken in order 'to keep
the "nigger" from getting besides himself, and to keep him in his
place.' "[35]

More than twenty years later Conrad reported that the Chicago
Defender was concerned, for it was being suppressed in the South.
It often was taken off the newsstands and halted at the post office.[36]

Such incidents were more likely to occur as the number of papers
and magazines continued to mount and because the black press was
the only one reporting the news of black America; except for crime
there was almost no news of it in the white press. Pride in his study
uncovered the fact that in one year—1902—almost one hundred newspapers were launched, beginning a long period of growth in numbers,
for about 1,400 were founded between that year and 1950.   ●

4. WORLD WAR II AND AFTER

THE YEARS BETWEEN the two world wars saw the strengthening of some papers and the decline of others, particularly in the late twenties and early thirties, when the economic depression had its effect. As usual it was the financially weak, not necessarily the least competent, that went bankrupt. But capable management did help the strong papers to become stronger, as did the beginning of the trend toward formation of chains and groups.

The most important newspaper founded between the conflicts was the Atlanta *World*, established in 1928 as a weekly. Within two years it became a semi-weekly and by another year a tri-weekly, and finally a daily in 1932. It now is one of three daily papers (see Chapter 5). It was the period, also, when several major serious magazines were launched: *Opportunity* already discussed, *Negro History Bulletin*, and *Journal of Negro Education*.

When the country entered World War II the publications that took a stand were accused of defeatism because they said black fighting men should be as well treated as white, just as others before them in the previous global conflict were charged with being seditious. Federal government efforts were made to quiet such papers as the *California Eagle* and the Pittsburgh *Courier*. What was considered unacceptable was no more than objection to what the publications considered undemocratic processes. The press was admittedly biased and made no pretensions of objectivity when it came to the need for equitable treatment of blacks.

After the war the black publications continued their demand for civil liberties, a policy which brought upon them new criticism, that of being leftist and even communist. One of the most vituperative critics was the late Westbrook Pegler, the sportswriter and later syndicated columnist. The black papers ". . . in their obvious, inflammatory bias in the treatment of news they resemble such one-sided publications as the Communist *Daily Worker* and Coughlin's *Social Justice*," he wrote.[1]

Some years after the war *Ebony* magazine examined the executives at the head of twenty-three leading papers, including some of those accused of disloyalty; most of them are being published still and retain their leadership. "Far from being parlor pinks," the magazine said, "most Negro publishers are arch-conservatives in their thinking on every public issue with one exception—the race problem. . . . The owners of the biggest newspapers have but two main missions—to promote racial unity and to make money."[2]

By the early and mid-1940's owners of black publications had to face not only the threat of war but also a rising enthusiasm for integration of the races, particularly in the world of education. The latter was a threat in one sense: blacks might drift away from their own press. On the issue of integration, despite the effect on circulation it could have in the long run, there was largely enthusiasm within the world of black journalism. The skeptics were mainly the more nationalistic black journalists, either remnants of the Garvey days or others concerned about the purity of the race. The large national papers were hopeful, reporting progress, editorializing, and carrying cartoons encouraging the idea of equality of some degree, certainly in education and job opportunities. But a few saw an outcome that would at least greatly weaken the black press. Among these was John H. Johnson, who in two decades was to become the head of a large and successful journalistic enterprise. He foresaw a decline in the press as a result of integration. He did not fear this result, but others did. There were dark forecasts about the disappearance of the press which created discomfort and argument (see Chapter 17). As it turned out, the fears were unnecessary but not illogical.

The rising interest and activity to bring about racial integration was a signal to editors and publishers that they must adjust their policies by reaching out for more black readers. A handful of whites joined some staffs; a few black magazines were put on newsstands that had not displayed them before. Existing quietly alongside the national papers and consumer magazines were a number of scholarly journals accustomed to subsidized living: *Journal of Negro History, Journal of Negro Education, Phylon,* and *Crisis* among the better known. They were not directly dependent on commercial support.

By 1947, two years after the end of the war, several papers hit

TABLE 4.1 ● Circulation Figures of Four Major Papers, 1940–69

Newspaper	1940	1947	1955	1965	1969
New York *Amsterdam News*	35,841	111,427	36,149	61,655	77,708
Pittsburgh *Courier*	126,962	286,686	159,238	56,733	61,548
Chicago *Defender*	82,059	161,253	107,841	69,867	33,320
Norfolk *Journal and Guide*	30,092	68,039	43,458	31,478	21,702

Source: Prepared by Robert D. Bontrager from 1940–65 figures in the *Ayer Directory;* for purposes of comparison the author has added 1969 figures from the same source.

their highest circulation figures. The accompanying schedule (see Table 4.1) shows this growth and the subsequent decline. The figures require interpretation, however. In the thirty-year interval, several of the big weeklies or semi-weeklies have added regional editions. One (Chicago *Defender*) became a daily with a weekly national edition; only the daily is included.

● SENGSTACKE, AND OTHERS

American white journalism has had its emperors and empires: Luce of Time Inc., within whose giant firm were magazines at first, then broadcasting stations and books; Hearst, father and son, heads of a huge combination of newspapers, magazines, news services, and film companies; Newhouse, who also heads a conglomerate of printed and electronic journalism enterprises; and the latest ruler, Lord Thomson, quietly acquiring scores of publications all over the world.

Proportionately, perhaps, black journalism has had just as many with what might be called the Murphy papers (the *Afro-Americans*) and the Scott papers (Atlanta and other *Worlds* as well as some not called *World*) and, largest of all, the Sengstacke Newspapers, which cover a large territory through various *Couriers* and *Defenders* (see Chapter 5). These are the publishers who saw the circulation rises and drops and the gradual rise of advertising volume and revenue to compensate.

John H. Sengstacke's relationship to the Abbott-Sengstacke family already has been recounted. When his uncle, Robert Sengstacke Abbott, selected him for responsibility in the organization he may not have foreseen the extent to which the empire would grow in the period after the first World War, minor as some of the publications in the group are today.

Sengstacke is a modest publisher, a model of neat appearance. Comparatively few mentions of him appear in his papers. His office on Chicago's South Side has none of the appearance of comparative luxury and spaciousness of that of the publisher of the *Amsterdam News* in New York, for example. He is a graying, low-voiced man who has been a quiet leader among black publishers, has twice served as president of their national organization, still heads the large advertising representatives firm, Amalmagated Publishers, Inc., and serves on various committees within the industry.

He was born in Savannah in 1912, and attended grade school in the Sengstackes' town of Woodville, Georgia. He first went to Knox Institute, then to Hampton Institute, from which he received a bachelor's degree, and next did graduate work at Ohio State University. Ottley reports that during his college days Sengstacke wrote his Uncle Robert what many a neophyte journalist still tells parents and friends:

"I am reading books on journalism, newspaper work, and taking

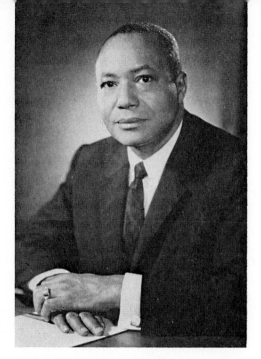

FIG. 4.1. John H. Sengstacke, president of the largest chain of black papers in the U.S.A., and head of several journalism, publishing, and advertising organizations.

a course in advertising. I am going to do some research work on the topic, 'Problems Confronting the Advertising Managers of Negro Newspapers.' "[3]

His first job was on the *Times* of Woodville, a paper his uncle's father had established and which Alexander Sengstacke, John's father, later renamed the *West End Post*. Young Sengstacke did various jobs—printing, advertising, and editorial.

After being at Ohio State he joined his uncle's firm in 1934, and has been in the organization ever since. In his early days at the Chicago *Defender* he studied at the Chicago School of Printing and also at Northwestern University, where he took business administration courses, applying what he learned to the *Defender* operations. In time he became a vice-president and treasurer of the paper and then general manager. Ottley reports that Sengstacke put the paper on a steady financial keel and developed the chain of which it now is the center. By and large his has been a financially successful tenure at the Robert S. Abbott Publishing Company, still the name of the publishing house.

Not every venture has been a success; few big publishing firms do not misfire now and then. He started a news and picture magazine, *Headlines,* in 1944 and made Louis E. Martin its editor and publisher and Frederick D. Sengstacke business manager. Small in format at first, it became newsmagazine size, was renamed *Headlines and Pictures,* edited in New York, and at one time had a circulation of 35,000. It ceased in 1946, the white newsmagazines being preferred.

***Powell and* People's Voice.** Among the other editors is one who has smothered his journalism activity in politics and marital as well as political troubles: Adam Clayton Powell, Jr. The principal journalistic work of the controversial churchman and Congressman was as editor of *People's Voice,* begun in 1942 in New York. While he was in that post Powell explained why he became a journalist as well as a churchman and politician. He had four reasons: from grade school years on he wanted to write; he wished to use the press to correct what he considered the false ideas held about the American black people; he wished to raise a militant voice in behalf of the black society; and he desired to employ the press as an educational force with the "new" black citizen aroused to demanding more democracy for his race.[4]

Chuck Stone, after he left the editor's desk of the Chicago *Defender,* observed that "Powell's weekly columns in *People's Voice* when re-read in the light of today's 'Black Power' militancy clearly anticipated these developments. Any one of those columns can stand alone today as a 'call to rally under the banner of blackness.' "[5] Stone also said that the paper, for tough, uncompromising militancy, brilliant editorial writing, and exciting layout "has rarely been matched." It was this toughness that earned some animosity for it. The paper began to run Richard Wright's novel, *Native Son,* now a classic of American literature, but so many readers protested that only four installments were printed. One objection was to the profanity in the realistic novel of poverty and crime in Chicago's black community, an objection which seems quaint today in view of the language in many a modern novel. Powell also invited criticism because he seemed to be timing the introduction of legislation in Washington, after his election in 1944, so that his paper got the story first.[6]

As he did during his career as representative of his Harlem constituency, Powell through his paper battled in behalf of the black people, which appears to be the main reason why, despite personal activities frowned upon by blacks as well as whites—luxurious living, intemperate language, boastfulness, failure to appear in the House or attend committee meetings—he continued to hold his power.

People's Voice was a tabloid weekly, somewhat imitative of *PM,* an adless daily in New York, but it sold space. Powell was not its only editor to gain national attention: so did Doxey A. Wilkerson, executive editor in 1945. Two years later Wilkerson left to become editor of the New York *Daily Worker,* the American Communist Party paper. When he departed Wilkerson said that the tabloid "is cowering before the witch hunters." It was playing, he said, the role of Uncle Tom to foes of the black people. But by then Powell had withdrawn and the paper was being directed by Denton J. Brooks, Jr., earlier of the Chicago *Defender,* and Max Yergan, once in charge of the Council on African Affairs. The new publishers placed *People's Voice* in support of Ben Davis, Jr., a black Communist Party leader. This policy brought suspicion upon it as being subversive. It ran into financial difficulties and ceased in 1947.[7]

James Baldwin, in his appraisal of the black press, published in 1948, found *People's Voice* "pretty limited," in its coverage, and its politics murky. But its exploitation of prominent blacks he considered pathetic, for the paper printed every detail of their lives it could uncover. He said the paper was full of warnings, appeals, and open letters to the government.[8]

Newman and Martin. When Gordon Parks, photographer, novelist, and man of many other talents, was broke in Minneapolis early in his career, trying to make a go of it in photo-journalism, it was Cecil E. Newman who helped him by giving him the somewhat unsuitable job of circulation manager but also the suitable one of official cameraman. Newman, then as now editor and publisher of the Minneapolis *Spokesman*, at first printed Parks' pictures to get the young man's work before a public, for he was unable to pay him, the paper then being in serious financial trouble. Parks paints a graphic picture of Newman and his paper's setting at the time, the late 1930's, in his book, *A Choice of Weapons.*

"Cecil was a small, brown-skinned man of perpetual motion and tremendous spirit," he wrote. In a cramped and disordered office Newman had to write the editorial, the sports, society, and general news and try to keep up with his bills. He could give his few employes little money, so he gave them what Parks calls "titles . . . of Herculean stature."

Times were better for Newman three decades later, but he had to engage in varied journalism activities first. Born in 1903, he entered publishing with the *Twin City Herald* of Minneapolis, from 1927 to 1934. For a year, during the same period, he also published *Timely Digest,* a magazine. In 1934 he became editor and publisher of the *Spokesman* as well as the St. Paul *Recorder*. He has served on many government bodies, such as the Citizen's Advisory Committee on Civil Rights of the Department of Agriculture, and has been active in various groups including the United Negro College Fund. He was cited by Lincoln University in 1957 for his journalism and civic activity.

Almost as well known in the world of Democratic Party politics as in black journalism, Louis E. Martin helped establish the *Michigan Chronicle* in the 1930's in Detroit, developing it into one of the major large weeklies. It now is part of the Sengstacke Newspaper empire, and Martin himself is editor of the entire assembly of Sengstacke papers, including the flagship daily in Chicago, and vice-president of the firm. In 1960 he was appointed deputy chairman of the Democratic National Committee. He returned to the newspaper business in 1969. For a number of years he has written a column, "The Big Parade," for his papers and for a few others outside the group. In it he comments on current problems of concern to the black citizenry, sometimes relying on an alter ego, one Dr. S. O. Onabanjo, "my learned Nigerian friend," to make his points. A graduate of the University of Michigan, Martin is a native of Shelbyville, Tennessee, having been born there in 1912.

● JOHNSON AND HIS EMPIRE

A major development in this period was the building not only of newspaper empires but also of large magazine companies (see Chapter 7). Head of the most ambitious of these firms is John Harold Johnson, who presides over the Johnson Publishing Company, with offices in the same area of the city as the Sengstacke Newspapers. Thus two of the most powerful black press firms operate in the same community.

Johnson, in contrast to the dignified Sengstacke, is bouncy and a bit bumptious. He likes to tell stories, has a shouting laugh. One incident he enjoys recounting occurred some years ago.

He was driving his car—one fitting to a man of his high income—on one of Chicago's major boulevards one day when he was stopped by a white policeman.

"Boy, does your boss know you're out in his car," the cop asked, suspiciously.

"He sure does," Johnson answered.

"Well, you'd better get it back to him soon as you can," he was warned.

"Sure will," the millionaire publisher of *Ebony* and other magazines assured him, and drove off.[10]

The success story of John H. Johnson probably is one of the few that is at all widely known about black publishers. It is a narrative that would have delighted Horatio Alger but it distresses both the blacks and whites who oppose the present American economic order. For Johnson represents economic success gained through use of all the procedures and methods embedded in the private initiative, private ownership system so characteristic of business in western society. He began with a pittance. After overcoming setbacks he persisted until today his company is one of the largest in the industry, regardless of color. In addition to publishing, he also owns cosmetic and insurance firms. He clearly has a vested interest in the U.S. financial system and apologizes not at all for it.

Johnson told a *Fortune* magazine writer, for an article about him and his enterprises, that his aim always has been to get himself into a position where he would own the building, not burn it down. "I don't want to destroy the system—I want to get into it," he added.[11]

And it is indeed a substantial building that he maintains a dozen blocks south of Chicago's Loop. In its oak-paneled lobby is red leather furniture with large plants standing about and paintings on the walls. On the floor above are the editorial offices of the four magazines, cubicles for chief editors and desks in a main room for writers and secretaries. Others of the 250 employes (in 1969 five were white) are in advertising, circulation, and other department offices, including a neat library nearby. Adjacent is another two-story building for storage and other uses.

The Johnson saga begins when he and his mother went from rural Arkansas there to visit the Chicago World's Fair of 1933. Like many other visitors, they decided to stay, the elder Johnson having died when the future publisher was six. They lived on relief for a time. But, as the *Fortune* writer reported it, in 1936 John Johnson, the student, gave a talk on "America's Challenge to Youth" at the annual honors convocation at DuSable High School, and was heard by Harry H. Pace, president of the Supreme Life Insurance Company. Pace encouraged Johnson to go on to college. He liked to help ambitious and talented black youths; another he befriended was Paul Robeson, whose later turn to communism must have distressed him. He gave young Johnson a part-time job. The future owner of *Ebony* attended the University of Chicago at the same time. At the insurance company offices he met various young black businessmen.

One day he was asked to work on the firm's house magazine. After becoming its editor he conceived the idea of a magazine containing articles of interest to the black population and about black citizens. Pace encouraged him, urging him to try to make a go of it without his help but said he could be turned to, as a last resort. Bank loans for black businessmen were much harder to get, in those days, than now.

The new publisher mortgaged his mother's furniture for $500,

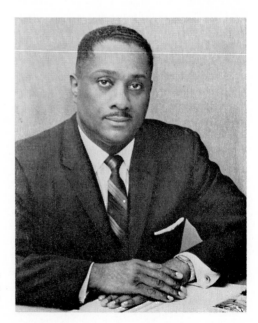

FIG. 4.2. John H. Johnson, editor and publisher of **Ebony, Jet, Tan,** and **Black World.** (**Ebony** photo)

so he could pay for his first direct mail advertising about his magazine, *Negro Digest* (since renamed *Black World*). That letter, sent in 1942, offered subscriptions at two dollars each and brought 3,000 subscribers. A first issue of 5,000 copies did not sell out. For one matter, distributors did not believe that the newsstands could dispose of a magazine of solely black appeal, a not unreasonable view in those days and still shared by many a newsstand operator. So Johnson persuaded thirty friends to ask for the magazines at the stands and thus create a demand. He then bought from the dealers copies not sold. But the second issue did not require such artificial sales stimulation.[12]

Circulation climbed steadily, helped partly by publication of a series called "If I were a Negro," containing pieces by Mrs. Eleanor Roosevelt, Norman Thomas, Marshall Field, Edward G. Robinson, and other whites. Some issues hit as much as 150,000 circulation, a remarkable figure for any black periodical of serious type and unusual even for a white periodical of the kind.

His first venture a success, Johnson now was ready to consider another, a black version of *Life*. In 1945 *Ebony* was born with the intention of emphasizing the bright side of black life and reporting success by black people in almost any endeavor.

The value of imagination and of luck was proved by what happened in the magazine's early years, as A. James Reichley tells it in *Fortune*. Johnson wrote letters to presidents of various large corporations, seeking entrée so he could sell *Ebony* as an idea and as an advertising medium. Presidents of black firms of any sort were not, at that time, accepted by white corporation counterparts, so Johnson received no encouragement. And black businessmen prepared to spend money on advertising were few and reluctant. Johnson's letter, however, did at last bring one appointment, this with Commander Eugene McDonald, president of Zenith, the radio set manufacturing firm. The commander, an Arctic explorer as well as a leading business executive, once had known Matthew Henson, the black explorer who worked closely with Admiral Peary in the 1909 journey to the North Pole. The publisher knew of the McDonald-Henson friendship and brought with him on his call a copy of the biography of Henson that had been autographed for the commander. As a result of this rapport, McDonald saw to it that the Zenith Corporation bought advertising space in *Ebony*. It became the Johnson firm's first big account and still is one of the major advertisers.[13]

Ebony went through a temporary decline to rise to new strength, and the rest of the Johnson empire was built gradually by the launching of *Jet, Tan Confessions, Hue, Ebony International,* and *Copper Romance. Negro Digest* was temporarily discontinued, and the last three were not successful ventures, for varying reasons. Johnson's method always has been to put out magazines with formulas and formats that have been used, often successfully, by white publishers with primarily white readers. His *Negro Digest* was suggestive of the *Reader's Digest; Ebony* is like *Life; Jet* much like a long-defunct miniature magazine called *Quick; Tan Confessions* (now just *Tan*) has much in common with *True Confessions.* Even his later *Ebony International* was in concept like *Life International.* Such imitativeness is normal in the publications world. Walter Goodman, writing in 1968, noted that Johnson, in his first years in mass journalism, declined to become "all hot and bothered about the race questions." He quotes the publisher as saying that the monthly picture magazine would "mirror the happier side of Negro life." The big money earned by entertainment figures and the lavish lives of some of them were played up, for example.[14] This philosophy *Ebony* has had until recent years; it was modified in the later 1960's from a somewhat Pollyanna-ish view to one of a more strident demand for the righting of wrongs against the race. The struggle for equality with rights finally has led Johnson to realize, apparently, that doing what whites strive to do in the world of business or entertainment perhaps is not the acme of accomplishment for people of the black race.

Perhaps because he smarted from criticism that he was too much concerned with making money and not enough interested in providing talented black writers with an outlet or with being an influence on the serious black citizens, Johnson revived *Negro Digest* just ten years after he had discontinued it. As the civil rights movement gained strength and the philosophy of black power, with its many interpretations and applications, could not be ignored by either whites or blacks, *Negro Digest* began carrying articles with such titles as "Negro Rights and the American Future." Promoting that magazine, which now began attacking white power as expressed through White Citizens' Councils and the like, the Johnson institutional advertising said:

> For more than 100 years, a native-bred philosophy not very different from Herr Hitler's has been preached in this country. With the upward thrust of the civil rights movement, this racist philosophy gains more strident voices. And these enemies of humanity are aided, perhaps unwittingly, by those whites who admonish Negro citizens to "go slow" and to be "more responsible" in the push for full and equal rights, as if Negroes had not gone slowly for a century and as if it is not precisely white America's disdain of its responsibility which has brought the nation to this terrible moment. . . . The enemies of Negro rights are both numerous and powerful, and many of them heard the cadences of Herr Schicklgruber's marching spirit and are hypnotized.[15]

By fall, 1965, *Ebony* was carrying articles by such outstanding liberal-minded blacks as Martin Luther King, Jr., Carl T. Rowan, and Kenneth Clark, in a number significantly devoted to the theme of "the white man's burden." Johnson began to give hard looks, often sympathetically, at the actions of rebellious black people, particularly youth. But the magazine did not lose its determination to tell success stories and it still speaks primarily to the middle-class black family which wants to be socially and financially successful.

● THE OTHER NEW MAGAZINES

John Johnson's early success with *Negro Digest* naturally led to the rise of competitors. One, the *Negro,* was similar in formula, but not so fortunate. Its publisher was not able to revive it once it had died. *Ebony* quickly inspired competition: *Color, Our World,* and *Sepia* came closely near its formula but only the last is still on the stands. Others, such as *Spotlighter,* which preceded *Ebony* by a year, were more cheaply produced but fell away after a few months or a year.

The post-World War II period also was one of establishment of a wide variety of magazines and of more small community papers. In the 1950's the larger papers were dropping back in circulation, the loss in sales revenue offset somewhat by the slightly increased success in selling advertising space. While not startlingly great, it was a reflection of somewhat better financial conditions for the American people, in which some blacks shared, and the first signs of impact of the developing civil rights movement, reflected in the New York-issued magazine, *Freedom.*

The specialized magazine and newspaper, although not new in black journalistic history, was by the 1960's a part of the general trend toward publishing periodicals dealing with special interests. There rose such titles as *Soul,* an entertainment paper, and *Pride,* a community magazine. The hairdressing salons had two: *Black Beauty* and *Beauty Trade.* The separatist churchmen brought out *Impact.* In the realm of literary and idea publications arose *Freedomways.*

What developed into the circulation leader of all publications for black readers was launched in 1965: *Tuesday,* a magazine supplement inserted in white newspapers in cities with large black populations. Within five years it had nearly two million circulation and was attracting a number of major advertisers (see Chapter 7). A women's service magazine, free of the confession tone, came forth in *New Lady,* was shelved for a time and resumed again with new funding late in the decade. A combination general discussion, fashion, job opportunity magazine was *Urban West.* Early in the 1950's, when the more general *Sepia* was founded, the same firm in Texas brought out three more or less similar confession-romance monthlies, *Bronze Thrills, Hep,* and *Jive.*

● THE COMMUNITY PAPERS

The 1960's in particular saw the beginning and sometimes quick failure of what virtually are borough or country papers begun in

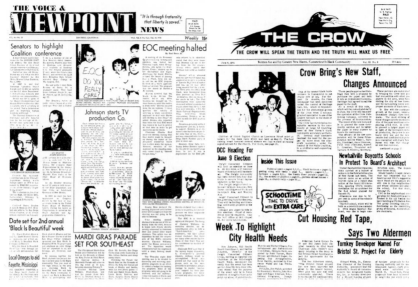

FIG. 4.3. Some of the new community weeklies established in response to the demand for more local news.

many sections of the nation, all stimulated by the hope of getting the now more readily available advertising of local merchants and big industries seeking personnel, or by the idea that the power of the press would further either a peaceful revolution or at least an improvement in the black condition. These bore such names as *North Shore Examiner* in Evanston, Illinois; the *Crow* and the *World,* both in New Haven, Connecticut; the *Bay State Banner,* of Massachusetts; and Atlanta's two rivals for the *World,* the *Inquirer* and the *Voice.* There also was the rise of the *Sentinel* in St. Louis, to challenge two long established weeklies, the *Argus* and the *American.* A few community magazines were born: *Echo,* of Milwaukee; *Philly Talk,* in Pennsylvania; *Proud,* in St. Louis; *Around the Town,* in Syracuse.

When the 1970's began, a few circulations were higher, but the rises were mainly in the magazines, not the larger newspapers, some of which fell lower. But advertising revenue was increasing. For there clearly was determination among some non-blacks to assist the black people to reach the place of equality of opportunity they had been struggling for or to meet the threats of destruction of the white society by correcting the conditions that led to unrest.

To say, however, that advertising revenue was increasing means little, for there was a long distance for it to go to give black publications assurance of a future. The discrimination against them by advertisers for the most part was continuing. The black newspaper or magazine, like any other, is at the space-buyer's mercy unless it has such clear command of its field that advertisers cannot do without it,

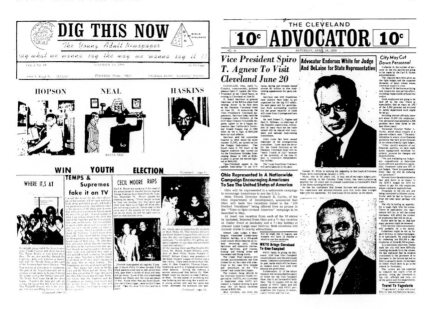

a rare situation in the black press, since the black market has been little understood or probed until recently.

Like other ethnic presses in the United States, during its history the black press has had to contend with some of the same basic obstacles facing the general press as well as certain peculiar to itself. The historians have shown that about 3,000 newspapers alone were established between 1827 and today, of which all but about 250 have ceased.[16] The number of periodicals begun during the same span of years is undetermined. It, too, must amount to many hundreds. Yet these relatively few publications exercised an influence far greater than one would expect from their numbers. That strength was possible because there were many causes for which they fought and for which many still do battle.   ●

5. TODAY'S NATIONAL NEWSPAPERS

WHETHER ON A NEWSSTAND in Harlem or in a drugstore in the black neighborhoods of the larger cities across the country, one is sure to find on sale, in addition to a local black weekly, at least one of the national black newspapers.

Generally newspaper publishers realize that the U.S.A. because of its large size does not actually have national newspapers as, say, does England. For there, as in many other smaller Western nations, the morning paper's final edition is received all over the country in time for reading at breakfast.

Therefore to call any black newspaper *national* would seem to be making exaggerated claims. But the use of the term can be considered accurate because virtually all black papers are weeklies, and several cover the black news of the country in about the same way as a weekly newsmagazine. In consequence it is possible for black papers to have more or less uniform distribution nationwide, albeit spottily, on their publication dates.

National black papers are of four kinds: 1) those with separate, regional editions but bearing one name, such as the *Afro-American,* which appears in Baltimore and sends separate editions to Washington, Richmond, and other cities and also has a national edition; 2) those originating in a particular community and sold widely in the country, an example being *Muhammad Speaks;* 3) those having a local edition but also one under the same name and intended for wider than local reading; this type is illustrated by the *New Pittsburgh Courier,* which has a city edition but also a national aimed at readers anywhere; 4) those known widely in the nation although they may have few subscribers outside their localities; an example is the Louisville *Defender.*

FIG. 5.1. These four newspapers are the national editions of the frontrunners among the weeklies and semi-weeklies. The **Daily Defender** publishes a national weekend edition; the **Afro-American** national edition appears in regional variations separate from the papers published for Baltimore, Washington, Philadelphia, Richmond, and New Jersey.

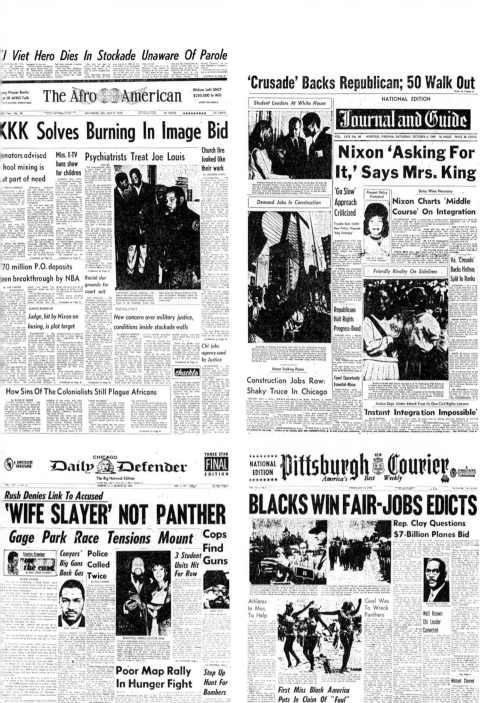

I Viet Hero Dies In Stockade Unaware Of Parole

The Afro ✺✺ American

Widow Left UNCF $250,000 in Will
(STORY ON PAGE 2)

BALTIMORE, MD., MAY 9, 1970   26 PAGES   ★★★★★★★★★   20 CENTS

KKK Solves Burning In Image Bid

Senators advised school mixing is not part of need

Miss. E-TV bans show for children

Psychiatrists Treat Joe Louis

Church fire looked like their work

70 million P.O. deposits

een breakthrough by NBA

Racial slur grounds for court suit

Judge, hit by Nixon on busing, is plot target

New concern over military justice, conditions inside stockade walls

Chi jobs agency's sued by Justice

chackle

How Sins Of The Colonialists Still Plague Africans

'Crusade' Backs Republican; 50 Walk Out

Student Leaders At White House

Journal and Guide

VOL. LXIX No. 40   NORFOLK, VIRGINIA, SATURDAY, OCTOBER 4, 1969   16 PAGES PRICE 20 CENTS

Nixon 'Asking For It,' Says Mrs. King

Demand Jobs In Construction

'Go Slow' Approach Criticized

Present Policy Protested

Delay When Necessary

Nixon Charts 'Middle Course' On Integration

Friendly Rivalry On Sidelines

Va. 'Crusade' Backs Holton; Split In Ranks

Republicans Halt Rights Progress—Bond

Mayor Seeking Peace

Construction Jobs Row: Shaky Truce In Chicago

Equal Opportunity Essential-Nixon

'Instant Integration Impossible'

CHICAGO
Daily Defender
The Big National Edition

THREE STAR FINAL EDITION

Rush Denies Link To Accused

'WIFE SLAYER' NOT PANTHER

Gage Park Race Tensions Mount

Cops Find Guns

'Country Preacher'
the cast
By REV. JESSE JACKSON

BLACK RADIO

Conyers' Big Guns Back Gus

Police Called Twice

3 Student Units Hit For Row

Poor Map Rally In Hunger Fight

Step Up Hunt For Bombers

Exclusive Report:

How Reformed Is The Bridewell?

Daily Defender Primary Endorsements

ENDORSEMENTS

NATIONAL EDITION
Pittsburgh Courier
America's Best Weekly

NEW

FEBRUARY 21, 1970

BLACKS WIN FAIR-JOBS EDICTS

Rep. Clay Questions $7-Billion Planes Bid

Goal Was To Wreck Panthers

Athletes In Miss. To Help

Well Known G'Leader Convicted

First Miss Black America Puts In Claim Of 'Foul'

Black Mafia

What Is It?

Militant Cleared

Mrs. King Raps Nixon

Black Count Questioned

Earlier in this century numerous papers sought national distribution and readership, especially in the days when they had reached the peaks of their circulation. But as they suffered a sharp fall-off in sales most contented themselves with area distribution or joined to become parts of groups or chains.

Today a few still print national editions, although not always so labeling them. The Chicago *Daily Defender* adds to its four-day tabloid a standard-sized weekly it calls its week-end edition. The Baltimore *Afro-American* and the *New Pittsburgh Courier* also have national editions, as does the Norfolk *Journal and Guide*.

● GROUPS AND CHAINS

A half dozen newspaper groups or chains exist today, running in size from the nine-unit Sengstacke Newspapers to the three-unit World group.[1] The advantages of any such unification include the possibilities of uniform policies, greater purchasing power than for a single paper, more circulation to offer advertisers, larger opportunities for staff members, and wider use of editorial matter. The disadvantages: possible lack of independence for local executives especially editors and writers, elimination of competition and possible reduction in news coverage and variety of editorial opinions, and reduction of job opportunities for staffs.

Largest of these associations of papers in 1970 was the Sengstacke chain, named for its publisher, John H. Sengstacke. The matrix paper is the Chicago *Daily Defender,* with editions Monday through Thursday and an equally large weekly, standard-sized paper called the week-end edition, for national sale. Five of the other papers—known with some others as the Pittsburgh *Courier* weeklies before Sengstacke bought them in 1966—are the *New Pittsburgh Courier,* Ohio *Courier,* Philadelphia *Courier,* Georgia *Courier,* and Florida *Courier.* The remaining three are the Shreveport (La.) *Sun,* Memphis *Tri-State Defender,* and the Detroit *Michigan Chronicle.* The New York *Courier* was part of the chain until sold in 1969 to the New York Courier Syndicate, Inc., in which Percy Sutton, Manhattan Borough president, has an interest.

The Sengstacke Newspapers comprise the largest association in terms of circulation as well. The Courier papers reach about 62,000, and the Sengstacke-owned others total about 165,000, thus the total for the combination is more than a fifth of a million.

The second largest combined circulation is that of the *Afro-American,* with its flagship paper in Baltimore and various editions for four other areas as well as the nation. In 1970 this group reached 134,000 circulation. Among the other multiple-unit papers of the same general size are the Post Newspapers, 50,000 circulation, serving Oakland, Berkeley, San Francisco, and Richmond; the New Leader group in Louisiana, 46,000, with papers in Alexandria, Baton Rouge, Monroe, and Lake Charles; the World (sometimes called Scott) group, 46,000, including the Atlanta *Daily World*, Birmingham *World*, and Memphis *World*.

● CHARACTERISTICS OF NATIONAL PAPERS

Bontrager, in a 1969 study of the use of black publications in a single community, selected five general characteristics of black newspapers, limiting himself, he pointed out, to those "most generally mentioned by scholars." These usually are the national weeklies discussed in this chapter.

"Negro newspapers," he wrote, "are protest-oriented; are typically suburban weeklies; are supplementary to the 'white' daily press; tend to be sensational; and have a high mortality rate."[2]

Although many of his observations are based on conditions of the 1940's and 1950's, all but one of Bontrager's list of characteristics still are accurately ascribed. The exception is the quality of sensationalism. Possibly these papers are sensational by comparison with general publications in the same cities, but by comparison with black papers in the 1920's to 1950's this press has toned down considerably. Because streamers and banners are used generously on front pages and tabloid size is increasingly popular the black papers often look more sensational than they are in fact.

The older papers, as already noted, were protest-oriented in their earliest days, but they were protesting about human slavery, brutal treatment of men, women, and children, and lynchings. Today the protests are over such matters as the failure of white groups to hire blacks for jobs they could hold, physical mistreatment by police and civilian groups, and discrimination in educational opportunities and housing. The national papers now look more like big city dailies than suburban weeklies, although the small weeklies fit the description just as before. More than ever the black paper is the second one in a household. And, among the smaller papers, the mortality rate has been high but it has not touched a major weekly in recent years.

Another characteristic, buried perhaps in Bontrager's point about the suburban nature of these papers, is that they are more and more stressing local news, a consequence of backing off from issuing papers for coast-to-coast distribution. This policy resulted from the need to carry news that the general press cannot accommodate, making it more certain that the black reader would continue to be loyal to his own papers. The desire for such local strength is supported by the circulation figures of the few papers that issue local and national editions.

The semi-weekly average circulation of the Baltimore edition of the *Afro-American* in 1968, for example, was 35,139; that of the na-

tional 26,055. The Chicago *Daily Defender*'s four-day daily product
averaged 36,614; the paper's week-end (national) edition was 32,841.
The *New Pittsburgh Courier* shows a slight advantage for the national
edition: the city edition was 13,372; the national, 13,634. It is not
possible to tell from circulation reports the breakdown between local
and national circulations in the instance of a large paper that sells
the same edition locally as well as regionally, such as the New York
Amsterdam News.

● VIGNETTES OF INDIVIDUAL PAPERS

The historical background of most national papers already has
been related. Events, however, have changed the nature of some of
these papers in recent years. They should be examined as they were
in the late 1960's and early 1970's.

Chicago **Daily Defender.** The mother hen of the Sengstacke papers,
a chain sometimes described by its enemies as an octopus, this four-day
tabloid strongly resembles the New York *Daily News* in its typography
and in its variety of feature content. For fifty years a standard-sized
paper, the *Defender* turned tabloid in 1956. It has city and home editions, as well as a national version; its title goes on the weekly version
for the nation including the word *Daily.* The week-ender is standard
size. Conceiving itself as an important source of national news about
black America, as indeed it is, the *Defender* carries considerable quantities of United Press International copy but also much Chicago area
and midwestern news of special interest to its readers and not often
to be found in the general press. Its editorial page strongly resembles
that of the New York tabloid but is in a different corner in point of
view. It differs largely in that it is moderate in its political position
and liberal on certain problems affecting the lives of blacks, such as
housing, equality in employment opportunities, and education.

Signed columns and a humor column fill the left-hand page-
opposite-editorial. The main editorial page has the unsigned essays
in the first two columns on the left, an Inquiring Reporter feature in
the middle alley, an editorial cartoon in the upper right side, and a
Washington column below it, i.e., a typical New York tabloid format.
The center spread which usually follows it consists of news and feature pictures also in the tabloid make-up pattern. Advertising of
food is supported with several pages of cooking copy, and sports copy
sometimes runs a half-dozen pages.

The week-end edition contains considerable copy not found in
the daily. Thomas Picou, managing editor of the daily, explained
to the author that both editions have their own sources and depend
little upon the syndicates. A letterpress product, each edition operates on a standard newspaper set-up. In the late 1960's the papers had

150 employes between them, one a white person. The facilities in the *Defender* building at 2400 South Michigan Avenue are well arranged. The news room on the main floor is directly beyond the entrance foyer, the editorial executive room is a series of small offices beyond, with the main administrative offices on the second floor.

The weekly national edition, more so than the daily, tends to carry greater quantities of editorialized and publicity copy, particularly in special supplements, such as career guides, wherein every college or business buying space also is discussed in editorial copy obviously emanating from the institution's publicity or public relations department. The regular pages of one issue, for example, carried a three-quarter column story about an oil company and its education plans, including considerable promotion of the company as such; it also offered, in the middle of an otherwise newsy page, a clearly promotional story about grass, the kind walked on, not smoked, coming from an acoustical firm. Hardly exceptional in American journalism are the many columns devoted to publicity for and gossip about entertainers.

Both the daily and weekly editions are heavy with advertising copy, much of it coming from local department stores and supermarkets. But many small shops and services also buy space; some of this is cooperative, that is, national firms and local outlets for their products combining in buying space.

The Atlanta Daily World. The nation's oldest black daily is a family venture like the *Defender,* long identified with the Scott family. As a daily it is the older of the two, having been made into a daily in 1932, whereas the *Defender* did not go on that schedule until 1956.

The Scott who founded it was William Alexander Scott, who, like Abbott in his decision to start his magazine in a depression, began the *World* in the same inauspicious times. It first appeared in 1928. Scott was not destined to remain with it long, for he was assassinated in 1934, when only thirty-one.[3] By then, however, he had developed something of a journalistic empire and also was engaged in real estate. He had contributed, also, a plan of having a staff in another city which gathered news for a local paper which was printed in the home city, in this instance Atlanta.

The Scott in charge thereafter was Cornelius A. Scott, a Mississippian born in 1908, and a former student at both Morehouse and Kansas universities. Under his direction the *World* has been consistently conservative on political issues. Lomax, in one of his books some years ago, called the *World* "the one exception" among the papers that generally have supported the black revolt. He labels it "highly-respected, rock-ribbed Republican" and notes that in 1960 it carried a double-column editorial asking, "Is This Type of Action Necessary in This Case?" in which it criticized students who had organized an economic boycott of white merchants who refused to hire blacks as anything but menials, although the shops were in the black neighborhoods.[4]

A standard-sized four-day paper, it is at the heart of the Scott group.[5] Much of its content therefore appears in the Memphis *World* and Birmingham *World,* including editorials, columns, and some news stories. The editorials in all papers frequently are on national rather than local issues.

The *World* has been the training ground for numerous black journalists who have gone on to prominence as writers and editors of other newspapers as well as magazines; some are known for their work as publicists. The paper as issued daily in normal times—it was undergoing a strike in the 1969–70 period—appears to have little news, but that is an erroneous conclusion, for its four copies a week should be matched against one issue of a weekly by each of the two other Atlanta black papers. It has maintained a fixed circulation of about 30,000 daily for a number of years.

Columbus Times. Columbus, Georgia, has been the setting for several attempts at a daily black paper, the earliest on record being the *Messenger,* begun in 1887, an outgrowth of what had been a weekly and then a semi-weekly. Briefly during the 1960's Vernon Mitchell, publisher of a weekly called the *News,* ran it on a daily schedule but soon reverted to the lesser frequency. After his death his widow, Ophelia De Vore Mitchell, widely known as founder and chief officer of a cosmetics firm and related enterprises, started a new paper, the *Times.*

Issued on a four-day-a-week basis, it first came off the press on October 21, 1970, in an eight-column format, offset printed. Emphasis is on interpretative and other features and major local news stories only. It contains considerable out-of-town copy of interest to its readers also, some of these materials coming from Copley News Service and Continental Features. Editorial opinions are forthright but kept to the editor's page. Advertising runs from 30 to 40 per cent, and is mainly local. It is too soon to draw fair comparisons with the two long established dailies.

The **Afro-American.** When the American Society of Journalism School Administrators made its annual award to a newspaper or magazine in 1969, it went for the first time to a black publication; the award had been made annually since 1946. It went to the *Afro-American,* "In recognition of the distinguished record of a newspaper which has served a predominantly black community and which has actively engaged in community service." The paper received nearly three times the vote of the second choice.

The strong vote for this paper, one of the few semi-weeklies in black journalism, was earned not only by the headquarters edition but also by the four others. The Murphy family continues to run the corporation, all of whose papers are standard sized and together command among the highest group sales. Like most other leaders, the *Afro* contains much to read, although its copy is more closely edited and its pages more carefully planned and coordinated than those of many of its rivals, if not as well printed. It gives considerably more coverage to foreign, especially African, news. Substantial stories received from UPI and its own staffers and correspondents report such major events in other countries as changes in government, new policies, and conflicts between them; the discrimination against blacks in South Africa and Rhodesia is emphasized.

Afro editorial pages are crammed with reading matter and cartoons, often offering as many as six editorials, supplemented by Roy Wilkins and other signed columns; the paper also allots far more space to letters than usually is found in black papers, although with so many editions it probably receives more as well. Service and opinion columns appear on the page opposite editorial: a Washington, a medical, and a poetry column, the latter not a common feature in most black papers. With its various regional or city editions it is possible to give space in the national version to news from those areas; this is supplemented with correspondence as well from Atlanta, Detroit, and other cities with heavy black populations. Society and sports occupy what seems like excessive space, although church and other special news is not slighted. And, once again, it must be noted that if this news does not appear here where then will it be printed?

A tabloid, four-page magazine section has humor material, games, a health column, a lonesome hearts piece, a comic strip, and other time-copy features. This paper for many years has generated many news and feature stories, such as a full-page illustrated one based on interviews with a number of wounded black veterans of Vietnam recovering in a government hospital. The *Afro* in recent years has conducted campaigns to get blacks to register to vote, to equalize teachers' salaries, for appointment of blacks to various city and state positions.

By providing financial support the paper has helped overcome discriminatory practices. Mrs. Elizabeth Murphy Moss, vice president and treasurer of the firm, reported to the organization that gave her papers the ASJSA award, that the paper was responsible for "financing the first lawsuit contesting the right of the Southern Railroad to jim crow colored passengers on all trains leaving Washington for the South." Another example of crusading was in the suit filed against the Maryland Art Institute because it had excluded black students; it also campaigned to open the graduate schools of the University of Maryland. It worked to make the Baltimore Public Library hire people of all races.

All editions—Baltimore, Washington, New Jersey, Richmond, and National—are printed in a three-story building in Baltimore, on a thirty-two-page press. The paper is nonunion throughout. The editorial staff in 1969 consisted of twenty persons, six of them white.

The paper's policy can be called moderate on national racial issues. Violent tactics by certain militants are ridiculed, constructive efforts at cooperation with whites are encouraged. An attitude of suspicion surrounds most comments on the Republican administration of the early 1970's.

New York **Amsterdam News.** Looking somewhat like the now defunct Hearst daily, New York *Journal-American,* with two or three streamers stretching across page one, the *Amsterdam News* now ranks as the standard black weekly with the largest circulation, in 1971 about 80,000. It is one of the few that has had an American Newspaper Guild contract with its employes; it was, in fact, the first to have an editorial union, signing the agreement in 1963. It also is known for its labor troubles, for it has had two strikes.

The paper is run by Dr. C. B. Powell, who as president and editor shares his time with his insurance, funeral, and loan service businesses. Dr. Powell has made entirely clear that he is interested in the paper purely as a commercial enterprise, an attitude that has earned him some dislike from idealistic blacks and appears to have kept the paper from achieving what has been accomplished by the determined crusaders in the black press world.

Today it represents mainly the conventional Harlemite or resident of some other black colony within New York City, but it does well by him, with many pages of news. Much of it is routine, to be sure, but most of it unavailable elsewhere, for the paper has the abundant New York field around it, and its competition is now reduced to numerous community papers and the now rebuilding New York *Courier.*

J. Kirk Sale explained in an article on this paper that while its union contract has raised the earnings of the staff it also hindered executives in getting a better quality of copy, such as interpretative stories on local issues, and even in covering ordinary events if overtime is involved.[6]

The *Amsterdam News'* political affiliations in recent years have been with the Democratic Party. Although it supported Eisenhower in 1952 it went on to urge voters to elect Stevenson in 1956 and Kennedy, Johnson, and Humphrey in succeeding elections. Lately it also has become milder in its news treatment. In the 1940's it was considered a sensational paper, printing much gossip and scandal. James Baldwin, among other of its critics then, cited its use of murder, rape, love-nest raids, and interracial war stories as well as accounts of social gains. He disliked what he called its "pathetic preoccupation

FIG. 5.2. The Philadelphia **Tribune,** one of the few bi-weeklies, is one of the oldest black newspapers, having been founded in 1884. The New York **Amsterdam News** has the highest circulation of a commercial paper. The Cleveland **Call and Post** and the Dallas **Express** are important moderate-circulation papers.

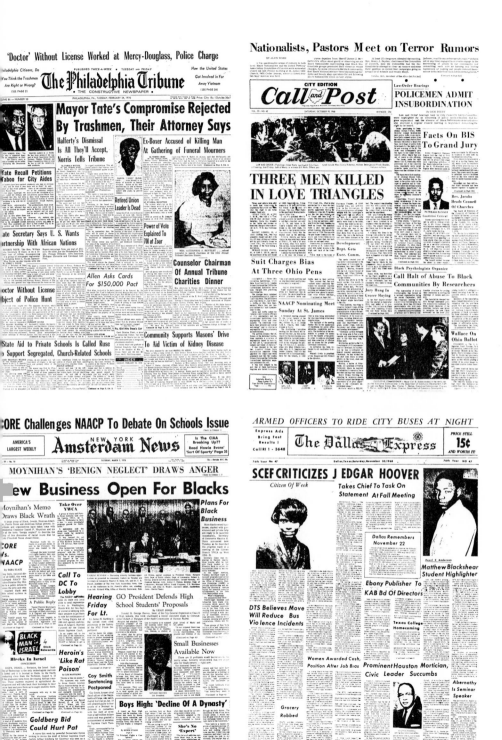

'Doctor' Without License Worked at Mercy-Douglass, Police Charge

Philadelphia Citizens, Do You Think the Trashmen Are Right or Wrong?
(SEE PAGE 3)

How the United States Got Involved in Far Away Vietnam
(SEE PAGE 38)

The Philadelphia Tribune
• THE CONSTRUCTIVE NEWSPAPER •

PUBLISHED TWICE-A-WEEK • TUESDAY and FRIDAY

VOLUME 86 — NUMBER 33

PHILADELPHIA, PA., TUESDAY, FEBRUARY 24, 1970

Price 15c (Outside 20c)

Mayor Tate's Compromise Rejected By Trashmen, Their Attorney Says

Halferty's Dismissal Is All They'll Accept, Norris Tells Tribune

Ex-Boxer Accused of Killing Man At Gathering of Funeral Mourners

Tate Recall Petitions Taboo for City Aides

Retired Union Leader Is Dead

ate Secretary Says U. S. Wants Partnership With African Nations

Power of Vote Explained To Tot al Zoar

Counselor Chairman Of Annual Tribune Charities Dinner

Doctor Without License Object of Police Hunt

Allen Asks Cards For $150,000 Pact

State Aid to Private Schools Is Called Ruse To Support Segregated, Church-Related Schools

Community Supports Masons' Drive To Aid Victim of Kidney Disease

---

Nationalists, Pastors Meet on Terror Rumors
BY ALVIN WARD

CITY EDITION
Call and Post

VOL. 23 — NO. 42

SATURDAY, OCTOBER 19, 1968

44 PAGES 20c

Law-Order Hearings
POLICEMEN ADMIT INSUBORDINATION
BY DICK PEERY

THREE MEN KILLED IN LOVE TRIANGLES

Suit Charges Bias At Three Ohio Pens

NAACP Nominating Meet Sunday At St. James

Facts On BIS To Grand Jury

Rev. Jacobs Heads Connell Of Churches

Black Psychologists To Organize

Call Halt of Abuse To Black Communities By Researchers

Wallace On Ohio Ballot

CORE Challenges NAACP To Debate On Schools Issue

AMERICA'S LARGEST WEEKLY

Amsterdam News
NEW YORK

Is The CIAA Breaking Up? Read Howie Evans' 'Sort Of Sporty' Page 35

SATURDAY, MARCH 7, 1970

15c — Outside N.Y. 20c

MOYNIHAN'S 'BENIGN NEGLECT' DRAWS ANGER

New Business Open For Blacks

Moynihan's Memo Draws Black Wrath

Take Over YWCA

Plans For Black Business

CORE vs. NAACP

Call To DC To Lobby

Hearing Friday For Lt.

GO President Defends High School Students' Proposals

A Public Reply

BLACK MAN in ISRAEL by Dick Edwards

Blacks In Israel

Heroin's 'Like Rat Poison'

Coy Smith Sentencing Postponed

Small Businesses Available Now

Goldberg Bid Could Hurt Pat

Boys High: 'Decline Of A Dynasty'

She's No 'Expert'

ARMED OFFICERS TO RIDE CITY BUSES AT NIGHT

Express Ads Bring fast Results ! Call RI 1 - 3648

The Dallas Express

PRICE STILL 15c AND WORTH IT!

74th Year No 47

Dallas,Texas,Saturday,November 30,1968

74th Year NO 47

SCEF CRITICIZES J EDGAR HOOVER

Citizen Of Week

Takes Chief To Task On Statement At Fall Meeting

Dallas Remembers November 22

DTS Believes Move Will Reduce Bus Vio lence Incidents

Women Awarded Cash, Position After Job Bias

Grocery Robbed

Matthew Blackshear Student Highlighter

Ebony Publisher To KAB Bd Of Directors

Texas College Seminar

Prominent Houston Mortician, Civic Leader Succumbs

Abernathy Is Seminar Speaker

with prominent Negroes and what they are doing," including in this comment also *People's Weekly*.[7] Two decades later, however, the paper is relatively sedate. Its news coverage is heavily local; a Brooklyn section with its own flag reading Brooklyn *Amsterdam News* is included. Yet much room is made for regular columns by Roy Wilkins, Floyd McKissick, and some of its own staff. Sports and women's interests are covered strongly; these are two staples of the national papers. Interpretative stories appear, but not as often as a paper of its size might provide. Editorially it runs to about the same views as the *Afro* and the *Defender*. It criticizes the Nixon administration but is uncharmed by the firebrands who seek to solve problems with fire-bombs.

The **New Pittsburgh Courier.** It was not always called that; the *New* is a recent addition, intended to create a different tone or image for itself. The word is hardly noticeable, however, in the nameplate; it is attached to the publishing company name but not the paper's in the masthead. The folio lines carry it. The *Courier* was not yet a part of the Sengstacke Newspapers when Baldwin wrote of it, but it was the only black paper to receive unqualified praise from the novelist in his 1948 appraisal of the black press. He granted that it had the reputation of being "the best of the lot" and called it "a high class paper."

Much like the *Amsterdam News* in its generous allotment of space to local news and features and to special pages as well as to columns, it varies from the other papers in that its national edition sometimes carries two sets of editorials, one in the specially prepared pages at the front and another set on the regular editorial page picked up from the Pittsburgh edition. This standard-sized page is flanked by another on which may appear columns by Roy Wilkins, Jackie Robinson, Benjamin E. Mays, and Bayard Rustin; most appear in both editions. Photographs are numerous; many, however, are no more than publicity shots provided by entertainers, motion picture producers, and food manufacturers.

Although for many years identified with the conservative viewpoint politically and economically, partly because of the presence on its staff of George S. Schuyler, one of the most able and articulate of the conservative black journalists, in recent years the paper has moved a little less cautiously on the racial issues of the day. Politely, for example, it called President Nixon's attention to failures to give blacks greater place in national developments, applauding black studies in the white colleges, and lamenting student activists.

Cleveland Call and Post. Pride, in expressing pungent opinions of the leading black papers in an article, once described the *Call and Post* as a paper that "provides bread-and-butter coverage." It is this concern for local news that has kept it a leading black weekly. At times the handling of such news has bordered on the sensational. A few sample headlines: a five-column two-liner reading: "Three Men Killed/In Love Triangle." The main streamer over the flag, one week, read: "Nationalists, Pastors Meet on Terror Rumors."

Editorially it has kept an eye on the local scene more than some of the other medium-sized papers; these often are elaborate and far more thorough than the usual opinion writing in these weeklies. Local columnists are featured as well as national writers. Much of the reputation for excellent coverage comes from the extensive society, club, women's, and entertainment pages and the generous use of pictures on them. Typographically the *Call and Post* is among the more modern papers, with a somewhat streamlined makeup for its standard-sized pages.

Mildly liberal politically and supporting Mayor Carl Stokes, the first black executive of a major city, the paper for years has played up the accomplishments of the black citizen. Editorials tend to be local; in general they are loyal to the Republican Party point of view.

The Philadelphia Tribune. A semi-weekly, the *Tribune* celebrated its eighty-fifth anniversary in 1969. It is the oldest continuously published black general newspaper in the U.S.A. Unquestionably one of the major papers, it is of professional quality, with an attractively planned front page. It provides detailed news coverage, the stories closely edited as a rule; often this reporting crowds the paper with many short news accounts. So many varieties of headline sizes and types are used that the pages beyond the first are not always easy to penetrate. It has standard-sized pages.

Society, sports, and youth materials supplement the several pages of general local news as does copy from syndicates. The editorial policy is hard-hitting but along moderate lines. It reflects the views of its late publisher, E. Washington Rhodes, who believed that such newspapers should crusade for black rights and set up various programs of aid to blacks in the Philadelphia area.

Norfolk Journal and Guide. Color generally has little place in the national papers, but the Norfolk *Journal and Guide* does use a tint in its nameplate on the front page and occasionally in advertising in its home edition. It is a quickly recognizable paper therefore, just as the *New Pittsburgh Courier* is easily spotted by its green tinted stock for the wrap-around pages. Like most of its peers, the *Journal and Guide* is standard size and has both a city and national edition at this writing but there was possibility of abandoning the latter. Both are newsy. A reader may be confused, sometimes, by the many small and large headlines but he must be impressed with the paper's tone of bursting with information.

The *Journal and Guide* carries much locally generated news as well as wire copy from United Press International and correspondence from numerous small mid-South towns. Pictures are used generously, but, as in so many papers, most are just head shots or of two persons shaking hands, or a line of men or women facing the camera. Special features, however, in which the black newspaper often is weak because of lack of staff to write such stories, are more numerous in this paper than usual, and are concerned with individuals as well as group activities.

Editorial pages contain standard materials but perhaps more of them: an Inquiring Reporter column, addicted to innocuous questions such as "Does a good salesman influence you in buying or do you think for yourself?"; syndicated columns by several staffers, humorous cartoons, a medical column, religious feature, from two to four other cartoons, some religious. Reproduction of all this material is not up to the quality of writing or quantity. Cuts often are blackish or washed out, retouching is amateurish. The firmness of the paper's editorial policies is not suggested by its sober presentation of news, especially off page one. Although editorials are few, they are forthright, a reputation the paper earned during the two world wars and has maintained since.

● THE MUSLIM AND PANTHER PAPERS

Although they are not conventional commercial newspapers, *Muhammad Speaks* and the *Black Panther,* two comparatively recent additions to the nationally distributed black newspapers, have come to major attention in the past few years. The first has shot to the lead in circulation over all other black newspapers (but not magazines), achieving the highest figure in the newspaper press' history, around 600,000 claimed by the publishers. The second, with only one-sixth of the Nation of Islam weekly's sales, nevertheless is able to note a larger circulation than any of the commercial publications, having by 1970 reached about 100,000 every week.

Both papers are tabloid-size and spokesmen for groups within the black society. They are not standard, national newspapers to be linked or equated with the *Afro* or the Chicago *Defender.* They are organs of groups, and cause or advocacy journals. Depending upon one's social and political outlook, they may be considered papers whose aim is a sharp, perhaps even revolutionary, change in the form of government of the United States. In the *Black Panther,* at least, it is apparently to be achieved through the use of force; many an issue contains pictures of guns on almost every page, including photographs of the party leaders carrying weapons, presumably only for self-defense. Nothing is said in the party's ten-point platform and program about how its ends are to be met, for the emphasis is all on the demands, which are typified by these quotations, printed in every issue:

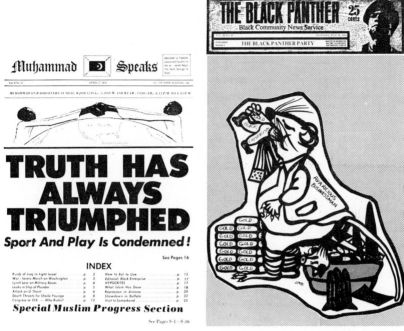

FIG. 5.3. These two weekly advocacy papers have the largest circulation among black newspapers. **Muhammad Speaks** is the voice of the Nation of Islam; the **Black Panther** is the official organ of the group whose name it bears.

We want freedom. We want power to determine the destiny of our Black Community. We want full employment for our people. We want an end to the robbery by the CAPITALIST of our Black Community. We want decent housing, fit for shelter of human beings. We want education for our people that exposes them to the true nature of this decadent American society. We want education that teaches us our true history and our role in the present-day society. We want all black men to be exempt from military service. We want an immediate end to POLICE BRUTALITY and MURDER of black people. We want freedom for all black men held in federal, state, county and city prisons and jails.[8]

The ninth point asks that black people be tried by a jury of their peer group or people from their black communities and the tenth states that the major political objective of the party is a "United Nations-supervised plebiscite to be held throughout the black colony in which only black colonial subjects will be allowed to participate, for the purpose of determining the will of black people as to their national destiny."[9]

The fifth point of a twenty-six-point "Rules of the Black Panther Party," also printed regularly, declares: "No party member will USE,

POINT, or FIRE a weapon of any kind unnecessarily or accidentally at anyone." Point sixteen, however, says that "All Panthers must learn to operate and service weapons correctly."

Muhammad Speaks publishes in all issues a Muslim program. Some demands are like the Panthers' but others vary or deal with different aspects, such as discouraging racial intermarriage. A major difference is that the Muslims—and their paper—seek "a separate state or territory of their own—either on this continent or elsewhere." Schooling is to be in the hands of Muslim blacks. The program is one for Muslims rather than all blacks, although the Muslim aim is to embrace all members of the race in the Nation of Islam.[10] Symbolic or actual pictures of guns, for either offensive or defensive use, do not appear in *Muhammad Speaks*.

By whose definition are these two papers radical or revolutionary? The overthrow of a government, either by force or in some peaceful method such as the ballot box, is considered a revolutionary act and certainly not strange in U.S. history. Publications that propose such a change, in any manner, can be called revolutionary. They are radical in the sense that they go to the roots of a situation. Although there may be nothing new in the socialism of the Panther Party, for example, it still is a revolutionary organ, as its tenets show.

The support for this at least militant press may be more substantial than is realized. A nationwide Louis Harris survey made in 1970 indicated that while "the vast majority want to work through the existing system," 9 per cent of the blacks of the nation consider themselves as "revolutionaries," a number exceeding two million, a mighty army, if suitably led and deployed. Thirty-one per cent of the nation's black people said that they believed only a "readiness to use violence" will ever bring them equality. That figure was 10 per cent higher than the one for response to a similar survey in 1966. Among the 31 per cent of the 1970 survey were black teen-agers who rely on violence, 49 per cent of them so declaring.[11]

Muhammad Speaks *Policies.* The Muslim paper developed from or alongside a miscellany of publications issued by the organization behind it, but it now is the dominant piece of journalism coming from the movement. Among these earlier publications was the *Messenger,* a magazine launched about 1960. It carried the name of Malcolm X as editor and printed mainly features on Muslim business activities, family life, school work, and other Muslim interests. Another, a tabloid, the *Islamic News,* came out in 1959; its one issue was devoted to a speech by a Muslim leader. *Salaam* was one of two pocket-sized magazines issued about the same time. Published in Philadelphia, it contained mainly pictures.

Mr. Muhammad Speaks to the Blackman was started in Harlem in 1960. Malcolm X has described the founding, noting that by 1959 the Nation of Islam was planning a paper. Malcolm had taken such preliminary steps as writing for the black press. James Hicks, editor of the New York *Amsterdam News,* published a column Malcolm wrote to express Muslim views. When that was taken over by Mr. Muhammad, as the Muslim leader, Elijah Muhammad, is called, Malcolm's writings were shifted to the Los Angeles *Herald-Dispatch.* He worked briefly at that paper after organizing a Muslim temple in the California city. Next he taught himself photography, then he began writing Muslim news stories and taking pictures of interest to the followers. Finally he found a printer and produced the paper. It was sold on the streets of Harlem, just as today much of its distribution is person-to-person in the black neighborhoods of the nation's cities.[12] It later became simply *Muhammad Speaks* and moved to Chicago. At one time it was edited by Dan Burley, the Chicago journalist (see Chapter 10). In its early years it was described by a critic as "a shallow publication, playing upon racial feeling in such a way as to be nauseous even to some Muslims."[13]

Printed in a modern, well-equipped plant in Chicago, the paper today trains and simultaneously gives work to blacks and hopes to employ more of them if it succeeds in its plans of going on a semi-weekly and then daily schedule. The building housing it contains the latest electronic production equipment (see Chapter 13). One-half the editorial staff of thirty-two are Muslims and "most top editors are trained in journalism." John Woodford, editor in 1970, is a Harvard graduate with previous news experience; the New York editor a Columbia journalism degree holder.

The present policies of *Muhammad Speaks* are easily enough discerned. Almost any issue makes clear that the paper is pro-Arab and anti-Israel, opposed to the U.S. participation in the Indo-China War, and to the Nixon administration's educational policies. It supports all Muslim goals, particularly achievement of black industrial and agricultural self-sufficiency and favors the present Cuban government.

The paper carries considerable copy, both text and illustrative, from various parts of the U.S.A. and the world bearing on its policies. Much of it is angled in line with those policies, such as defense of blacks and exposure of police brutality toward them. It shows sympathy with the aims of the Viet Cong and supports the efforts of Africa's underdeveloped nations to gain strength and stability. It does not neglect straight features about progress of individual blacks in serious occupations.

Muhammad Speaks was one of the first publications to uncover a movement to do genetic testing on blacks in the belief that people of a "lower social class" are more given to criminal behavior. The paper dubbed this plan "Nazi-science" in a story provided by its Washington bureau.[14] It is stimulating to go through the paper because of the large amount of original news coverage, specially written features, and orderly plan of content. Another world opens

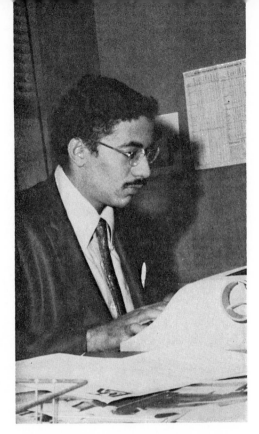

FIG. 5.4. John Woodford, editor of **Muhammad Speaks,** weekly newspaper of the Nation of Islam. (Chester Sheard photo)

before the reader who is not of the Muslim order. Most of the advertising is from small merchants in the Chicago area but the volume of it is misleading at a glance, for much of it is announcing speeches on radio by Elijah Muhammad or presents his views, in that form, on some current issue. The paper gives the impression of being newsy with its punchy headlines; now and again it presents treatment of some topics in depth, such as a several-part article on "The Black Policeman."

This paper's high circulation figure requires closer examination. Loyalty to Islam is an important factor, as is the sales organization. The Muslim vendors are told to sell all copies and unsold ones are not accepted for credit. These salesmen regularly canvass the black neighborhoods and dispose of the paper to steady buyers. The loyalty is exemplified by a Waterloo, Iowa, subscriber's letter, which said, after noting that he was sending his renewal by special delivery, "I find it unbearable to rely on whitey for my only source of news." L. F. Palmer, Jr., a Chicago black newsman, gives 498,000 as the paper's press run (apparently in 1969) and thinks, therefore, that it must have a circulation of "well over 400,000."[15] *Time* magazine reported its circulation in 1970 at 400,000. The publishers claim 600,000. Whichever the figure, it is five to six times greater than that of the largest commercial black newspaper.

The **Panther** *Growls.* A black intellectual has observed to the author
that the Black Panther Party needs money; its paper, therefore, is
a means to raise it. He insisted that many of its sales are made to
whites—especially the "white Negroes," as he called them, who want
to know what the Panthers are saying. The street salesmen in New
York and other big cities therefore go to places were interested whites
would congregate: Central Park in New York rather than Bedford-
Stuyvesant, for they can dispose of many in such spots. The informant
is borne out by the content of the paper, for it says what militant
whites and blacks appear to want to read. To please militants white
or black, the *Black Panther* publishes mainly opinion articles, some
from its party branch correspondents, others from party officials. Its
news content does not stand comparison with that of *Muhammad
Speaks,* either in importance, variety, or manner of presentation. Its
front page is a satirical cartoon; its back page, likely as not, another.
Inside most pages contain two or three reports each about what is
going on in the party branches or a half-page message from "Big
Man," deputy minister of information of the party, or material reprinted, with full credit, from white newspapers, usually stories of
white attacks on blacks: "N.Y. Pigs Frame-Up Leaders of International Women's Day Actions," reads a headline, whose story sat on
a two-column picture of a gun. Near it was a cartoon of a group of
black men, women, and children carrying guns, knives, and dynamite
sticks as well as a sign, "All Power to the People." Below it ran a
statement: "There is something that you should remember: we have
a human right to kill in defense of our lives."[16]

Facts about the paper's operations are not easy to come by. Party
officers and staff members are secretive. It is produced in California,
with an all-black staff working in Berkeley. Its top editorial official
is the black writer-in-exile, Eldridge Cleaver, who not only is editor
of the paper but also minister of information of the party's central
committee. A Black Community News Service also is offered by the
party, but appears to be only the *Black Panther* itself as an "alternative to the 'government approved' stories presented in the mass media
and the product of an effort to present the facts not stories as dic-
tated by the oppressor, but as seen from the other end of a gun."[17]

Perhaps the paper is more rhetorical overkill than revolutionary
intention. Its language, at least, is a different if not an altogether
unknown element in journalistic literature. *Newsweek* once described
the *Black Panther* as a "handsome tabloid weekly." By comparison
with some of the smallest black papers it is attractive, for it uses
one color, changing from week to week, on its outside covers and
its center spread. It also prints photographs dramatically, often using
shocking scenes of mistreatment of blacks. The content, however,
makes the publication as much a magazine as a newspaper.

Its tone is reminiscent of the revolutionary journalism in the
U.S.A. in the days when the International Workers of the World

(IWW) were active, early in the century. Its attitude brings adverse criticism from groups to both the right and the left of it. One strong anti-war organization printed in its own paper a protest from certain members against the *Panther*'s "rhetoric of hate, violence and destruction." They went on to complain that "Issue after issue celebrates killing and threats of murder. . . ."[18] But in the next issue there were defenders, including an officer of the peace group in question, who said, "I consider housing conditions where children are bitten by rats to be violence . . . the failure of our country to eliminate starvation and malnutrition to be violence. . . . A large proportion of black people are victims of this violence. . . . Who are we to quibble about the violent rhetoric of some black people when we acquiesce in the institutionalized and overt violence to which many blacks are daily subjected?"[19]

In implementing its policies the *Black Panther* unremittingly prints articles and cartoons opposing the U.S. intervention in Indo-China, condemning the police anywhere in the nation, and opposing Zionism, and supporting the Arab as well as the Cuban causes. These views coincide with those in *Muhammad Speaks,* but are presented far more bitterly. Lacking is the social program of the Nation of Islam, which *Muhammad Speaks* supports with special sections and numerous illustrated features.

The *Panther* has strongly influenced the Young Lords Party, essentially a Puerto Rican group whose followers live and work in New York City. It publishes a bi-lingual bi-monthly, *Palante,* subtitled Latin Revolutionary News Service; it is a direct imitation of the Panther weekly, for it has the same format, similar typography and layout, and some of the identical gun-laden cartoons. It praises the Panthers and repeats their philosophy, even to the itemized list of demands.

● NATIONAL PAPERS AND THEIR STANCE

The position a black paper or a chain or group of such papers should take in the racial turmoil of today is one of the major problems facing the owners and publishers (see Chapter 7). Here it is enough to note that the large newspapers that support the ideal of justice for black citizens in all matters are impatient, both with the white community and with the tactics of violent militants. Those that are cautious, noncommittal, or silent are experiencing circulation problems. The highest circulations of all are held by the two papers that take strong stands.

Time magazine reported the jump of *"In Sepia"* Dallas, a forceful tabloid, from a circulation of 5,000 in 1965 to 22,500 within a few years; by 1968 it claimed a verified, controlled circulation of 35,000. An older rival, the Dallas *Express,* lost almost half its circulation in that period and since has remained at about 5,000, verified by the Audit Bureau of Circulations, until 1969, when it descended below 3,000. The *Express* is a revered paper, more than seventy-five years old. The politically and socially conservative Atlanta *Daily World* has a circulation of around 30,000 that varies little from year to year, in a time when other papers in its locality have shown increases and when it faces keen rivals in two brisker, more socially liberal papers. The situation appears to disturb its publishers, since Standard Rate and Data Service in reports issued in 1969 and 1970 notes that "after three requests, the publisher has failed to file circulation statements on SRDS forms."

The competition from the white press insofar as that press has stepped up its coverage of the more prominent racial issues of the day, and the rising popularity of several black magazines of national distribution, such as *Ebony, Sepia, Soul! Illustrated, Jet,* and some of the new community periodicals, such as *Philly Talk* and *Proud,* have pushed the national papers somewhat out of the race to cover countrywide racial stories and caused them to bear down harder on the local scene.

Writing about the national newspapers, L. F. Palmer, Jr., says that "the end of the national black newspaper is clearly in sight."[20] He is supported in this by John Jordan, then acting publisher of the Norfolk *Journal and Guide,* who is quoted as saying: "We can't afford field men any longer, and transportation is too complicated and expensive. It is virtually impossible to provide adequate coverage of the national scene anyway."[21] Palmer also brings to the point the statement of an unnamed black editor in Chicago who observed that the four black-oriented radio stations there reach more listeners in an hour than the black paper has readers in a month. Just how such a general statement was arrived at is not made clear. Nor does it indicate the depth of attention for each. On the other hand, minds can be made up and action taken quickly through the impact of broadcasts in contrast to the slower effects of reading newspapers.

● THE BLACK DAILY

In writing about the newspapers serving a group of citizens which for years has constituted about 10 per cent of their country's population, one would expect to be able to report that there are many papers that come off the press from five to seven times a week. But today only three daily newspapers are being published. A few black papers have gained attention as dailies over the years, but the daily has been a losing investment for most black publishers.

With around 1,800 dailies for whites, including several for the business and other specialized worlds, the few for black readers is surprising but understandable. In the history of this press there

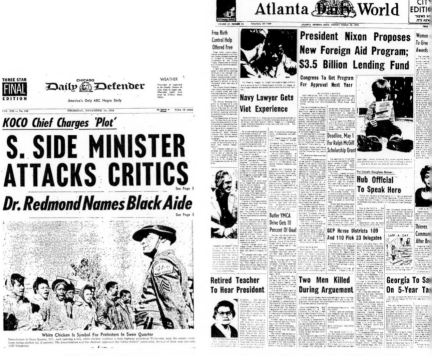

FIG. 5.5. These two papers are the leading black dailies. The Chicago **Daily Defender** is issued four times a week, plus a weekend national edition; the Atlanta **Daily World** is a four-day paper.

has been no time when more than three or four dailies were issued in the same period. More than a half-hundred have been attempted but today there are only the Chicago, Atlanta, and Columbus, Ga., papers. Perhaps the black society in America does not want or need more than two or three such dailies. But this is a physically large country; white papers, although their coverage of black citizens and their activities and interests has improved, still handle only the more obvious stories and, in many communities, do not cover even those.

Pride, the historian of the black newspaper, reported in 1950 that forty-five black dailies had been published in the preceding century, of which he had been able to identify forty-four.[22] Such papers naturally were issued in communities with large black populations. New Orleans had seen several efforts, as did Dayton, Ohio, and Washington, D.C.; others were founded in Cairo, Illinois; Knoxville, Tennessee; Roanoke, Virginia; Newport News, Virginia; New York City, and Muskogee, Oklahoma. Since 1950 a few more have been attempted; all but one are gone.

An early daily usually considered the first was the New Orleans

Tribune. It began as a tri-weekly in 1864 but soon was converted into a six-day daily. Published in both English and French, it also was known as *La Tribune de la Nouvelle Orleans.* Because it was the voice of the state's Republican Party it was considered influential. Allan Morrison, of *Ebony's* staff, has recorded that it campaigned for weekly wages for ex-slaves; was highly critical of certain Southern representatives in Congress; asked for the ballot for freedmen; and foresaw persecution of blacks when Federal troops were withdrawn from the state.[23] It was too early, perhaps, for a crusading paper to succeed in New Orleans, and its owner, Dr. Louis Charles Roudanez, a physician, had to suspend its publication in 1868; he revived it but it ceased permanently in 1869.

Reasons for Failure. Black dailies fail mainly for economic reasons. Raising sufficient capital is one problem, making a sufficient profit to manage the always increasing costs is an even more formidable one. Until recent years profits were difficult if not impossible to make because of the comparatively low literacy rate and the small incomes of black readers. Advertising income could not absorb costs; circulation income, while high, had a ceiling. These obstacles have existed for years, and only now are lessening. That they persist, even if slightly less overwhelming for some papers, is all the more to be regretted because by now more well trained and able writers, advertising personnel, and others needed for staffs might be attracted if there were more dailies offering adequate salaries.

Chuck (C. Sumner) Stone, who was editor-in-chief of the Chicago *Daily Defender,* once advised the National Newspaper Publishers Association members to "go daily" because "as long as all Negro newspapers are weeklies, we can never compete as equals in a society controlled by daily newspapers. . . ."[24] This advice was logical, but it did not show how to finance such dailies.

In addition to Stone's motive there also is, in a day of electronic journalism, the need to communicate more often with readers than weekly or even semi-weekly. Not only to provide information unobtainable elsewhere but also to set before readers points of view rarely found in the general press, a strong daily press for blacks is desirable.

The way publishers sometimes move into the costly area of daily black journalism may explain the failures as being more than economic. At times it is merely well meaning but inexperienced activity. This point is illustrated by the Washington *Daily Sun,* brought out in the national capital in 1968. Eugene Melvin Garner, a Washington lawyer, published it first on October 30 as a morning daily tabloid. It became the city's only black daily. Clearly Washington is a rich market, for the population is predominantly black. If a black daily can be sustained in any American city, it would seem to be in Washington. The *Sun* sold for seven cents a copy. Within less than two months it was showing signs of hasty production. Changed to standard size, it was far from comparable to the other two black daily papers of the country or its semi-weekly competitor, the *Afro-American*. Some editorials obviously were no more than news releases. Numerous technical errors appeared: pages were misnumbered, headlines garbled. Almost all headlines, where there were any, were in typewriter capitals; only front page streamers were easily read. The *Sun* was produced by offset. When not carefully used that method can produce an amateurish-looking paper. The entire edition offered six pages. United Press International and Negro Press International copy was used but little original material appeared except on page one. Almost no hard news was reported on inside pages; advertising occupied one page.

It was no surprise, then, when the *Sun* soon set permanently.

A few publishers have started papers or continued some well established national ones as semi-weeklies. Both the Washington and Baltimore editions of the *Afro-American* come out twice a week; the Tampa (Fla.) *Sentinel* and the *Philadelphia Tribune* both go to their readers every Tuesday and Saturday.

But for all its life the American black newspaper press has been essentially a weekly type of journalism, made up largely of separate, independent papers. A successful daily is an exceptional publication. Publishers now appear to be more interested in groups and chains of papers.   ●

6. LOCAL NEWSPAPER VOICES

COMPARATIVELY, the black newspaper is a small one, even if it is one of the national weeklies or bi-weeklies discussed in the preceding chapter. Alongside two Japanese dailies, each with a circulation of more than 8,500,000; two Russian papers with in excess of 7,500,000 apiece, and one British paper with 5,000,000, no U.S.A. newspaper of any persuasion is in the running. The largest American paper, a daily, reaches only 2,100,000. Thus the approximately 600,000 of *Muhammad Speaks* hardly makes that a large paper in comparison with these multi-million sheets on other continents. Certainly no individual black paper is comparable in size to the individual large dailies in the U.S.A. or outside. And no standard, commercial black paper has even 100,000 circulation.

The largest regular black paper existing as a commercial venture, the New York *Amsterdam News,* has a circulation of about one-half of one per cent of the black population of the nation. The largest white paper, the New York *Daily News,* has the same circulation-population ratio in the white world. The other larger black papers do not continue the parallel. Only a few dozen command circulations above 25,000 a week. The great majority of the approximately 225 black papers of the various frequencies range in circulation from a few thousand to under 25,000, a situation much confused in recent years by the rise of the often unaudited free circulation or controlled publication or the trend toward combining free and paid circulation.

The black newspaper, then, is for the most part a local voice, with mainly a local outreach, for even the national newspapers have their core circulations in the communities from which they spring, issuing city and other localized editions separate from those for wider distribution. A good many retain the tone of personal journalism so common in the nineteenth century in the press as a whole. For in some towns and cities the black community newspaper office, like the newspaper building of the country village of the past, is the gathering or meeting place for black residents. The readers bring their problems to the proprietor. This practice is especially common among black people because many have nowhere else to go. A church or club may provide a haven, but such institutions are not often prepared to advise on such practical matters as taxes. If the owner wishes, the paper can crusade for its readers, for he knows many personally.

At the same time they discharge this social function, the small papers nevertheless are business operations. For many years they have been speaking out loudly for the liberties due black citizens. Such leadership has been accentuated in recent decades, chiefly because of the increased interest in the life and culture of the Afro-American by both blacks and whites. What the early papers said is becoming better known because of the attempts made in recent years by the microfilm makers to recall from long forgotten files some of the early publications. The historians someday may have a better idea of the black life of the nineteenth and twentieth centuries by reading the black papers, large and small, now being preserved far better than they were. An anonymous prophet wrote in 1955:

> Negro editors may not know it as a body, but it is one of the inescapable truths of our time that the Negro weeklies of today will be prized possessions of the future and will be religiously sought out for the record of the Negro's thinking, his movements in a flexible society, and his manner of encountering a rebuff. . . . The editor may go unheralded and unrewarded in this hour but the perennial monument to his name is a carefully preserved . . . file of his daily labors.[1]

● THE MELANGE OF FORMATS

That future researcher will find a melange of formats, styles of writing, and viewpoints when he examines the community weeklies that exist in the shadows of the larger national papers. He will learn that in Texas, for instance, in the 1960's there existed a group of vigorous if not always well produced papers, some energetic in aims, others clumsily written and edited, and still others sedate and substantial in their news coverage. Clustered near major cities in other states weeklies will turn up, some commercial, some mere political tracts. In Chicago *Daily Defender* territory, for example, the historian will find the tabloid *North Shore Examiner,* a bi-weekly, covering news of the black residents in the suburban towns along the Lake Michigan shore north of Chicago, such communities as Evanston, North Chicago, and Waukegan benefitting. The Illinois political papers that may be unearthed bear such names as the *Plain Truth, Voice of the Black Community, Afros Expressions,* the *Black Rapper,* and the *Black Truth.* Ethel Romm, in her study of the underground press, calls these "the street corner press." The *Black Truth* claims a circulation of 30,000 but the others run only a few thousand each.

The rationale for many a community paper was described by Lesley Kimber, publisher of the Fresno *California Advocate.* His paper, with a circulation of 8,000, was established in 1968 "to bring out the positive things," he told a Sigma Delta Chi group.[2] The white papers, he said, print only such black news as crime rates in the black community. "Financially," he said further, the paper "has been a disaster but it has been a gratifying experience to see how the people of West Fresno have responded to our efforts."

The publishers of these papers, devoted as they are to being local voices, were encouraged to launch their publications by the improvement in living conditions of some of their potential readers during the 1960's and early 1970's. Both employment and income were up for the black population. Thirty-two per cent of all nonwhite families earned $8,000 or more in 1968; eight years before 15 per cent had earned that amount or more, wrote Daniel P. Moynihan, counselor to President Richard M. Nixon, in his controversial report.[3] He also noted that "Young Negro families are achieving income parity with young white families. Outside the South, young huband-wife Negro families have 99 per cent of the income of whites."

Employment, the report said, likewise changed dramatically in the decade. Although blacks continued to have twice the unemployment rates of whites, the rates were down for both groups. "Black occupations improved sharply. The number of professional and technical employes doubled in the period 1960–68. This was two-and-a-half times the increase for whites." That such figures should be used with caution was emphasized by a black member of the Federal Reserve Board, Andrew F. Brimmer, who in 1970 noted that "the rate of decline of poverty for whites has been substantially faster than the rate of decline for nonwhites."[4] But what a publisher must regard is that there has been a decline.

Small paper owners are particularly affected by the level of education of their potential readers. The education of black people improved in the 1960's. Selecting the situation as it existed in 1968, the Moynihan report notes that more 3- and 4-year-olds among black children (19 per cent) were in school than white of the same ages (15 per cent) and only 2 per cent fewer (49 to 51) blacks aged 18 and 19 were in school. The number of black schools and colleges rose 85 per cent between 1964 and 1968; in the latter year 430,000 blacks were enrolled. The report admitted, however, that only 16 per cent of black high school seniors have verbal scores at or above grade level.[5]

Such information encourages the entrepreneurs of newspapers. But a larger audience is no guarantee of publishing stability. The publication must win the support of enough of that audience to survive. For a time it appeared that the black press was headed for serious problems of survival (see Chapter 4), but since the civil rights movement and the black revolution against many white institutions, several of the smaller local voices have gained strength and been joined by dozens of newcomers.

The importance of these local voices is pressed home to the white community by such incidents as the effective boycotting by black citizens of institutions in their neighborhoods which they believe treat them unfairly, in which activities they usually are aided by their own papers. One example is described at length by D. Parke Gibson, a prominent black public relations and advertising man. Philadelphia residents conducted a campaign, which he calls an economic withdrawal, against various oil companies and food chains. Gibson notes that "the consumer campaigns . . . received little, if any, publicity in the white-oriented media." But they did receive wide exposure in the black media. Finally, one of the white papers, the *Evening Bulletin,* was chosen for "selective patronage" because it had no black truck drivers or blacks "employed in any numbers in sensitive positions behind a desk in the editorial or business departments." It took seven weeks, but the company complied by hiring blacks.[6]

Involvement or cooperation with such activities increases the element of danger in publishing a black community paper. Although black journalism never has been exactly a placid occupation, it might be thought free in these times of the sorts of hazards which haunted the early publishers, whose plants were burned or who themselves were murdered. The local voice is stilled by violence even today, however. The Associated Press in 1969 reported the murder of a forty-five-year-old Jackson, Michigan, publisher. The victim was Charles Cade, owner of *The Jackson Blazer,* a weekly. He was found dead in his apartment, with the words "Black Niger [*sic*]" scrawled in blood on two walls. The paper's editor, James J. Murphy, called the slaying racially motivated, as the bloody words would indicate.[7] The *New Pittsburgh Courier* later carried a story from Jackson quoting the prosecutor's opinion that Cade's murder was not racial. Yet the paper reported thirteen sniping incidents in the city of 5,700 people in the preceding three months. In another incident in Jackson a white boy was slain in a racial fight with a black. Later, an elderly white man was killed when, as an insurance collector, he went into an apartment house said to be occupied by armed blacks fearing a raid on the Black Panther Party.[8] But why anyone seeking revenge should murder Cade was not made clear.

A somewhat different and less vicious incident occurred at the Atlanta *Inquirer* in 1968. The paper experienced what can be called editorial highjacking. Its publisher, Jesse Hill, Jr., charged that while the editorial copy was on its way from the editorial offices to the printer another editorial was put in its place. The original editorial endorsed a certain political leader and attacked another. The replacement was one dealing with the Democratic convention in Chicago, the publisher said. Before the switch was discovered 26,000 copies of the paper had been run and many distributed. A new batch of the same number was printed, with an editorial entitled "Inquirer Sabotaged," again endorsing the candidate.[9] Earlier the candidate's office had been firebombed.

Eight months later the offices of the *Voice,* a nonprofit paper in Plainfield, New Jersey, were hit by a firebomb. Only minor damages were reported.[10]

● POLICIES OF LOCAL PAPERS

Some local papers have their credos and platforms just as do the larger nationals like the Chicago *Defender* and the *Afro-American,* expressing somewhat similar aims. One such is the Jackson (Miss.) *Advocate,* a weekly of about 5,000 circulation founded in 1939 by Percy Greene, still owner and editor. During Negro Newspaper Week in 1969 an editorial declared, with evident pride, that "despite sometimes bitter and unreasoning opposition, the paper has not missed one single edition since it began publication. He went on to say:

> The policy, purpose and program of the Jackson Advocate was stated in an editorial on the front page of its very first edition. The policy, purpose and program of the Jackson Advocate, as then stated and which has remained unchanged to this day, is to gain for the Negro citizens of Mississippi the uninhibited right to vote; and the right of political participation; and to help in the creation of an atmosphere, within the state, in which responsible white and Negro citizens can work together for the betterment and benefit of all the people of the state.
>
> The unchanging position of the Jackson Advocate on the question and issue of Civil Rights, may be seen in the seven-point Civil Rights program, for the improvement of relations between the Negro and white people of the state, which follows here, published first in a 1944 edition of the Jackson Advocate, a considerable time before the beginning of the contemporary and current Civil Rights movement.[11]

The seven points deal with equality in education, upgrading of Alcorn and other black colleges in the area, admission of black students to surrounding white colleges, interracial athletic competition, election and appointment of blacks to local and state boards, elimination of all discrimination in public transportion, and removal of all restrictions against voting by black citizens.

The idealistic yet practical statement of policy, purpose, and program of this paper is not in most ways typical of the slogans and platforms regularly printed by some of the other local voices, particularly in its length. For example:

Madison (Wis.) *Sun:* "From rising to setting sun—all over the world, our policy is truth, righteousness, justice and charity for all."

New Haven (Conn.) *Crow:* "The *Crow* will speak the truth and the truth will make us free."

Memphis *World:* "The Memphis *World* is an independent newspaper—non-sectarian and non-partisan, printing news unbiased and supporting those things it believes to be of interest to its readers and opposing those things against the interests of its readers."

It may not be unduly cynical to oberve, however, that, as with certain white papers that announce such policies, they are violated in some instances, simply perhaps because newspapers are products of the fallible human mind. The fidelity to their ideals may, also, be a matter of interpretation. The Mississippi paper, for example, applies its aims in its editorials in ways which, from another point of view, can be considered inconsistent with them. It has editorialized against northerners coming to the South to take part in civil rights activities, and called school integration hopeless several years before the federal government actions of 1970 appeared to be canceling gains toward educational integration. Black power it called, in 1968, "just another part of the scheme to widen and continue to promote hatred in the minds and hearts of Negroes toward white people and is lock, stock, and barrel a part of the communist scheme for using the Negro in its revolutionary plan to overthrow the present government. . . ."[12]

● THE GROWTH IN PAPERS

As many as thirty new small papers were founded during the second half of the 1960's alone; undoubtedly this figure is a conservative one because thirty is the number the author was able to identify; others are reported to have been established and have not as yet been verified. In addition are the scores of little publications that can be dubbed newsletters for areas within some of the same communities. They are born in large numbers; many die, but a few continue here and there in their own modest formats. Among the new, smaller standard or commercial papers, that is, the weeklies or bi-weeklies that seek to be community news organs and not shrill street-corner political papers, a number have survived. They exhibit a briskness of tone and a forthrightness of attitude and policy. Because of them it is possible to say that a new force has been added to the small city black press. It may be the result of a greater push toward commercial success but it also has been in the direction of providing for opinions not so often heard in this journalism since the nineteenth century days of strong protest.

The growth of papers is illustrated by events in Philadelphia and New York. As a result of a project undertaken by a Temple University journalism graduate a dozen small community papers and newsletters were started in Philadelphia.[13] It began in summer, 1968, when Miss Kitty Caparella, a Temple senior, became interested in the hostile attitudes in the black community near the campus. She edited a supplement to the *Temple University News* that called attention to the situation and tried to explain the source of the resentment, such as displacement of residents by university expansion. She decided that a community paper might open communications lines.

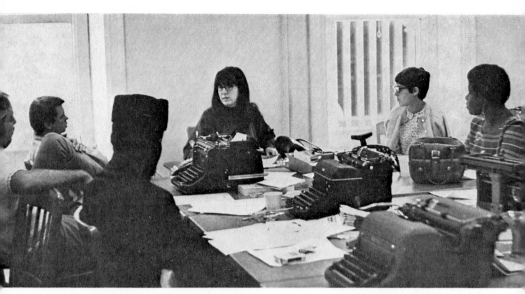

FIG. 6.1. Temple University journalism students in Philadelphia coached staffers of a small community newspaper, **Dig This Now.** Residents were given training in reporting, editing, and other skills during a ten-week program. (Jay Lamont photo)

Miss Caparella won the support of a black activist neighborhood group, the Morroccos. She taught its members basic techniques of newspaper journalism and guided them in producing an eight-page tabloid, *Dig This Now,* billed as "Philadelphia's Only Teen-age Newspaper." The University assisted by allowing use of the *News* offices as a training center, its staffers and some journalists from downtown papers serving as volunteer instructors. A dozen neighborhood people became trainees and were given five dollars a weekend to cover transportation, meals, babysitters, and other expenses resulting from spending Friday afternoons and Saturday mornings in the ten-week program.

By mid-1969 a dozen other publications were being issued, all inspired by the first, such as *It's What's Happening,* a sixteen-page duplicated publication which lasted for a time with Temple's help. It, too, was produced with the aid of both youngsters and adults. One graduate of the program put her training into effect by launching a newspaper crusade to rid a street of twenty tons of rubbish, with university cooperation. But some of the new publications soon died for lack of financing. *Dig This Now* was still being published in early 1971.

In New York, beginning in summer, 1969, the New York *Times* sponsored workshops which resulted in publication by that fall of a four-page weekly community paper, *Transition Press.* It served the Corona-East Elmhurst section of the city, printing poetry as well as regular community news and feature stories.

Minority group members are being attracted by such papers as these to journalism as a career. Funding has come from other sources than universities, although these have been active in several parts of the country. The New York project was funded by the Times Foundation. A second paper was being planned for another black section of the city in 1970.

● THE DEATH OF PAPERS

The experiences of owners show that keeping these new papers alive is a serious problem. It is virtually impossible without heavy political, academic, or other financial support that must be available for several years or until the paper catches on sufficiently to acquire the revenue from advertising needed for survival. New papers sometimes are launched in the expectation that the recent desire to make black enterprises go will shorten the waiting and operating loss period, but this assumes management abilities not always available.

In the author's city, Syracuse, New York, two black weeklies were attempted in recent years which illustrate the methods and experiences of similar papers in other parts of the nation. These case histories point up the hazards of venturing into publishing any kind of paper unless one can bring ample capital and experience, hazards which are especially great if the publishers are persons whose motive is bringing more power to their communities' black residents.

The *Home Town News* and the *Liberated Voice* represented this motive in their own ways. The *News* was begun by Chris Powell, a former band leader who had grown up in central New York. He told a black journalist interviewer that he considered himself a revolutionist and not a journalist. He brought no journalistic training or experience; he had grown up in the city's ghetto, he knew his people's problems, and he felt deeply the mistreatment of American blacks. His interviewer, Larry Sampson, mentioned that the weekly had been criticized for lack of professionalism and general technical deficiencies. Powell's answer was one to be heard from others who defend such often inescapable weaknesses.

"He argues," Sampson wrote, "that journalistic rules established by the white society, by the white press are only beneficial to the white press. He believes that the black press must not be content to imitate the white press. . . . [it] must establish its own rules if it isn't to be subdued by white interference."[14]

The paper was published during 1967–68 as a twelve-page tabloid, sometimes with three covers. It sold advertising space to a few large and small Syracuse stores and a few national accounts, such as Royal Crown Cola. Printed by offset, it carried a miscellany of material. Pasted up for reproduction were cartoons and news stories clipped from other publications, including wire service stories lacking proper credits. Similar papers elsewhere, such as the *Plain Truth* of Champaign, Illinois, were drawn upon. Also in it were helpful hints to consumers as well as book reviews, an editorial, and locally written columns. The editorials included attacks on Syracuse blacks in public office as being only Uncle Toms. On the Vietnam war the paper took a firm position of opposition to U.S. intervention. Powell used every opportunity to crack out at local manifestations of racism and bigotry, often publishing reports of Syracuse events ignored by the city's two large white dailies, although aside from some such exposés there was little original news. The *News* petered out in fall, 1968, when Powell became seriously ill. The *Home Town News* had been largely a one-man operation and when that one man was incapacitated the paper could not survive. The publisher died in 1970.

While the *News* was being published another paper for the city's black citizens was begun. The *Liberated Voice* was founded by one of Powell's assistants and another young man. They were 24-year-old college graduates, Elwood Berry and Harden J. Southall. They succeeded in getting backing from an executive director of the local Organization of Organizations, an assistant business administrator of the school district, and two citizens active in the black community. Southall and Berry, both black and enthusiastic, divided the major responsibilities, Southall becoming publisher, Berry editor. The paper appeared as a tabloid in July, 1968, with a press run of 10,000 and was sold for fifteen cents. Also an offset printed weekly tabloid, it was far more modern in typography and layout than the *News* but similarly entranced with revolutionary slogans. Yet it attracted a few advertisers from among the leading department stores as well as small, exclusive specialty shops.

Somewhat contradictorily and irregularly it carried Whitney Young's and Roy Wilkins' columns as well as one by Julius Lester and several local black writers, including the editor. Berry was an energetic young man but like his partner equipped with little practical journalistic experience on either the business or editorial side. Berry had been for three months assistant to Powell. Southall had worked briefly as a reporter for the white evening daily in Syracuse. They had met at a campus rebellion at Colgate University. Southall was reporting it; Berry, as he put it later, was there "to aid and abet it."

Both the *News* and the *Voice* had moved into a journalistic vacuum, so far as Syracuse-originated black journalism was concerned. The black community had not had a newspaper of its own since J. Luther Sylvahn launched a standard-sized paper, the *Progressive Herald,* as a bi-weekly in 1933 and kept it going for twenty-five years, changing to a weekly but not being able to survive television's effect upon advertising. But the two new papers had to compete with the large national weeklies purchased by many of Syracuse's 20,000 blacks.

In what turned out to be the final issue of the *Liberated Voice,* December 11, 1968, Berry and Southall told the story of their attempt, entitling it "The Birth, Death and Resurrection of TLV." There never was a resurrection, however. Berry went into educational work; his partner went to other climes.

The community paper trend did not die, however, for in 1970 a Buffalo publishing firm entered the Syracuse market with a weekly section wrapped around its Buffalo-Rochester paper, the *Challenger*. For that matter, black journalism for a time was looking up in a new way in Syracuse when a community magazine, *Around the Town*, was begun in 1969 (see Chapter 8). The Buffalo tabloid, established in 1962 and unrecorded in most directories of black papers, operates with a small editorial staff, largely volunteers, for its Syracuse edition. For a time a Syracuse University journalism student with background in black communications was editor while working for an advanced degree. In its early stages at this writing, the Syracuse *Challenger* has reversed the order of things by having more advertising than such papers usually can obtain at first, but finds difficulty in covering the news of the black citizens for lack of staff.

Certain lessons were learned by the publishers of the two new publications from the recent Syracuse failures. The two militant papers were strongly attractive to sympathetic whites. Berry admitted that the bulk of readers and advertisers were white and that the black community would not or could not support his *Voice*. Neither paper did much, however, about covering the community and did not think it important until too late. For fear, perhaps, of seeming too dependent upon the white establishment no attempt was made to enlist the help of black students in journalism classes at nearby colleges, although white weeklies as well as the dailies give such students practice to mutual advantage.

The publishers of the *Challenger* and *Around the Town* realized, on the other hand, that black opinion papers are available in Syracuse via organizations such as the Black Panther Party and the Nation of Islam. The *News* and the *Voice* too often sounded much like the *Black Panther*. Both those local tabs also were riddled with spelling, grammar, and composing errors and often marred by verbose, shoddy writing.

Newspaper failures are not restricted to central New York, of course. Around the country similar failures have occurred for many of the same reasons. The papers given to serving chiefly as advocacy journalism have failed just as readily as those that were unprofessional as journalism; death has been practically certain for those that combined advocacy with sloppy writing and editing and inefficiency in business methods. The exceptions have been papers subsidized to keep them going no matter what the public reception; usually these are training grounds rather than commercial ventures.

Some of the new community papers have their counterparts in that journalistic phenomenon that rose in the 1960's, the underground press, which in tone and appearance both the *Home Town News* and the *Liberated Voice*, the latter especially, resembled. In their business operations some black papers experienced the uncertainties and obstacles of the underground press and like many of the latter offset-produced tabloids, appeared for a year or two and then departed.

The tone of anarchism and nihilism to be found in some underground papers is echoed in some of the extremist local voices. Both groups of publications, with some exceptions, have the same tentativeness, the same insecurity, the same shrillness of tone. Both are deeply concerned with the right to try to raise the black people to first class citizenship, along with other goals. Both types are essentially opinion papers, voices of protest.

Protest papers, as has been shown, are nothing new in black journalism. If *Freedom's Journal* were to be revived today, with slavery gone and material conditions better, even if not satisfactory by any means, it would not last perhaps even the short time it did. The successful and influential black local voices are those that seek not only to arouse their readers to do something about the injustices of the day, but also are service papers that give readers a substantial budget of news and facts that support opinions.

● THE CONVENTIONAL WEEKLIES

The quasi-revolutionary paper just described is one type of usually small and insecure publication of the present. The other is the more or less conventional paper unfavored with advertising, ill-supported by readers (perhaps for lack of money), published where there may not even be enough possible readers, or produced by an owner seeking influence in a community. Often papers combine these circumstances. In Rochester, New York, is a bi-weekly, *Frederick Douglass Voice,* once the *Rochester Voice.* Douglass, it will be recalled, published the *North Star* and *Frederick Douglass' Paper* from that city. This present-day publication asserts its intention of carrying on in his tradition.

The story of its life is that of so many other small black papers, past and present. Most of the time since 1934, when it was founded its owner, Howard Coles, has done other kinds of work for a living, and so has his wife.

The organization of the paper is not as simple as was that of Douglass' a century before. Thirty-five years after the paper was founded, Coles and a daughter did most of the work, aided only by two part-time helpers, one with graphic arts training and the other a community college student who wrote and handled subscriptions. To this extent there is a resemblance to Douglass' enterprise. But he did not have, as have the Coles, the occasional help of Rochester Institute of Technology photography students, usually whites who take pictures to supplement those from the owner's own camera, earning class credit with their prints. Whites also have contributed articles to the paper.

The paper is standard sized, six or eight pages an issue. Like an increasing number of black papers, this one is printed by offset. A plant in Geneseo, New York, not far from Rochester, is used. The

Voice has both paid and controlled circulation; boys distribute it to routes and are paid a flat rate.

Circulation varies from 8,500 to 9,500 an issue in a city with a 65,000 black population. About 350 copies are sold at a five dollar subscription rate. With such a plan the chief revenue source is advertising. In the early days several large companies bought space, such as the Rochester Gas & Electric Company, a large furniture firm, big coal companies, and one food chain. Lately its advertisers are mainly local merchants, although its masthead claims affiliation with a firm of national advertising representatives which went out of business many years ago. The local accounts number between fifty and ninety, all but 5 per cent are white. Coles in 1968 complained that black business does not support its press. " . . . whenever they have a cause, they yell for the black press, but have a community gathering with an invited speaker and you can be sure the black press won't be represented on the platform," he told his interviewer.

To put organizational backing behind the paper, the Frederick Douglass League was formed; the paper is its official organ. The League's activities are not clear. The paper's office is in the heart of one of the two main black neighborhoods, in a storefront shop. In many ways it is like numerous other small journalistic efforts. Typographically it is somewhat uneven, but the picture reproduction is effective. Editing is not thoroughly professional. For example, many stories appear without headings or only small, unattractive ones. Little news is printed, although the owner seeks to appeal to Buffalo and Syracuse as well as his own city. But there is considerable relevant opinion (not labeled as editorial, however) on the problems of blacks in the area.[15]

● VIGNETTES OF INDIVIDUAL PAPERS

Descriptions and evaluations of certain papers in this local voice group are even more essential for them than for an understanding of the national newspaper scene. For the national papers have received some attention elsewhere, but these local voices have won little notice from commentators on the black press. Because it is necessary to be selective, many worthy publications have been passed over in what follows. The papers included are considered representative by the author. To provide geographical balance, they have been selected from different areas of the nation. These also will reflect some of the local variations in journalistic fashions and black concerns.

The Cleveland Papers. Cleveland, a major black population center widely known for its black mayor, Carl B. Stokes, has since 1913 been served by one of the most competently written and edited quasi-national weeklies, the *Call and Post* (see Chapter 5). Its editor and publisher, William O. Walker, who in 1970 was honored for his fifty years in black journalism, has long been numbered among the leaders in his profession.

In spring, 1969, Cleveland heard rumors of a new local voice, a paper to be established by Walker's nephew, who had left his uncle's paper, where he was an advertising executive. This publication turned out to be the Cleveland *Advocator,* a small tabloid which did not appear regularly until nearly a year after it was first issued. It contained, in four to eight pages, a few news stories, several news features, some space for sports and women's material, and an editorial page emphasizing the local angle. Pictures had a prominent place. Advertising ran from about 45 to 55 per cent. Early 1970 found the paper with more stability, after a rise in space sales. But it still was far from its much larger rival in coverage and had no consistent or discernible editorial or news policies and left much to be desired as a printed product. Although the *Advocator* was not to be taken seriously as a competitor for the almost sixty-year-old *Call and Post,* it at least was another local voice. In a day when one-newspaper cities are the norm, the rise of any sort of competition, for any racial group's benefit, is important.

Competitive Atlanta. One of the most competitive black newspaper cities is Atlanta. As the white papers, two large dailies, drew closer by combining their business operations, the black publications multiplied. This deep South metropolis has one of the nation's two black dailies, the *World,* and two lively weeklies, the *Inquirer* and the *Voice.*

The Atlanta *Inquirer* grew out of reaction to the highly conservative *World.* A group of students and teachers founded it in 1960. It became a crusader, so much so that the late Louis E. Lomax, the black author and journalist, credited it with persuading hospitals that once were all-white to change the policy of not allowing black doctors to practice. Vigorous in writing tone, appearance, and in policy, the *Inquirer* is standard size with one of the larger circulations among the local voices, 33,000. Its slogan is "To seek out the Truth and report it without fear or favor." It also prints in one front page ear the statement, "On Guard for Human Rights 24 Hours a Day." Its editorials are moderately phrased but broach many subjects; on some news stories it has more penetrating coverage than its daily rival. It uses none of the usual columnists but works a coeditor hard; Ernest M. Pharr sometimes writes a major portion of the first page. In other respects it is conventional, having the usual special pages for sports and other interests. It is financially successful and has won honors for its community service.

The Atlanta *Voice,* begun in 1965, has a strong editorial page stance, relying often on sarcasm in its editorial essays. Space is provided for the Wilkins and other syndicated columns as well as for local writers; these, too, offset the *World*'s viewpoint. The *Voice* provides the usual entertainment, sports, and other such pages. It

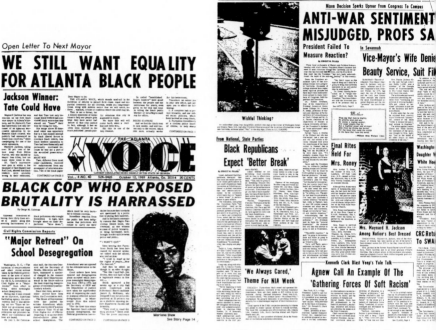

FIG. 6.2. Atlanta has two weeklies in addition to the **Daily World**—the **Inquirer** and the **Voice**, both founded since 1960.

calls itself the "Largest Circulated Negro Weekly in the State of Georgia," the dubious English of which deflecting attention from the fact that its figures are not available. This paper has three front pages: two are printed tabloid size.

It may appear that a city able to support three black papers must be in more need of such a press to help solve its racial problems than most other cities. That is not the situation in Atlanta, which has the reputation of being moderate in its racial attitudes. It is not the city teeming with efforts to solve its racial problems that has no black press, however. It is the city that is so rigid, so unprogressive, that lacks vigorous black papers. When little hope for reform appears possible a publisher fears that he will not obtain support for a local journalistic voice.

The Milwaukee Weeklies. Like Atlanta, Milwaukee has a lively black weekly press, and perhaps for the same reasons: a bold civil rights movement has joined both black and white portions of the population and considerable news has come from their actions. A few years ago as many as five black publications were issued, four newspapers and one magazine: the Milwaukee *Courier,* the *Greater Milwaukee Star,* the *Gazette*, the *Sepian*, and *Echo* magazine. By the end of the 1960's both *Gazette* and *Sepian* were gone.

The *Courier* is an outspoken paper, militant short of extremism, exciting in tone and treatment of the news, but making room for moderate columnists to provide other viewpoints. It makes dramatic use of photographs, printing many and at times offering a full page of newsy ones. Despite its emotional, often strident voice—created by use of large headlines as well as realistic and simple words in them ("Dirt Floor Shacks are Black Homes" appeared over a rent strike story)—the paper succeeds in selling advertising space to major banks and supermarkets. Its growing circulation of 4,324 is small but supported by an ABC audit.

The rival *Greater Milwaukee Star*, in tabloid size whereas the *Courier* is of standard eight-column format, also is a paper of strong policies. The policies appear in the news columns through selection of events to be stressed. Once a semi-weekly named the Milwaukee *Star Weekly News*, it is less dramatic-looking than the older and more general *Courier* but claims a far larger circulation, about 24,000; it defines its area as Beloit, Kenosha, Racine, and Madison in addition to Milwaukee. A special effort is made to cover the activities of young people, especially with pictures.

Echo, a community magazine, was fighting to keep going in 1971 because the funding of a large activity of which it was a part was cut (see Chapter 8). It provided Milwaukee readers with literary and art work by workshop students as well as opinions on local and national subjects.

Black Journalism in St. Louis. St. Louis, with four black weeklies and a city magazine, is richer in its black journalism than most U.S. metropolises. Best known is the long-published *Argus*, a solid, news-centered paper founded in 1912. It is crammed with local coverage, considerable free publicity for one black enterprise or another, special features, and columns. Its advertising runs unusually heavy for such papers, about 50 to 60 per cent; its circulation is approximately 6,000. A substantial paper, for some years it has made a specialty of running interpretative stories on racial issues.

Not as old as the respected *Argus*, having been founded in 1928, but still among the older papers of the Midwest is the St. Louis *American*. It is smaller, about half the number of pages, with around 25 per cent of the space sold to advertisers. Crime gets big play on the front page and elsewhere, usually in a heavy, two-line-deep head across the page. Major local stories are handled. Many columns appear inside, but only one, during much of 1970, was by any of the usual syndicated writers, in this case Bayard Rustin. Others are locally written. Sports runs heavy, sometimes to three pages.

The third paper, the *Sentinel*, was opened in 1968 and like the other two is an eight-column standard-sized weekly. Loud and forceful

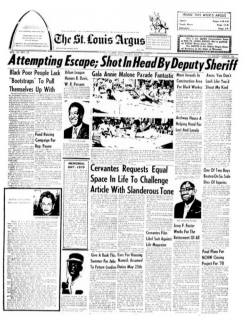

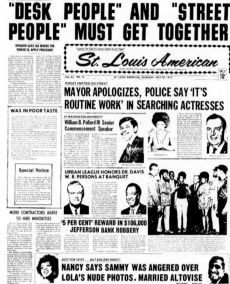

FIG. 6.3. Competition is strong in St. Louis, with three paid circulation weeklies vying for readership. The **Argus** was founded in 1912, the **American** in 1928, and the **Sentinel** in 1969. A fourth, controlled circulation paper is the St. Louis **Mirror**.

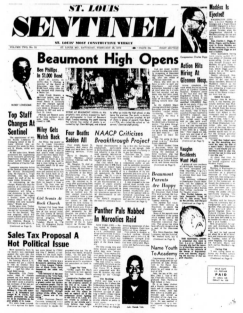

but not as heavy with crime news as the *American* or as thorough in coverage locally as the *Argus,* it gives more room to national wire news than they. Its editorials are less punchy than those of the two other papers, but it goes in more for crusades. It claims a circulation of almost 25,000, more than three times that of either rival.

The fourth weekly, the *Mirror,* founded in 1956, has a controlled circulation of 51,000. Although it has a newsy front page, little more than advertising copy appears on the rest of its 8-column pages.

Proud, an ably-written and edited city magazine, was begun in 1970 (see Chapter 8).

Big Texas Rivalry. The closely related cities of Dallas and Fort Worth provide the black population of the northeastern corner of Texas with great journalistic variety. For from these cities come two standard-sized and two tabloid-sized weeklies of considerable difference in quality, survivors of a group of seven available in the later 1960's. Those that continue are the Dallas *Post-Tribune* and the Dallas *Express,* both eight-column papers, and in Fort Worth the oddly named *"In Sepia" Dallas,* Fort Worth *Mind,* and the *Bronze Texan News.* All are read in both cities. These five exist in a state with important black papers in other communities; the semi-weekly Houston *Informer* is one of the major papers in the Southwest and the weekly *Forward Times* of the same city and the San Antonio *Register* have substantial followings, the former having close to 30,000 ABC circulation.

The Dallas *Express* is one of the oldest papers in the country, founded in 1892. The late president of the publishing company, Carter Wesley, was a leading black publisher. A newsy-looking paper, with an orderly and attractive editorial page, it actually has little hard news, much space being given to local publicity copy. Conservative, it avoids controversy and clings to conventional appearance. It is old fashioned in its advertising policy, with accounts of the Madame Judah variety as well as ads for skin problems, wigs, and gospel records; considerable national space also is sold. Its circulation has fallen sharply in recent years and in 1969 was below 3,000.

Its rival, the *Post-Tribune,* is of post-World War II origin, having been founded in 1946, and has more than seven times the *Express'* circulation, about 20,000, also ABC. They are much alike in kinds of news carried, special pages offered, and types of advertising accounts accepted. Although it embraces Fort Worth as well as Dallas, the latter city is favored by the *Post-Tribune.*

Both these standard-sized papers are made to seem sedate by the pennysaver called *"In Sepia" Dallas.* A controlled-distribution tabloid which claims a 35,000 verified circulation, it contains more news than most papers of its type, black or white. Some is written in a lively style, yet the whole is a mishmash of promotion copy for advertisers and the strong political opinions of its owners. Much copy is cluttered with exclamation points. A bit more carefully edited but still poor technically is the other tab, *Bronze Texan News*, established in Fort Worth in 1966. Preoccupied with crime news, which sometimes comprises most of the news stories on page one, the paper's editors have made it a catchall for miscellaneous copy, often badly printed by the offset process. Advertising in both tabloids is in high quantities from local markets, theaters, restaurants, and other neighborhood sources.

Thus to the outsider the three standard papers should overshadow the tabs, for they can give the reader far more information for his money and the sense that he is reading a well-established and traditional type of paper. But, as in some other cities, the discontent of some persons in the black community give the new, small papers that appear to be mere pennysavers or freely distributed advertising sheets a following that in calmer times they might not earn. An unedited letter in the *Bronze Texan News* makes clear what some readers want in their community papers in these times:

> . . . The Negro community has long been in need of a newspaper to speak out for justice in our area. There has been a concensus [sic] of opinion among certain individuals that the black community was satisfied with the status quo. This was due to the fact that most of the Negro publications devoted most of their time to the social page and to who did what to whom last Saturday night. Our Negro press had never taken a stand for the true principles of democracy and free speech until your publication began to write editorials that were enlightning [sic], and beneficial to the community. The most important aspect of this contribution was the fact that you took a stand on what you believed was right for the entire community. This took courage and fortitude on your part. The "Establishment" is a cruel and demanding adversary. These people have a way of restricting [sic] and removing individuals who "rock the boat". . . .[16]

The West Coast Scene. One of the few studies of black community journalism has been made by Professor Jack Lyle of the University of California faculty.[17] His book consists of about one-third background on the news media, mainly newspapers, in the U.S.A. in general, and two-thirds examination of the total press in Los Angeles, drawing upon various studies. In the chapter titled "The Negro and the News Media" he points out, as one of his general statements about this ethnic press, that megalopolis has within it not only geographic communities but also communities of "interest" or "mutual identification." Ethnic groups are included here.

"The Negro's community is very apt to be both geographic and ethnic," he observes, and goes on to say that the "prejudice-enforced relationship of geography to ethnic group is a growing source of tension."[18] As ethnic groups break out of geographic isolation, therefore, the whites object to the arrival of the blacks in their territory.

To comprehend the Lyle report we should know that at the time (1966) more than a half-million black citizens were living in Los

Angeles County, most of them in the largely black areas which he describes as "the southern quadrant of the central city which includes the Watts area." At the time he was writing the bulk of his book, he said, there were three weeklies for the black readers of the area, the *California Eagle,* the *Sentinel,* and the *Herald-Dispatch.* On record for the time, however, were the *News* and a fifth, *United Pictorial Review,* the latter described as a controlled circulation publication of about 70,000. These Lyle does not mention. The three he discusses were somewhat different papers; their characteristics are described. But the *Eagle* was suspended later the same year after an unsuccessful attempt to maintain it when Loren Miller, a national NAACP officer and lawyer, was appointed to a judgeship and had to sell the paper. The new owners could not make it go. A full-sized weekly, with much attention to civil rights coverage, it generally supported Democratic Party candidates. It had 27,000 circulation.

The *Herald-Dispatch,* founded in 1952, is a considerably different type of paper, judging by reports on it, for it is much in the news despite a small circulation of only 3,100. Lyle writes that much of its content bordered on racism, that there has been an off and on relationship with the Black Muslims. It has sporadically attacked the black "establishment" (meaning the NAACP, the Urban League, and other groups) and labeling them as Uncle Tomish. It generally endorsed Republican candidates at the time. In summer 1964, its offices were bombed by persons still unidentified. A paper of standard size, it mixed objective news reporting and writing with editorializing, according to Lyle's report on it at his time of writing. He also noted it was carelessly prepared, with many unprofessional practices, such as lack of proofreading.

The *Sentinel* he reports to be the dominant paper in both circulation and size, and perhaps the only profitable one. Considerable advertising and fifty or more pages a week were characteristic. Its 1966 circulation was 39,811; after a slight loss for a few years it was up to 41,482, audited by ABC, by 1970, confirming Lyle's point about its dominance. A moderate paper, although strongly outspoken on civil rights, it supported the Democratic Party and in Lyle's opinion was professional in its techniques, having as its editor a professionally trained newsman. Founded in 1934 by the editor, who also is publisher and owner, it today stresses local crime as well as political news at the local and national levels. The owner-editor, Leon H. Washington, Jr., received his original experience on the one-time rival, the *California Eagle.*

Lyle then draws on a study of the three papers—the *Eagle, Herald-Dispatch,* and *Sentinel*—made in 1963. This research revealed that seven of every ten persons interviewed reported reading the *Sentinel,* one out of ten the *Eagle* and one of every seventeen the *Herald-Dispatch.* He questions the methodology, however, because of an educational imbalance he believes existed. The reading of the white press, the distrust of the city's general press, are reported. The

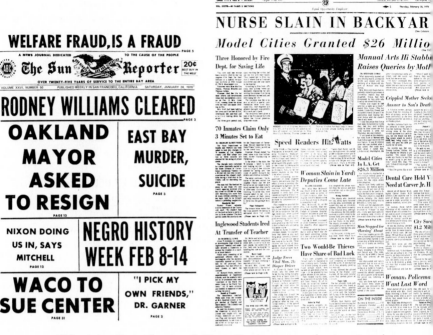

FIG. 6.4. Two of several West Coast papers, the Los Angeles **Sentinel** and the San Francisco **Sun-Reporter.**

black population read the white papers little and expressed itself as dissatisfied with the coverage of black news in them.

Why the *Sentinel* was read is explored; among the findings is the important one that these citizens want news, not just local news but black news. The press was strongly endorsed as comprehensive and accurate. But there was criticism as well. The *Sentinel,* so went the most often registered complaint at the time, was too sensational— too much crime and sex news displayed too prominently. Relationships to advertisers also came into question; there was skepticism about independence from them. It also was accused of overpublicizing some black citizens and ignoring many others.[19]

Frederic C. Coonradt, of the University of Southern California journalism faculty, who analyzed the coverage of the Watts riots of August, 1965, by two black newspapers and one black radio station in Los Angeles (the *Sentinel* and *Herald-Dispatch* and KGFJ), concluded that the three media "seem to be, in their separate ways, more mirrors of the thinking of various elements of that community than leaders in the community's thinking."[20] The *Sentinel*'s attitude in the crisis was "impatient, perhaps, but not violent," he added.

Unlike many other black papers of any size, the *Sentinel* belongs to several publishers' organizations, the black National Newspaper

Publishers Association and the white California Publishers Association.

Soon after 1971 began, Chester L. Washington, publisher of two Los Angeles community papers, *Central News* and *Southwest News,* announced purchase of five new weeklies for "approximately $1 million": *Southwest Wave, Southwest Wave Star, Southwest Topics Wave, Southside Journal,* and *Southwestern Sun.* The combined circulation, to be "well over 200,000," would make the group the nation's largest among the small weeklies.

Los Angeles is not alone in producing influential California black papers. San Francisco and surrounding communities have several substantial publications, including the *Post* and the *Sun-Reporter* in the big city, and three other *Posts,* in Richmond, Berkeley, and Oakland, and the *Voice* at Oakland. None equals the Los Angeles *Sentinel* in circulation, the largest being the Oakland *Post* with 20,000. The four *Posts,* however, make up a group whose 50,000 circulation is sold as a whole to advertisers.

Begun more than a quarter of a century ago, the tabloid-sized San Francisco *Sun-Reporter* is a newsy, generously illustrated paper run by a physician, Dr. Carlton B. Goodlett. He has guided the paper to a position where it supports local NAACP activities but also defends the rights of the Black Panther Party members. The paper has considerably more intellectual appeal than many others, with space for book reviews, the arts, and news from Africa. Advertising comes from both national and local sources. It includes two pages of classified notices. Crime is played down, local black organization activities emphasized. An ABC circulation has held steadily in recent years betwen 8,000 and 9,000.

A New York Voice. New York City's black journalism some day may inspire book-length treatment. Only one local voice is being reported here, for it differs from others elsewhere and may forecast a trend. This different voice is that of the *Manhattan Tribune,* a weekly tabloid with a racially-mixed staff which first appeared in 1968. Although not owned solely by blacks, its contribution to black journalism cannot go unnoticed.

William Haddad, white, and Roy Innis, black, designed the paper as a means of providing a realistic laboratory for young blacks and Puerto Ricans seeking journalistic experience. An advisory board including some noted journalists aids in its training work.

Attractively and modernly designed, the paper is typographically much in advance of most others aimed at Harlem. It emphasizes background stories on urban problems, race relations, and education, rather than spot news. Much space is devoted to human interest features as well. Better written than many a purely commercial paper, it uses photographs in the manner of picture magazines, giving it a strong periodical tone. Story topics are of broader than minority interests at times. Both national and local advertising are taken.

Haddad, at the time of the founding, was a director of the Urban Coalition as well as a one-time Pulitzer Prize-winning reporter. Innis was director of the Congress of Racial Equality and holder of strong views on social justice for his race. The two divide the responsibilities and print their views on an issue, which may be directly opposing, side by side. Innis, in an interview soon after the paper appeared, explained the paper's viewpoint:

"Half the problem in this country is semantics," he told James F. Fixx. "The press isn't objective; too many times what it's trying to do is not clarify things but cloud them." He cited as an example "the white reports about blacks. You get nothing but a reflection of white ideals because the only reports you read are about that part of the black community that is trying to live by white ideals."[21] His paper, Innis said, would do correctly any story which the staff thinks isn't being done correctly. That staff is about half-and-half racially. The paper has the financial backing of the U.S. Research and Development Corporation, of which Haddad is head.

In Detroit and Kansas City. Another paper serving a large black population is the *Michigan Chronicle* of Detroit, a weekly with a circulation larger than most of the other black papers, about 60,000. One of the Sengstacke publications, it exists in a city which has a larger percentage of black inhabitants than New York, Chicago, Philadelphia, and Kansas City. Because its circulation is so heavily concentrated locally, it emphasizes Detroit events but includes material, such as columns found in other papers of the Sengstacke chain, not obtainable from nearby rivals by readers. Standard in size, it is a physically big paper because of its heavy advertising schedule.

Also reflecting local interests is the Kansas City *Call,* a weekly which gives an unusual amount of space to religious news, as generally is true of papers in Missouri and other Southwestern and Southern states, regardless of color. Printed by offset and standard sized, it is strong on local stories but tends to de-emphasize national news. Local topics are treated often in the editorial pages, a practice that over the years has given it the reputation of being a fighting paper. Columns dominate less than in some other papers; an unusual feature is a section of book reviews.

● **CAMPUS LOCAL VOICES**

Like local voices within local voices, several dozen newspapers are issued at black colleges and universities and generally owned by the institution. W. E. B. Du Bois, in his days at Fisk, edited that university's paper, and many another black journalist who became a professional broke into the field of journalism through such a publication.

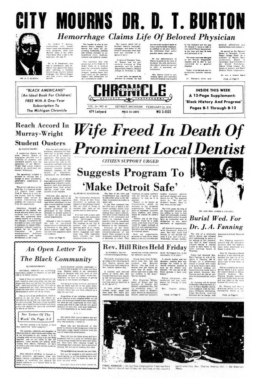

FIG. 6.5. The **Michigan Chronicle** has one of the largest circulations among black newspapers.

Some of the better known papers issued on black college campuses include the *Maroon Tiger* of Morehouse, the *Paineite* of Paine, the *Famuan* (formerly the *Florida State A. & M. News*), the *Virginia Statesman* at Virginia State, and the *Gold Torch* of Central State. As will be noted in the biographies of black journalists, several of the more prominent did their first journalistic work on their college papers (see Chapter 10).

In many ways typical of these generally orthodox papers is the *Famuan,* for like college publications everywhere it takes a critical attitude towards the institution's administration and deals with national topics, but lacks the bitterness of the black paper on a white campus. And, like its white counterparts, it now is less of a bulletin board than it was several decades ago, and to some extent given more to opinion than informative journalism.

The *Famuan* serves an as open forum for the campus at Tallahassee, but it does not have easy going, for it lacks paid advertising and depends upon university subsidy. A recent editor complained that the paper was unable to obtain motion picture house advertising, although those theaters buy space in the white college papers published in the same area.

Many of these papers are tabloids. Unless, as few do, they have a substantial journalism program in the curriculum they are likely to be amateurishly written and edited. Nevertheless, they give students an outlet and a measure of experience.

What is recent in campus journalism is the black paper for black students who study at white colleges or universities. Usually such a campus already is served by a university-sponsored paper, but at a few the black student groups have wanted their own publications. From such desires have come *Blackout* at the University of Missouri; *Our Choking Times,* Ohio State; *Black Voice,* Syracuse; *Vindicator,* Cleveland State; *Black Fire,* San Francisco State; *Black Watch,* Kansas State; and the *Colonial* at Stanford.

In at least one instance—Wayne State University—black students gained control of the paper for all students. *South End* is the official daily serving a campus population of about 33,000, of which 11 per cent was black in 1969. During its first year under black editors, beginning in 1967, and in a second year with a predominantly black executive staff, the paper became vigorously militant. One slogan was: "Year of the Heroic Guerrilla."[22]

Among the earliest of the independent, black campus papers at white institutions was *Blackout,* published by the Legion of Black Collegians at Missouri, in the fall, 1969. The Legion, asserting that there have been "no news media representative of black opinion," that there "is now an urgent need for consolidation," and that "Blacks comprise one of the largest minorities on campus," set up a newspaper committee to produce *Blackout.* Although unprepossessing physically, if its first issue is typical, its purpose was clear enough. Duplicated on legal-sized sheets, it sold for ten cents. Poorly reproduced, most of the line drawings were hardly discernible, and some of the text was obscure as well. The paper contained little news, and as to be expected with any advocacy publication, a maximum of opinion. Two stories had news value. The rest was subjective pieces or literary materials. One of the latter was on the Black Panthers. Several were critical of the university, one beginning: "The University of Missouri, alias 'Little Dixie,' is a society of racism." The literary content—a book review, a list of new black books, and several poems—occupied three pages.

The *Vindicator* was published in early 1970 as an eight-page tabloid financed by the Cleveland State University Student Affairs Committee. It serves a campus of 13,000, of whom 300 are black. Its reason for existence, its editor explained to the Cleveland *Plain Dealer,* is that "there is no other now-existing student publication that has included the black life style in its scope of news coverage." Another statement by its editor, Ronald E. Kisner, shows that black students, like many white ones, overrate the college publication as a training ground. He told the *Plain Dealer:* "There is a great demand for black journalists. I see the *Vindicator* as a vehicle through which interested students could get basic training in journalism and then go into professional media."[23]

Black Voice, a semi-monthly tabloid published since 1968 at Syracuse University, began as a duplicated newsletter; by 1970 it was being printed offset. It emphasizes news events, offers a news feature or two, poetry, and photographs. It is not sold to the public; its staff is not announced; it is withheld particularly from whites on campus, and has a strong separatist tone in its content. Its editors want it to be a communication medium for black students alone.

● **NEWSLETTERS AS LOCAL VOICES**

Although some newsletters have grown into larger community papers, most are variations on the local newspaper that exists undoubtedly by the hundreds among clubs and other groups. Although physically an unimpressive publication often, sometimes it is newsy and well-edited.

Most of the newsletter editors follow the common pattern of one or two columns on a letter-sized sheet, with a printed standing heading but the rest produced on a duplicating machine. Sometimes drawings are cut on the stencil as well as in the text, embellishing what might be a dead-looking publication. One of the more professional newsletters in black journalism is an offset-printed monthly issued by the Greenwich Village-Chelsea branch of the NAACP since 1962. Produced on both sides of three legal-sized sheets, it has branch news on page one in one column and another column devoted to messages from the branch president. The inside pages carry reports of meetings, results of money-raising campaigns, brief news stories, and reprinted articles from other black publications. A few inches of advertising space are sold. Most of the material is prepared on a typewriter and reproduced from such copy.   ●

7. THE BLACK MAGAZINES— THE FRONTRUNNERS

MAGAZINES of any kind generally are divided into two broad groups: consumer and specialized. The first are the large-circulation periodicals of broad appeal, aimed at anyone who can read and containing something for almost anyone. The others are magazines that deal with all kinds of special interests—cats and caterpiller tractors, music and the milk industry, plumbing and party-making. In a twilight zone between them are magazines that while somewhat specialized make such a mass appeal that they belong with the consumer group; among these are the newsmagazines, women's and men's publications, and the shelter periodicals for home lovers.

The black magazine industry is subject to the same divisions. Although numerically there are relatively few in each area, the patterns are the same. It is made up of a dozen or so consumer books (magazine industry people talk of these publications as books), such as *Ebony, Tuesday,* and *Soul! Illustrated;* several more are in the twilight zone, like *Jet* and *New Lady;* and about half a hundred that are truly specialized and are dealt with separately in the next chapter.

The frontrunners occupy that position not because they are necessarily better as magazines but chiefly because, being generally consumer-aimed, they have larger circulations, more advertising revenue and volume, and broader influence than the others. Furthermore, there is reason to say that the modern black magazine of general circulation is coming to symbolize the black press whereas in the past black journalism was dominated by the newspaper. But newspaper distribution, slightly improved as it has been in the late 1960's and early 1970's by the creation of more papers rather than rise in circulation of the established ones, is overshadowed by the steady growth of the magazines.

Yet the story of the black consumer magazine has been one of success for only a few, and those in relatively recent times. Beginning with the *Colored American* in 1900 failures were frequent until recent decades (see Chapters 2 and 4). For a time such magazines as *Bronze*

World, Color, Our World, and the *Urbanite* hoped to stay in the consumer field but failed. Some clues to their failure are to be found in the story of one of the longer-lasting, *Our World.* Expensively produced, lavish with tinted inks and printed on high quality paper, it was a rival monthly to *Color* and *Ebony* when it was begun in 1946. Subtitled "The Picture Magazine for the Whole Family," it attempted to penetrate the black market.[1] It evidently hoped to ride on the popularity of the white leaders, *Life* and *Look,* but too little of that popularity rubbed off.

Nevertheless, *Our World* managed to reach a circulation of 251,599 in 1952, an achievement for a magazine of the sort today and even more so for one of that time. But as with various white magazines that reached high circulations (the original *Coronet* and all the Crowell-Collier publications reached boxcar figures running into the millions but failed nevertheless) it is possible to have too much circulation. Such a situation comes about when too many copies must be printed and distributed in ratio to the advertising revenue and circulation earnings collected. And in 1955 *Our World* went bankrupt, having lost 100,000 circulation as well as precious advertising accounts because it could not sell more space.[2] A brief effort to salvage it failed.

Another attempt at a general consumer magazine was the *Urbanite.* *Life*-size but otherwise not *Life*-like, it was issued monthly for nearly a year in 1961 from New York. Announced as a magazine aimed at comparatively affluent blacks with $5,200 to $15,000 incomes, it attracted quality advertising—book clubs, cigarettes, and record players—but not enough. Contributors were among the best known writers at the time, such as the authors James Baldwin, John O. Kellens, and John A. Williams and the playwright Lorraine Hansberry. John Ciardi, poet and teacher, also wrote for it, one of the few white writers to appear. Evidently the economically elite group was too small or not interested in the intellectual fare the *Urbanite* offered.

● THREE COMPANIES DOMINATE

Dominating the general magazine field of black journalism are three companies; together they are responsible for issuing what might be called the frontrunners among the black magazines in the sense that they have the largest distribution or sell the most advertising space. Since the possibilities for exploration of black history, culture, personalities, art, and the existing condition of the black people have no limit, it is likely these firms will continue to flourish and may, in time, be confronted with competitors.

The three firms are the Johnson Publishing Company and Tuesday Publications, Inc., both with headquarters in Chicago, and the much less widely known Good Publishing Company of Fort Worth, Texas. Johnson and Good have four magazines each; two in each firm are directly competitive for advertising and circulation. Johnson scarcely recognizes Good as a competitor, the circulation and advertising gap between them is so great. But if one compares the Good performance with that of any publishing establishment other than Johnson or Tuesday it can be seen that it holds an important place since it reaches a substantial group in the black communities and has a somewhat different formula for its publications than do the other two big firms.

● **THE EBONY STORY**

The Johnson output is led by *Ebony,* a picture monthly usually containing about 200 pages. Like *Life* and *Look,* it offers considerable text in addition to numerous pictures, and thus is not merely a photo collection to be riffled through quickly. Since 1968 it has been in the select group of around sixty U.S. magazines that have more than one million circulation (there are approximately 20,000 U.S. magazines of all types). *Tuesday* also is in that group, although its circulation method is different and somewhat unorthodox.

The first Johnson magazine was what now is titled *Black World,* then *Negro Digest.* It did well enough to encourage John H. Johnson, its publisher, to attempt *Ebony,* which was born in 1945 with the intention of emphasizing the bright side of black life and reporting successes by black people in any endeavor. This philosophy it has had until recent years, when the struggle for righting of the wrongs against the black race in America demanded its cooperation more heartily. At the beginning *Ebony* was a mild, moderate picture monthly. Then, to boost newsstand sales, it was changed into a somewhat sensational publication. Sexy articles, cheesecake pictures, and other come-ons shot the circulation to a half-million. But its success did not last, for an economic recession hit the country in 1954, cutting the circulation by 20 per cent. Moderation again became the tone, to get the book back into black homes. The earlier pose had been given it by Ben Burns, a white journalist who thought moving it into the girlie magazine realm would give it heavy newsstand sales. And he was right, it did.

But what Burns did not anticipate was opposition from religious people, whose use of black newspapers and magazines always has been important to this special press. Johnson wanted his magazine in black homes, for without such an audience much advertising cannot be obtained. With the content changed, *Ebony* then was able to add a substantial home circulation. It now notes that 70 per cent of its circulation of 1,250,000 is in subscription copies. And it has been able to obtain many advertising accounts of a type vital to consumer publications.

With the rise in black militancy and the impression upon the black society made by groups such as the Black Nationalists and the Black Panther Party, *Ebony* has become more outspoken in behalf of quicker improvements in the living conditions, educational opportunities, and vocational acceptance of blacks. The change—still not enough to convince the would-be revolutionaries who read *Black News* in preference—is reflected in such articles as "How Racists Use 'Science' to Degrade Black People" by Carl T. Rowan, and such editorials as the one against no-knock drug raids. The extremists do not see these articles as clearly as they see an editorial warning blacks against being lured into violence to bring about their revolutionary aims. They are disdainful, also, of the success stories in each issue.

Walter Goodman quotes an unnamed New York photographer "whose sympathies lie with SNCC" who is "particularly scornful of 'all those flukey jobs they write about, like the cat at IBM who's making seventy-five hundred dollars a year. What the hell are they telling me, man? Everybody *knows* if he was white he'd be making twelve thousand.' "[3] A comparison of issues a decade apart however, shows that in 1970 room had been made for more aggressive writing in behalf of the race.

In edging into their changed position, however, the editors are running into a new sort of trouble. A reader in Isle of Palm, South Carolina, wrote this complaint:

"I'd like to protest the insults I receive every time I read it. Not an issue goes by but that you refer to the Caucasian race in the most insulting terms . . . Whitey, Charley and Honkie. . . ." The writer goes on to say that he feels "we are all Americans, not black, white, yellow or red," and accuses *Ebony* of preaching bigotry and violence.[4]

And a Canadian reader calls the magazine discriminatory because whites are excluded from it. "For you to be proud that you are a black man is just as wrong as for me to be proud I am a white man. We are men," he wrote, adding: "You are the ones now giving importance to the colouring of the skin, the very crime you condemn the whites for."[5]

But *Ebony* goes on, gaining in circulation steadily at a time when some of the largest white magazines are cutting theirs for economy reasons.

Jet, Tan *and* Black World. The other three magazines from the Johnson firm are *Jet,* a peppy, pocket-size weekly, shy on advertising but long on news nuggets which sometimes are original coverage and always tightly written; *Tan,* a sensational, somewhat squishy women's and confession publication, like the white *True Confessions* as it was back in the 1940's before it became something of a service magazine for the white workingman's wife who now is a person of comparative affluence; and *Black World* (called *Negro Digest* until 1970), the maverick of the family because it is firmly militant in behalf of the black citizen whereas the others strive for impartiality *(Jet)* or confine themselves to more conventional relations of human beings (*Tan*). *Negro Digest,* the first in the group, was begun in 1942 and discontinued temporarily in 1951; *Tan* was started in 1950, and *Jet* two years later.

Jet was modeled after the midget or less-than-pocket size of the original Cowles magazine, *Quick,* and remained about four inches by six inches in size until 1970, when it was enlarged to roughly five by eight inches. At founding it sold for fifteen cents a week. Ben Burns, then executive editor of *Ebony,* added the editorship of *Jet.* Edward T. Clayton, associate editor of *Ebony,* was made managing editor of the new little book. Owner Johnson explained its function: "to provide Negroes with a convenient-sized magazine summarizing the week's biggest Negro news in a well-organized, easy-to-read format. . . ."

Jet was not, as sometimes thought, the first black newsmagazine. In 1925 appeared a *Time*-size one with the unlikely name of *Heebie Jeebies.* Published in Chicago, it had departments but also some fiction. P. L. Prattis, a widely known black editor, was its president and editor. It may have been the first.[6]

During the recession period of the later 1950's *Jet* lost heavily in newsstand sales, although it had the benefit of more exposure than either *Negro Digest* or *Tan.* But it came back. The early issues carried sensational titles ("Ten Ways to a Mink Coat") and this tone has been maintained, as in an article headed "One of the Sexiest Men Alive, Says Miles Davis' New Bride." Along with such copy have gone hard hitting crusades against injustices to which blacks have been subjected. Alfred Balk has pointed out that *Jet* brought the Emmett Till and Montgomery bus boycott stories before the country and "it probably saved Jimmy Wilson's life by publicizing the now famous $1.95 theft case."[7]

Robert E. Johnson (not related to the owner, John H. Johnson), an editor whose brisk personality is reflected in the magazine's punchy style, has seen *Jet*'s circulation approach a half-million in the early 1970's, and a small lift in its advertising revenue because of inclusion of a table of popular music in each issue, thereby attracting record and tape company copy. But Johnson is most proud of the exclusive articles he runs. He notes stories overlooked or ignored by the white press. At a meeting of the Chicago Headline Club in 1969, for example, he asked the members of the audience of eighty-five to raise their hands if they had heard or read the statement made by President Lyndon B. Johnson in 1968 about the report of the National Advisory Commission on Civil Disorders, known familiarly as the "Kerner report." In March of that year the president, at a White House conference with members of the National Newspaper Publishers Association, had said: "I think that the most important thing in the report is the conclusion that it reaches about the cause of our problems in this country evolving primarily from white racism." He also

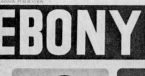

**HOW RACISTS USE 'SCIENCE'
TO DEGRADE BLACK PEOPLE**
By Carl T. Rowan

**Have Black Models
Really Made It?**

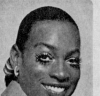

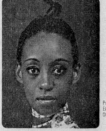

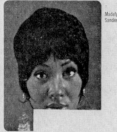

Princess
Elizabeth
Of Toro

Madelyn
Sanders

MAY
'70
60c

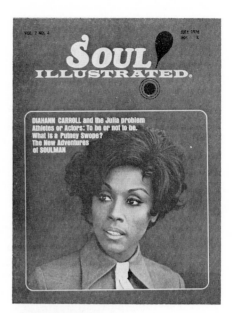

VOL. 2 NO. 4   JULY 1970 NO. 1

DIAHANN CARROLL and the Julia problem
Athletes or Actors: To be or not to be.
What is a Putney Swope?
The New Adventures
of SOULMAN

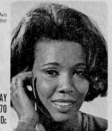

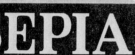

**SHIRLEY
CHISHOLM**
The 'Fusion Bomb'
of Congress
tells it like it is

JUARY, 1970 50¢   The Action Magazine

**HOW PHONE
MOLESTERS
GET TRAPPED**
What you can
do to help

NE HUNDRED
IVISIBLE BLACKS
ets, explorers,
ventors, scientists. . .
hored by history books
cause their skin
s the wrong color

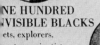

**THE MILLS
BROTHERS**
43 years and
still swinging

CALVIN HILL:
They call him
Super Rook

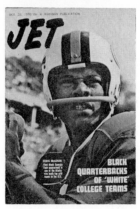

BLACK
QUARTERBACKS
OF 'WHITE'
COLLEGE TEAMS

FIG. 7.1. Among the large consumer magazines sold on newsstands or by subscription, **Ebony** leads in both advertising volume and circulation; **Sepia** is the only direct competitor. **Jet** is a newsmagazine, and **Soul! Illustrated** combines entertainment and social purposes.

said: "I think it's the most important report that has been made to me since I've been President."[8]

Only one member of the audience raised a hand; there was a sprinkling of black journalists in the group but the only hand was that of a white. Bob Johnson's point was that here was an important statement by the president, especially in view of the accusations against him of silence concerning the report. And it had been overlooked or ignored by the white press.

The early issues of *Tan Confessions,* which was *Tan's* original name, contained articles entitled "Is the Chaste Girl Chased?", "Love in a Choir Loft," and "I Took My Mother's Man." Circulation bounded to 300,000, but as with the early *Ebony* some black readers objected to the tone of the confessions magazine. After all, it was not in line with Johnson's announced aim for the black race: "to help the Negro have greater dignity." The title was shortened and it became more of a service magazine, but not entirely free of the come-on appeal; today the old type of material is subdued and conveyed largely as fiction. Fashion and food articles and such general magazine content as "Why Teens Run Away from Home" and "Make Every Penny Count" are to be found. Personality pieces are side by side with short confession-type stories.

Tan has outlasted several other attempts with the same original formula, such as *Negro Romance* and *Bronze Confessions,* by other publishers both black and white. In fact, it outlasted a sister publication, *Copper Romance,* which Johnson began in 1953. But it has steady competition from a trio of monthlies published by the Good firm.

When *Black World,* still called *Negro Digest,* was reborn in 1961 it returned to its original formula, from which it had drifted somewhat in the late 1940's in an attempt to appeal to a wider audience. It now was interested in new literary horizons. Material on black culture, history, and personalities, especially serious artists and writers, appeared and continued to do so for the next decade. Among the titles in the revived version were "FEPC is Not Enough," "Black Metropolis Revisited," "The Negro's Escape from Freedom," and "Brazil: Study in Black, Brown and Beige." The growing dislike among some black Americans for the word *Negro* finally led the magazine's editors to make the name change in May, 1970. Hoyt W. Fuller, managing editor, briefly recounted the magazine's past in the announcement of the change and wrote about "the new black spirit" and "Black Consciousness." He reported that "many of those who read *Negro Digest* and approved it wondered why, in the new age, it did not make the extra step which would have brought it into full harmony with the times. 'Change the name,' they urged." Fuller went on to say that the editors agreed it was time and revealed the new title—*Black World.*[9]

There have been other Johnson company ventures. *Hue,* the

same size and shape as *Jet,* was started as a monthly, partly to provide a place for copy left over from the others. Another motive was to see if money could be made with still another pocket-size newsstand periodical. It emphasized entertainment world doings of the black society, reached 150,000 circulation, and then went weekly. But like the experience of *Jet,* the new little magazine never commanded enough advertising, its size preventing it from using standard plates. It also brought in too little circulation revenue. The newsstand diseases that hit most large magazines in the 1950's and 1960's brought about its demise. Another unsuccessful Johnson publication was aimed at Africa, *Ebony International,* intended for English-reading Africans. It lasted only a few issues, running into political and ideological complications as well as high production and distribution costs.

● THE GOOD IMAGE

In any of the four magazines issued by the Good firm in Texas the image of the black person is different from that portrayed by *Ebony,* particularly through three that look and sound alike: *Hep, Jive,* and *Bronze Thrills,* whose kinship with the Johnson publications is largely through *Tan.* If *Ebony* can be called the flagship of the Johnson fleet, *Sepia* is Good's leader, although for financial purposes in recent years has been put into a publishing company of its own bearing its name. The Good commander is little known outside Texas, however. He is George Levitan, a white man who depends upon a black staff to produce his magazines and operates a substantial plant in Fort Worth. Levitan, who dresses in big-hat Texas fashion, joins with black publishers at their meetings. By the specification that ownership must be black (see Chapter 1) the Good magazines may not qualify as black journalism, but they meet the requirements in every other way and cannot be ignored because of their influence.

Like *Ebony, Sepia* is *Life*-size, if not as thick with pages as either. It has only a fraction of the *Ebony* circulation (roughly 65,000 to *Ebony*'s 1,250,000), relatively little advertising, and sometimes one hundred fewer pages in a comparable seasonal issue. Superficially it looks like any picture magazine, and, while less susbstantial than *Ebony* in content, has more substance than its outward appearance would indicate. Begun in 1955, it consists largely of simply written articles that emphasize human interest. Medical angles are popular. One piece called "Is Your TV Set Killing You?" was not about the violence or low quality of material shown but about the radiation poisoning supposedly emanating from color sets; another was titled "Sickle Cell Anemia: The Black People's Disease." As with *Ebony,* public affairs topics were avoided for some years but gradually are in view through such articles as "Blacks Kill Blacks," a report on Biafra, and "George Wallace: A Racist Covets the White House."

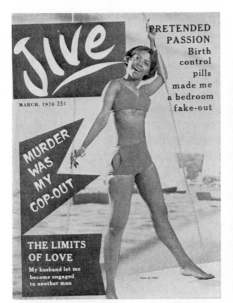

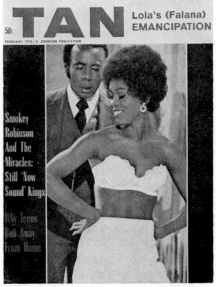

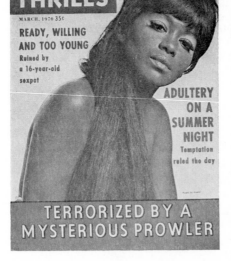

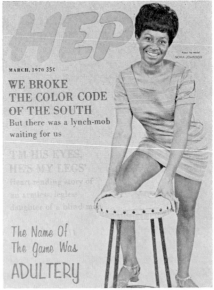

FIG. 7.2. These are confession-romance consumer magazines. **Tan** is a Johnson publication; the other three are from the Good firm in Texas.

Sports and entertainment world figures are prominent copy. "Wanted: Black Talent; Apply Hollywood" was an article springing from the success of Diahann Carroll. There are also book reviews, Washington news reports, and historical and biographical pieces calculated to engender pride in black accomplishments.

In the magazine business, if one of a group of competitors shoots far ahead of the others, advertisers tend to move from the others into the pages of the leader, a logical and practical step if an advertiser is to get the most exposure for his money. *Ebony,* as noted, has vanquished all its rivals except *Sepia* which, therefore, has accomplished something in being able to survive. It has a comparatively successful formula, although in a group with three other popular content magazines it is bound to benefit from the operations of a large firm. That formula is to be less sensational than its companion magazines, to be timely, to offer a variety of content, and to avoid high costs by doing comparatively little color printing, by using inexpensive printing paper, and little promotion, and to venture cautiously into fundamental social issues.

Bronze Thrills is reminiscent of the early *Tan.* Under a general heading of "I Confess," which has run for many issues, one finds articles titled "Held Together by Sex" and "She was Ready, Willing and Too Young." Designated as true love stories are tales called "Afraid to Love, Afraid to Lose," "Terrorized by a Peeping Tom," "A Den of Homosexuals," and "My Husband Was Only a Shell." Models pose for the photographs, a true confessions magazine technique to impart reality. Some stories are from the male angle, a device white periodicals of the sort avoid, since women are the assumed sole readers. Yet there are articles exhibiting a broader interest than these, or at least a great sense of social responsibility, even if only one every few issues. One such dealt with blacks in the Peace Corps (how can we tell Africans how to live when we can't ourselves?).

The other two Good magazines, *Jive* and *Hep,* also monthlies, are uniform in size with *Bronze Thrills* (newsmagazine dimensions) and have various staff members in common as well as almost the same advertising copy, since most advertisers buy space in them as a group. *Jive* is a confession book also but adds some short editorialized news paragraphs, a teen-agers page, an astrology section, a sermonette, and advice letters. *Hep* is devoted to "The Lowdown on Sepia, U.S.A.," to quote its subtitle, and much copy similar to the *True Story* type of the Macfadden days. Much show business news, some hard news coverage, picture stories (one of an interracial marriage in two prominent families), many short news accounts of general interest, and a lot of attention to blacks in sports make up its formula.

These Good magazines operate much as *Tan* does except that they are aimed at an older audience, the young adult and adult women, whereas *Tan* aims for the young girl and young housewife. The stories deal more with sex than with love (the *Tan* staff says the opposite of its content) and a somewhat lower reading ability is expected of the readers. By their twentieth years *Jive, Bronze Thrills,* and *Hep* had toned down their advertising somewhat if not their editorial contents, which still emphasized sex. Still being used in 1970 were the types of advertising bordering on pornography; advertising largely banished from the major black papers and consumer magazines other than those issued by the publishers of *Jive* and her sisters: lucky stones, nude photographs, filmed sex, girlie calendars, stag records, "Hard-to-Get French Items," a "Privately Printed" magazine, and desire-promoting potions, drinks, and creams. Gone were the battery-run dildoes and other devices, including life-size "playmates" named Eve or Candy. *Hep,* while providing some of the usual copy, added more unsexy human interest material—articles about a handicapped girl and the problems of interracial marriage.

Each Good periodical hovers between 50,000 and 65,000 circulation. All four appeal to the lower economic middle class women, the rock music set among the young, and the lonely, apparently sex-starved housewives or working women of any age or situation. They attract little of the class advertising that the Johnson magazines or *Tuesday* have commanded. The implications of these magazines' content may be that such reading matter satisfies certain impulses and provides a safety valve. Or that it develops an appetite for that kind of material which never satiates some readers and therefore will keep the magazines alive. From the viewpoint of the person who wants the black press to fight for the rights of the black citizens and to turn black people's interest in the direction of having pride of race and culture, these confession magazines (and not excepting the Johnson *Tan*) are just so much waste or soporifics which let the reader wallow in self-pity and enjoy the lubricious. Whether readers who turn to these periodicals would be willing to walk on picket lines or take part in demonstrations and protest marches or any other such social action one cannot say; here is another instance where thorough research into what the black population reads would be valuable. Who, specifically, are the readers of these magazines, by economic and educational levels? Why are the books liked? What action do readers take on either the reading matter or advertising?

On the other hand these confession and romance periodicals may be far more realistic than the *Ebony-Black World-Soul! Illustrated* types. Why should black citizens be expected to be any freer of problems about man and woman or family relations than any other group of humans?

● THE TUESDAY SUPPLEMENT

In white journalism such publications as *Parade* and *Family Weekly* and scores of locally produced variations are not accepted

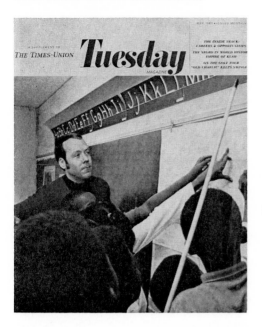

FIG. 7.3. **Tuesday** is a monthly consumer magazine, distributed through insertion in white newspapers.

by the organizations of the magazine industry, such as the Magazine Publishers Association and its subsidiary, the Magazine Advertising Bureau, as regular members of the periodical world, but are left to the newspaper business. For many millions receive them each week as part of their daily newspapers and cannot buy them separately. When one opens such a publication, however, one finds more or less the same sort of content as is in a general magazine of more orthodox method of distribution, only less of it: articles on public affairs, puzzles, contests, picture stories, human interest features and the usual soup, soap and salve advertising.

Tuesday is one of these newspaper magazines, so called because for years the black weekly in America was delivered on a Tuesday. The second (or third) day of the week, then, is newspaper day to many a black family, and when W. Leonard Evans, Jr., *Tuesday*'s publisher, launched the magazine in 1965 he gave it this significant name, although by 1970 few if any of the twoscore newspapers distributing it did so on the named day. A monthly supplement to white papers published in large cities with distribution to black communities, it lays claim to the largest circulation of any black newspaper or magazine, about 2,000,000. Physically like *Parade,* it is picture magazine size, and is to be found in large dailies in Chicago, Cleveland, Dallas, Minneapolis, and other major cities. It puzzles whites to be told this, for most do not see *Tuesday* in their copies, since the supplement is inserted only in those that go to the black residential areas. However, it goes to the entire circulation of at least two of the papers each month. About 128,000 copies go to colleges regularly. The magazine was scheduled to go semi-monthly in April, 1971, with a circulation of 2,300,000. *Tuesday at Home* was the name given to a new magazine to be inserted alternately with *Tuesday* in white papers also, and distributed beginning in Spring, 1971. Its appeal was to the world of the "Black Homemaker" of median age 38 and of "a high purchase level."

Evans has a specific goal for his publication, and realizes its economic potential and that of the black society. "We are poor individually, wealthy collectively," he said in the third anniversary issue, pointing out that the black income when added up represents $32 billion annually. His solution for the inequity he explained thus:

"The solution is simple enough, if men of good will and honest concern are willing to invest their time, their money, their talents and knowledge. And they must, for time is running out in our black communities. When there is no hope there is despair. And we have seen too vividly in recent years the product of despair. *Tuesday,* for one, refuses to believe that despair is necessary. There must be hope for our people, our communities, our nation, our world. We believe these few ideas and proposals can help provide a solution. Once the black communities become economically profitable like others in our nation through the utilization of their creative and intellectual capacities then, and only then, will the true meaning of freedom be realized."[10]

In attempting to carry forward its founder's ideals, *Tuesday* is giving its readers an objective, attempting to create a particular concept of themselves or at least something to which to aspire. Its subjects generally are serious, although there is the usual magazine content on fashions and food; in this magazine, of course, it is soul food. But articles on "The Negro Cowboy," a series of thirty on the great men and women of black descent, on achievers in the law, the arts, city affairs, sports, education, and other activities generally have been of high quality. It gives space to important Washington news and has a travel column. Like *Ebony, Tuesday* has been able to obtain advertising from major white firms and also like the Johnson magazine it seeks to be positive in its editorial approach. It therefore has earned the contempt of blacks who criticize the black press because it supports what they call the establishment.

Also like the Johnson firm, Tuesday Publications is diversifying. Adding enterprises is a settled practice in American publishing: some major companies issue not only their magazines but also own broadcasting stations, book publishing companies, and in a few instances such unrelated enterprises as lighting fixture manufacturing companies. Johnson is in the cosmetics, book, and insurance businesses. *Tuesday* also has gone into book publishing.

Although launching a general consumer magazine and maintaining it is one of the most expensive ventures in American journalism, another entry into the black consumer field appeared in fall,

1969: *Black America.* It began as a bi-monthly, apparently with the hope of being sustained by the promotion possible through the Miss Black America beauty contests and a fashion model agency in Philadelphia. Newsmagazine size, with generous use of color printing and high quality paper, it prints articles on social problems, service topics (food, home, fashion), and personalities. Its editorial views are moderate. While it seeks for general appeal, its content is heavily tailored to women's interests.

● NEW MAGAZINES FOR WOMEN

Community newspapers are by no means the only new elements in black journalism. Born in the late 1960's and early 1970's have been numerous community and special interest magazines and several large consumer magazines involving considerable financial investment and risk. Prominent among the latter have been two for women: *New Lady* and *Essence.* Each is unlike anything available for black women previously.

New Lady, clearly a women's service periodical of the *Good Housekeeping* variety, is not as new as it seems. Begun originally in 1966 in California, it managed three issues, and then was suspended because of inadequate financing. Three years later, with the help of the Ford Foundation and Opportunity Through Ownership, each of which provided loans of $70,000, it was revived. Staff members visited the offices of *McCall's* and *Redbook* for briefing on their duties; Select Magazines, a distributor, undertook to put it on the stands in nearly one hundred localities. Early in 1970 its executives reported a paid circulation of 100,000, obtained through the efforts of various organizations, such as the National Council of Negro Women, National Association of Negro Business and Professional Women's Clubs, and youth groups and sororities.

The theory behind the formula was expressed by Warner Beckett, the publisher, who came to his post with public relations and marketing experience. "Our magazine attempts to fill a void for the black woman," he told an interviewer at the Los Angeles *Times.* "All of the other popular women's magazines are edited for the Caucasian woman." Beckett believes that the black woman has her own special needs and is a special individual. About 80 per cent of the staff is black. Few of the top editorial staffers have had professional journalism experience or training. The editor is a former postman, the managing editor has been a free lance writer and once worked on a black weekly community newspaper. Copy is accepted regardless of the race of the writer.

The magazine's content, offered in an eight-by-ten-inch format, in general is in the familiar patterns of women's magazines—a few short stories, a children's page, articles and departments on fashion, cooking, medicine, personal care, dieting, and like topics, and per-

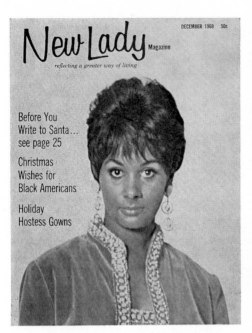

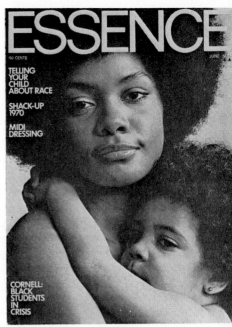

FIG. 7.4. **New Lady** and **Essence** appeared in 1969 and 1970. Both are women's service and glamour magazines, with som[e] social concerns.

sonality pieces about successful black women, therefore offering what editors like to call an opportunity for reader identification. Editorials are not used. After a few issues articles dealt with racial subjects, the views of Rap Brown or the viewpoints of black activists on campus or of other rebels, perhaps in answer to a reaction represented by a letter to the magazine saying:

"Your magazine is 'nice.' How come you don't tell it like it really is, that the black people are starving and losing their lives in the streets every day. I don't see anything about the Panthers or their activities and why don't you use Kathleen Cleaver for a new black lady. Your black lady doesn't even have a natural. Black people are involved in the serious struggle to live every day. That's what you should be printing."[11]

Advertising, slim in the first year but expected to pick up, was from major firms advertising beverages, floor coverings, bakery products, and household supplies. Such accounts are in strong contrast to the other magazines aimed at black women except the more recently begun *Essence*.

Technically the magazine is better produced than all the others excepting *Essence*. Fashion and food materials are in full color.

Except for occasional typographical errors the printing is superior. The fiction, however, is much like the shallowest in the white women's magazines. Black characters use language the reader of *New Lady* presumably abandoned long ago, if she ever spoke that way. Art work does not match the photography in quality. Much of the major copy is staff written, perhaps for reasons of economy and because high quality material by and about the interests of blacks is difficult to find. The editors announced their search for contributions and planned to pay reasonably well for them.

Its rival, *Essence,* was launched in spring, 1970, with considerable advance publicity, more than heralded *New Lady*, which was located far from the publishing center of the nation. *Time* and *Newsweek, New York,* the trade press, and NBC's "Today" show helped launch it. With Gordon Parks, the photojournalist, novelist, music composer, and cinema producer as editorial director, it began on a formula of providing handsome color photographs of fashions and food, numerous articles on current black issues, some aimed particularly at women (the problem of black men sometimes preferring white women, for instance), fiction and departments of the sort common to white women's magazines—home, recipes, and personal care. Newsmagazine size but looking larger because of its many bled pictures from cover to cover, *Essence* is an odd combination of defiance of the capitalist order ("Cornell in Crisis" is sympathetic enough with the black students to disturb persons who remember the photograph of the armed young men leaving a campus building) while presenting advertisements for some of the symbols of decadence—cosmetics and expensive clothing. An article entitled "Five Shades of Militancy" would have pleased the letter writer to *New Lady*, for it dealt with Kathleen Cleaver, among others, and gives understanding, if not encouragement.

The most glamour-filled black magazine on the market was conceived in 1968 when a white executive of the Shearson, Hammill firm of Wall street brokers encouraged a trio of young black businessmen to launch *Essence.* After considerable delay raising $1,500,000 (part of the backing coming from Playboy Enterprises), receiving briefing from various New York magazine publishing people at Time Inc., *Psychology Today, New York,* and *Newsweek,* as well as advertising executives, the entrepreneurs were in business. They are Cecil Hollingsworth, who had a graphics consulting firm; Ed Lewis, a financial planner for the First National City Bank at the time, and Jonathan Blount, an advertising salesman for the New Jersey Bell Telephone Company. All were in their twenties at the time the magazine was launched.

More than three-fourths of the twenty-six-person staff is black; one of the few whites is the executive editor, Barbara Kerr. Ida Lewis, editor-in-chief since the second issue, was a free lance writer for ten years before joining the magazine, contributing to *Life, L'Express,* and other French publications while living in France for five years. During the NBC program Miss Lewis was asked about the magazine's audience. She replied that seven-and-a-half million black women between the ages of eighteen and thirty-four are potential readers. The name was chosen out of hundreds of possibilities because black is the essence of all color.

These new magazines for women appear in a far different economic and social climate than did some of the early attempts, such as what is noted by Penn as the first publication for black women and children, *Our Women and Children.* Like so many other early black periodicals, it was edited by a man of the church, in this instance the Rev. William J. Simmons, who also was president of the State University at Louisville, Kentucky, where the magazine was published beginning in 1888.[12] Much later came other attempts. One, *Designs for Gracious Living,* was started in Cleveland in 1964; out of Los Angeles in 1963 came *Elegant* and *Elegant-Teen,* the first a bi-monthly for women that used color and ran to about one hundred pages an issue. In three years it was moved to New York City, went on a monthly schedule, stressed fashion, and promoted modern living. The one for younger people was a monthly. Neither survived to see the end of the decade.

● THE SOUL PUBLICATIONS

Two publications that are magazines in content although one is issued on newsprint and superficially looks like a tabloid newspaper are *Soul* and *Soul! Illustrated,* begun in the 1960's and now gaining a considerable consumer response.

In scope like *Variety* but written without the latter's special English, *Soul* is for the black entertainment world every other week and calls itself "America's Most Soulful Newspaper." Printed with three covers, in the manner of the early *Downbeat,* almost all content is bylined and has a magazine tone. Much play is given to the big names in black show business and musical life, such as the departure of Diana Ross from The Supremes and the assumption of her place in the trio by Jean Terrell (a cover and three pages for an illustrated interview on the former, cover and four pages on the latter); a feature on Tammi Terrill at her death in 1970 took up the largest cover, the first four inside pages, and another at the back, with many pictures of the young singer and a detailed story on her health troubles during her career.

Not all these depth pieces are on entertainers. A cover and more than three additional pages once were on the Rev. Jesse Jackson, the militant leader of the Chicago Operation Breadbasket plan.

Soul was begun on a budget of $11,000. Four years later the

figure was $24,000 and the publication was being distributed in fifty-
two cities with an unaudited circulation of 150,000.[13]

Soul! Illustrated's original function was conceived by its publishers to be to tell it like it is "in this world through the eyes of the
black man in the performing arts. . . . Reporting how he made it
. . . what his contributions are. The black man's philosophy and
the advice he gives to others is the basic theme," to quote a publicity
announcement from the company, which also publishes *Soul.*

The formula, when the magazine was launched in 1968, was to
offer features, such as in-depth biographical articles on important
black artists. From there the plan was to branch out into the political and sports worlds and offer material on fashions and food.
The plan is being carried out. The July, 1970 issue, for example,
contains an article about "Diahann Carroll and the Julia Problem,"
dealing with the discussions about how faithful to black life Miss
Carroll's television program is; another, "Athletes or Actors: To be
or Not to be." Books, records, plays, and movies are reviewed regularly. The magazine was financed out of the profits of *Soul* and by
1970 was claiming an unaudited circulation of 250,000. It is well
printed, using color moderately, but so far has been unable to command much advertising.

Soul! Illustrated content smacks a bit of *Playboy* because of its
cartoons, a selection of content that is likely to make it of more interest to men than women, and a general ruggedness of layout and
makeup which gives it a masculine tone. These characteristics relate
it to an abortive black imitation of Hugh Hefner's bunny magazine
attempted in the early 1950's. Called *Duke,* it went in for nudes.
But one of the problems, it appears, was finding suitable black girls
to pose. At that time Hollywood and the entertainment world in
general had little interest in black entertainers and there was no investment in a career, perhaps even the contrary, for the young women
at the time.

● THE RESPONSE

What is the reception for these black consumer magazines? Are
they preferred to white periodicals? If so, which are preferred and
why? Little research has been undertaken to answer these and many
similar questions. The few studies reported are perhaps of less significance than they might ordinarily be because the climate of opinion within the black society in America is both confused and rapidly
changing.

A thesis written at West Virginia University recorded the results
of an attempt to "investigate the use patterns, and to some extent,
the effects of the mass media on the residents of a metropolitan Negro

ghetto."[14] The research tool used primarily was a public opinion survey based on a questionnaire and personal interview with one hundred black residents of Pittsburgh, Pennsylvania, in 1967. The researcher learned that *Ebony* was read by most of the persons interviewed and received by more than one-third of those taking a magazine. Two-thirds of the respondents received other magazines; none received a weekly newsmagazine.

Part of a report by Dr. Jack Lyle on the media in Los Angeles indicated that most of his respondents read some magazine regularly, with a median number of three. *Ebony* led the list of black magazines. The only other black periodical scoring substantially was *Jet*.[15]

Two later studies produced at Syracuse University in 1969, one a master's thesis and the other a doctoral dissertation, produced similar information about two different groups of black residents of Syracuse (see Chapter 16).[16]

The two Syracuse studies and that of Allen indicated that broadcasting received far more attention from the groups of respondents than did printed matter.

Such studies, while their purposes and findings go far beyond the matter of response to black magazines, since they deal also with the black newspaper and the accessibility of black and white publications to readers in this ethnic group, and many other aspects, help to explain why *Ebony*'s circulation is so much larger than that of any other publication issued by black publishers (except *Tuesday,* which is not a separately bought periodical). *Ebony*'s dominance also explains its selection for more intensive study than any other current black magazine. Research was conducted into it, for example, by a graduate student at the University of Michigan in 1967 which resulted in a careful analysis in depth. Paul M. Hirsch was concerned with the nature of the magazine's readers. He wrote: "It has been suggested, throughout this paper, that the Negro middle class consists of several factions which disagree over a variety of questions . . . in short, our study of *Ebony* has been a study of within-class differences." He also discussed the magazine's "editorial ambivalence and occasional self-contradiction," which he believed came about in an attempt to "please all segments of its audience."[17]   ●

8. THE BLACK MAGAZINES— THE SPECIALISTS

Name a human special interest and at least one magazine is available for it, whether it may be ecology or entomology, space travel or slenderizing. At least this is so in the U.S.A.

Publications usually feed interests and respond to them. Such a policy exists in black publishing, but it is restricted by the racial differences or special circumstances. Blacks do not need a magazine of their own when their special interest is mining or gardening. But they do need their own in areas where they are physically different, have cultural differences from the nonblacks, cannot obtain white services, have been forced into their own groups, or have special problems of little interest to nonblacks and so not worth much space in the white journal.

Black business, for example, supports two periodicals for black beauty salon operators. The special reasons are clear enough. Until recently black women did not have the services of white establishments in some areas, and still do not in some places, partly because of prejudice and partly because white operators were not trained to handle their hair. Enough women patronize the black-operated beauty parlors to support a trade press. Whenever for some reason a large number of blacks could not join whites in an activity they developed publications of their own—there are or have been journals for black doctors, dentists, lawyers, journalists, religionists, and other professionals.

Some specialized black periodicals came into being because of prejudice. Black society's more substantial house organs, sometimes confusingly called industrial publications, come from insurance companies. Black firms were founded because white companies refused policies to blacks on various bases, such as uncollectibility of premiums or greater risk because of the way many blacks had to live (their dwellings being more vulnerable to fire). Thus a black agency logically issues its own magazine for its clients or its agents.

The black specialized periodical (it sometimes has newspaper format but magazine content and vice versa; the majority are magazines, but both types are included in this chapter) is most often a scholarly, political, or literary journal, an organ of an organization, or a business publication. The rest are no less specialized but simply fewer in number.

The militant or radical spirit so strong in the U.S.A. at this writing has given rise to several new publications, some of such wide following and impact that they are of national significance. But most of the special interest publications go on in their small circles, known only to their little groups of readers albeit influential among them, as has been the way of such periodicals for many years. And if the readers influenced are themselves key individuals in society the outreach of this specialized black press is important. When Roi Ottley wrote about the black press in *Common Ground* magazine in 1943 he said he knew of 239 religious, fraternal, literary, labor, school, fashion, picture, and theatrical periodicals. To these he apparently added what he called quality publications, specifically naming *Phylon, Crisis, Opportunity,* and the *Journal of Negro History.*

The variety, if not the number, is as great as ever. Many of the 239 are no more, but the staying power of the specialized books is greater, on the whole, than that of the consumer type. No consumer book is as old as many of the specialized. The argument can be made that many of the special interest publications are subsidized to keep them alive, whereas the consumer periodical usually must make its own way economically. That is true, but subsidizers sometimes tire of steady losses, so there is an element of uncertainty as well for the publishers and editors of the specialized magazine.

● **THE MAJOR SPECIALIZED JOURNALS**

Usually because of their long service, certain magazines in this group stand out as influential and significant. Out of any list of those existing in the 1970's should be selected *Crisis, Phylon,* the *Journal of Negro History, Freedomways,* and the *Journal of Negro Education.* Several more which have not been as favored with noted editors or as many distinguished contributors deserve attention as well: the *Journal of Human Relations,* the *Quarterly Review of Higher Education,* and the *Journal of Religious Thought,* for example. Several more begun only in the late 1960's and not yet tested by time are potentially of greater importance—the *Black Scholar, Amistad,* and the *Black Politician,* for instance.

Usually a publication serving as an organ of a group is looked upon by the public as less than authentic journalism, not to be equated with a commercial magazine. Somehow it seems to be something less than professional journalism. To be sure, many organization publications are amateurish propositions. A reflection of this attitude is in the wariness of advertisers, who cite it, among other reasons, for not buying space. A number of periodicals serve as examples in the white world's journalism. The well-written and edited *Junior League*, the *Rotarian*, the *Jaycee*, and the *Kiwanis* magazines are not lush with advertisements. Only a few organization publications have been able to override the handicap. *National Geographic* is one; *Boy's Life* is another.

In the same situation is the black world's journalism. *Crisis* and *Phylon*, for instance, are not on the newsstands, are financed by institutions and organizations, and have been unable to command advertising revenue of consequence. Yet they and others like them have published some of the best literary and scholarly work in black journalism.

The Crisis. This magazine has been seen in an earlier chapter through the career of its noted founder, W. E. B. Du Bois, but only in its early years.

Crisis, began in 1910, was edited by Du Bois during its first thirteen years. Among its contributors has been Langston Hughes, whose poetry first appeared in a magazine in 1921 when "The Negro Speaks of Rivers" was published in *Crisis.* Others in its pages have included Ann Petry, the novelist, Countee Cullen, Jesse Fauset, and Claude McKay, now coming to fuller appreciation as black poets or playwrights.

The idea for the magazine came from George Wibecan, a black newspaperman in Brooklyn. He found the name in a poem by James Russell Lowell called "The Present Crisis." The first version of the *Crisis* was sixteen seven-by-ten-inch pages and used as its subscription list that of *Horizon,* an earlier magazine run by Du Bois. The one thousand copies of that first issue more than paid for themselves.[1]

Circulation rose steadily, a fact which must have given the first editor considerable satisfaction, for he started the *Crisis* without encouragement from associates. A friend, Albert E. Pillsbury, then attorney general of Massachusetts, had written him: "If you have not decided upon a periodical, for Heaven's sake don't. They are as numerous as flies."[2] The rise in sales was at the rate of one thousand a month until by 1918 it was selling more than 100,000.

The reasons for the increase reflect the changes in black middle-class life in America in those years. Du Bois aimed the magazine, as it is directed to this day, toward a well-educated group of readers, then a small minority. Its position in defense of the rights of the black soldier during World War I raised its circulation far above normal. Furthermore, the black citizens were more unified than they had been for some years and certainly more so than they are in the later years of the century, where there are many conflicting opinions over ways to achieve justice and improved conditions for living and working. The *Crisis* then was also much less a house publication for the NAACP than it is today, and something more of a literary vehicle. It was talked about because of its controversial writings by its first editor. What it said then is little different from what appears in today's militant journals; it was avant-garde in those years; it insisted that segregated people are kept inferior, that skilled and professionally trained Southern blacks should move north and that those without skills or some money should stay home. Du Bois also pleaded for social equality and attacked whites for their insults to black demonstrators. He became militant enough to advocate killing of "white invaders" of black homes.[3]

The depression years, however, put a halt to the magazine's growth for the time being. It also was affected by Du Bois' resignation, the NAACP officers finally tiring of his constant use of the magazine to criticize the organization. It also suffered from Du Bois' attacks on some members of the black press. He criticized their English, bringing upon himself sneers at his academic background. The black papers were flamboyant in style in those days and too much in contrast to the serious tone of the magazine.

When Du Bois left, Roy Wilkins, who later was to reach national prominence when he became executive director of the NAACP, became editor. By 1934 the circulation had dropped to 8,500. But it came through the stress under Wilkins' editorship, his earlier journalistic experience coming into use at this important time (see Chapter 10). As the organization gained new strength under Walter White as its head, its magazine began to climb once more and by the 1950's was again up to 60,000. In seven more years it went to 121,000, thanks to the civil rights movement. Its editor in 1970 was Henry Lee Moon, who succeeded James W. Ivy. In the meantime it went through two changes of physical appearance: pocket size from 1949 to 1970; and newsmagazine size beginning that later year. Unlike most organization periodicals, the *Crisis* does not go automatically to contributors but only to members of the association who subscribe or others who pay the subscription charge.

In its present larger format it is bright and readable in both typography and writing; editorials and articles on current racial issues and news of NAACP activities are presented attractively and consistently. Perhaps it has more the character of a house organ today than in its first decade, but certainly less of this tone is present than during the 1950's and early 1960's.

Du Bois today might be unhappy with some policies of the magazine. In recent years it has taken a moderate social position, opposing militant radicals who resort to physical violence to achieve their ends. "Dissent, protest and militancy, yes," a 1968 editorial declared. "Intimidation, disruption, suppression of free speech, extremism and violence, no!"[4] The social and political content, so controversial in Du Bois' days on the magazine, still is stimulating if not inflammatory.

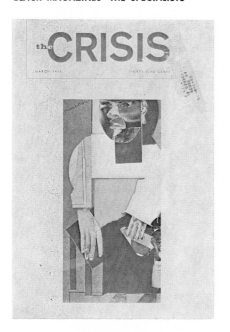

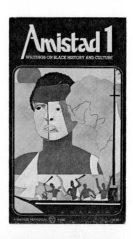

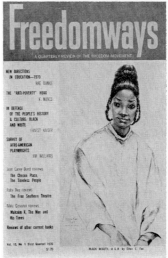

FIG. 8.1. With both literary and public affairs emphasis, these are among the more scholarly but still popular black magazines: **Amistad** is a new magazine-book; **Crisis**, although an official NAACP organ, has had a distinguished record since its founding in 1910; **Freedomways** is one of the struggling quarterlies.

The *Crisis'* experience with advertising sales is typical of that of many another serious black magazine serving a special purpose. It began selling space in 1914, but revenue came slowly. By 1918 the amount earned reached nearly $6,000; it doubled by 1919. But again it fell off and was only a dribble thereafter. In 1969 a firm of representatives was engaged and a few accounts obtained; others were expected during 1970.

Of so much historical value was this magazine that in 1969 two firms began reproducing many of its back issues. The first fifty years were sold in a set for $1,450, the volumes in the sizes of the original magazines. The first thirty years also have been brought out by another firm, selling for $1,950.

● PUBLIC AFFAIRS AND LITERARY MAGAZINES

The revolutionary spirit, violent and nonviolent alike, has turned to the magazine no less than to the newspaper as an outlet. Carolyn Gerald, a Philadelphia poet and free lance writer, reported in 1969 that she could list as many as thirty "revolutionary" journals which appeared (although not all survived) between 1966 and 1969. She divided them into types: a) those with local contributors and readers; b) those produced on college campuses by black student groups; and c) those which have appealed or seek to appeal to the black community as a whole.[5] *Soulbook, Black Dialogue,* and the *Journal of Black Poetry* were cited. The first three she considered magazines of the black literature, written by and for blacks, noncommercial, irregular in publication frequency, carrying only a little advertising, and possessing overlapping editorial boards.

Black Dialogue, Miss Gerald wrote, "provides a good study in the growth and development" of a revolutionary journal. It was begun in 1965 by a group of students at San Francisco State College. In the years since it apparently has come out four or six times a year and offered political writings, illustrations, and literary work of increasing breadth, dealing with national as well as local issues. *Soulbook* is described as more militant than *Black Dialogue.* It subtitles itself the "Quarterly Journal of Revolutionary Afro-America," also was begun in 1965, and likewise on the West Coast, at Berkeley. It, too, publishes poems and short stories as well as political and cultural articles. Miss Gerald cited as its theme "throwing off the shackles" and the call to arms for the revolution.[6]

Also a mid-1960's product, the *Journal of Black Poetry* differs in that it is concerned with one literary form supplemented with illustrations. But the revolutionary aim comes through. Tributes to Malcolm X and to revolutionary heroes abound.

Although almost all such revolutionary journals are unknown to the great majority of black and white citizens and appear to be of interest only to a small minority, Miss Gerald was of the view that "they are an important index of the measure and meaning of the sixties." They exist, she thinks, "as one manifestation of that intense looking inward to see what we really wanted." She may be right, if one remembers the place in literary and journalistic history occupied today by the *Masses* and various other small literary and political magazines of the first half of this century.

Black Theatre, which Miss Gerald mentions only in a note, reflects the black revolution as seen by the dramatist. Subtitled "A Periodical of the Black Theatre Movement," it is eight-by-ten inches and printed on low quality stock. Issued by the New Lafayette Theatre of New York and edited by the theatre's director, Ed Bullins, it first appeared in 1968. Its scope is broader than the stage, however, for it carries poetry and line drawings. Interviews with LeRoi Jones and others, an article by Bullins rejected by the New York *Times* as well as a radio interview with him and another black theater playwright which never was aired, have appeared.

A handsome, new and expensive scholarly magazine came from San Francisco in 1969 not long after Dr. Nathan Hare, director of black studies at San Francisco State College, resigned from his post. Dr. Hare, joined by Robert Chrisman, also formerly of the college faculty, late that year brought out the *Black Scholar,* to be devoted to "Black Studies and Research." They announced that its issues had within their pages "the most weighty and meaningful black thought we could summon." Thirty persons lent their names as contributing and advisory editors, including Lerone Bennett, Ossie Davis, Vincent Harding, Chuck Stone, Carlton Goodlett, Alvin F. Pouissant, and John O. Killens.

The magazine's intention, under Hare as publisher and Chrisman as editor, was to be issued monthly and, according to *Newsweek,* sought "to unite the black intellectual and the street radical." Its first few issues contained considerable rhetoric as well as evidences of scholarship, revolutionary aims, and doctrinaire opinions. Early issues contained such articles as Earl Conrad on Harriet Tubman, Shirley Chisholm on "Racism and Anti-Feminism" and Robert Staples on "The Myth of the Black Matriarchy," a few poems, and drawings.

Four years earlier, at Harvard, the Association of African and African-American Students launched a quarterly, *Harvard Journal of Afro-American Affairs,* which up to 1969 turned out to be an annual. Its personality was still to be established at this writing.

The *Black Politician* is novel in its field. A quarterly founded in 1969, it takes as its purpose to fill "a need in the classroom and among the public for a single authoritative reference source on the political tendings in the black community. . . ." Published by the Center on Urban and Minority Affairs in Berkeley, it is edited by Mervyn M. Dymally, a state senator from Los Angeles. Early issues announced that the *Black Politician* would be bi-partisan and cover "the full spectrum of political thought now current in the black community." No revolutionary fervor is detectable in the first few issues. One article is about American Indians, describing their conditions candidly; another is on President Nixon and the American blacks, written by a White House research assistant.

Few black magazines have attempted to duplicate the formula and general format of the journals of opinion of general appeal, such as the white ones called the *Nation,* the *New Republic, Commonweal,* or *National Review.* One that has done so and managed to survive since 1961 is *Liberator,* a monthly founded by Daniel H. Watts, an architect. Like one of its white counterparts, the *Nation,* which for a decade was banned in New York City schools because of supposedly anti-Catholic articles, *Liberator* also has been embroiled in controversy, although of a different order. On one occasion both Ossie Davis and James Baldwin resigned from its editorial board, charging anti-Semitism. Made up along opinion magazine lines, with editorials, articles, poetry, and reviews, it has the same modest following as what are called the butcher-paper weeklies. Much of its readership is from the revolution-minded. Typically, also, it has little advertising. It uses photographs, which such publications usually do not, and these plus the occasional art work give it a livelier appearance than its sober articles promise.

Watts has been quoted as saying that he became so aggravated with both the white and black press in their handling of black news that he began *Liberator* as a "voice of the Afro-American."[7] "The white press," he went on to say, "constantly covers only one side of the Negro community—that of degradation. Financially well-off Negroes are rarely given exposure by white media." Watts' comments about the black press as well, and his views echo those of other critics (see Chapter 16). The black newspapers might serve the race better if they went out of business, he once said, because they do not give the true picture of events within the black community.

The presence of literary material, not usually found in the white magazines of similar formula, like the *Progressive,* also a monthly, has provided one more outlet for the black creative writer who until lately has had few places in which to publish short stories and poems about what goes in within the black society. *Liberator* includes fiction but does not present itself as a magazine of literature, only as one charged with offering opinions. Black journalism has few entirely literary publications, a genre that has gone out of fashion on the larger publishing scene. Usually, as in *Liberator,* poems, novellas, plays, and poems are printed alongside current affairs articles, but the proportion of purely creative work is greater in such periodicals as *Amistad* and *Freedomways,* two of the better known.

Uptown Beat, a quarterly issued by the East Harlem Writing Center in New York, qualifies as a literary publication that comes from the grass roots, as does *Echo,* a Milwaukee community publication discussed later in this chapter, for both print drawings and creative writing by members of writing and art workshops. Begun in 1968, *Uptown Beat* gives space to new writers and artists and provides opportunities for designers. Since it lacks outside support, it cannot pay contributors; the editorial and production duties are performed by volunteers or done at cost. A somewhat unusual aspect, it is reported, is that much of the content first is exhibited on bulletin boards of community centers and theaters. Like *Echo,* it is affiliated with a workshop; this particular group was begun in 1967 by Gayle Greene, a writer and teacher. Much of the magazine's content is drawn from the workshop, but some copy is contributed by writers in Europe and Africa.[8]

Bearing the subtitle, "Quarterly Review of the Negro Freedom Movement," *Freedomways* grew out of the efforts for freedom from injustice and discrimination that reached a peak during World War II and soon thereafter. It was continued by such activities as the bus boycotts of the mid-1950's in Montgomery, Tallahassee, and other cities, the student sit-ins, the work of CORE, NAACP, the National Urban League, the Southern Christian Leadership Council, and many other groups. First published in early 1961, it has remained a quarterly of distinguished but not stodgy format. Like the typical scholarly and literary magazine published anywhere in the world that has not been underwritten by a government, a foundation, or a millionaire, *Freedomways* always has been in need of dollars. It continues to appear only because of the devotion of a small group of persons who believe it deserves to live.

Shirley Graham, widow of W. E. B. Du Bois and herself a writer, was its first editor. Working with her was Mrs. Esther Jackson, managing editor from the beginning; Miss Graham is now on the advisory board. During the years after 1961, as Ernest Kaiser, another staff member, has summarized them up to 1966, the magazine introduced many black writers of poetry, short stories, and articles. It was deeply concerned, as it continues to be, with racial events, issues, and problems in and outside the U.S.A. Certain black leaders have been featured, such as Louis E. Burnham, onetime editor of *Freedom* and an associate editor of the white weekly, *Guardian,* as well as a public speaker and organizer. Du Bois, whom Kaiser has called the godfather of the magazine, also has been written about considerably in *Freedomways;* the magazine has become something of a repository for new material about him. Particular attention has been given to Africa and also, and more originally in this journalism, to the black people of Latin America and the Caribbean. Much of the fourth issue of 1969 was devoted to the American Indian, as another American minority group.

Kaiser, a contributing editor, evaluates the magazine thus: "over its first five years, the evidence is overwhelming that *Freedomways* has done a tremendous, almost unbelievable job as a critical review, a stimulus and direction-giver of the freedom movement and as a publishing outlet for young and developing and reputable unknown Negro writers." He also found shortcomings. Not enough such writers were published; "the language of the magazine is too sanitary, not earthy enough as a fighting people's organ," and there is not much humor.[9]

Still abiding by its formula expressed in the first issue, it now has a circulation of about 7,000 and carries a few pages of advertising, depending for its income mainly upon various types of sources. Mrs. Jackson, the managing editor, lists them as benefit concerts, theater parties, house parties, individual contributions, sales of greeting cards, art, books, and other materials. "Occasionally," Mrs. Jackson reports, "we receive a legacy or an editor receives a foundation grant for a special issue."[10] But the magazine suffered a serious loss in 1970 of

the sort that can knock one of these literary-cultural affairs magazines out of existence. *Freedomways* suffered $25,000 in damages when
a fire burned a building part of which it used in its greeting card
business and for its mailing service. The magazine could not afford
to pay the premiums to cover it with insurance.

Since Miss Graham resigned as editor and moved out of the
country *Freedomways* has not had an editor. Editorial responsibility
rests with Mrs. Jackson, John Henrik Clarke, the history professor
and author, Ernest Kaiser, and J. H. O'Dell, all working in any ways
they can to keep the magazine going.

The black press published its first bookazine or magabook (a
regularly issued periodical bound like a paperback book) in 1970
when *Amistad* was launched as a literary-cultural affairs publication.
Although it prints material that could just as readily have appeared in
Freedomways or *Black World*, it is depending upon its format to get
it into black studies classes; it is issued infrequently enough (thus far
as a semi-annual) to serve as a textbook. Its professional backing also is
somewhat unusual. Random House, a major book firm, published
it through its paperback subsidiary, Vintage Books, and also undertook to distribute it. One of *Amistad*'s coeditors is Charles F. Harris,
a Random House senior editor; the other is John A. Williams, the
novelist.

Robert Bernstein, Random House president, explained at the
magazine's launching that it hopes to become a quarterly and that it
"will be a great step forward in helping black people to know and
understand more about themselves and in helping white people
know and understand more about blacks."[11] The editors agreed
and added a practical angle. In the first issue they said: "The word
Amistad means friendship in Spanish. The Amistad Mutiny of 1839
stands for revolt, self-determination, justice and freedom. With these
meanings always firmly in mind, we have designed this publication
primarily for use in college courses in literature, history, sociology,
psychology, education, political science and government, and the
arts."[12]

Exceeding three hundred pages, its first issue carried articles by
Vincent Harding, professor of history and sociology at Atlanta University; C. L. R. James, visiting professor of political science at
Northwestern and other universities; and Calvin C. Hernton, an
essayist. These and other contributions dealt with James Baldwin,
black history and the slave trade, and Southern white writers. The
fiction consisted of three short stories, two by George Davis and
Oliver Jackman, recording first person experience, and one by
Ishmail Reed, whose unusual approach may be judged by the title
of his, "D Hexorcism of Noxon D Awful."

A clue to the new magazine's racial attitude came in a statement
by Williams, when asked if it would be open to white writers. "We'll
handle white, black and pink writers if they deal with the problems

of the black or third world," he answered. "We feel they're all linked."[13]

● THE SCHOLARLY JOURNALS

To some extent magazines in the political and cultural affairs group also are scholarly, some more than others. Certainly *Freedomways*, with its strong emphasis on history, thanks to John Henrik Clarke, its chief associate editor, offers results of important scholarly work. And *Black World*, which for so many years under its old name of *Negro Digest* was much broader in its appeal than now, is printing scholarly work along with the hortatory and argumentative.[14] In recent years a number of new scholarly journals have appeared, some lasting only a few quarters.

The *African Scholar*, a quarterly that considered itself a "Journal of Research and Analysis," and was published in Washington, appeared in the late 1960's. A quarter of a century earlier came the *Negro Quarterly*, from the Negro Publishing Society of America, Inc., in New York. First issued in spring, 1942, it carried articles concerning "The Negro Author and His Publisher," by Sterling A. Brown; "Negro Education and the War," by Doxey A. Wilkerson, the black newsman and editor once connected with the New York newspaper, *People's Voice;* and "Slavocracy's System of Control," by Herbert Aptheker, who in the 1970's is taking a place as an authority on black history from a Marxist viewpoint. The magazine did not continue.

But by no means did all of the scholarly journals go the same path. On the contrary, certain of these serious magazines of research and theory have a greater longevity than any group in black journalism with the exception of the religious and fraternal and for the same reasons: they are subsidized by organizations and often go automatically to those who hold membership. The better known are the *Journal of Negro History,* the *Journal of Negro Education,* the *Journal of Human Relations,* the *Negro History Bulletin,* the *Journal of Religious Thought, Phylon,* the *Quarterly Review of Higher Education Among Negroes,* and the *Negro Educational Review.*

Patrons of a large public or college library who wander among the shelves that hold current periodicals soon are struck by the sameness of the scholarly journals of the various disciplines, particularly in the social sciences. The black journals of this type, except for the word *Negro* in some titles, are not immediately recognizable as different from the majority because the familiar scholarly journal format is followed. Since they usually are subsidized and need not compete on the newsstands with such glamour books as *Soul! Illustrated* and *Essence,* their covers often carry their tables of contents or little more than the logotype plus a few titles and the symbols of the associations sponsoring them. Inside are from one hundred to three hundred pages set in solid type, with article titles breaking the bleak pages or a poem filling an empty space at the end of an article. News notes and book reviews give the last few pages a little more variety. The devoted reader—a college professor, a researcher, an independent scholar—is not disturbed by the blandness. He wants the ideas and facts, not entertainment. He would resent pictures, jokes, and other ingredients of the typical newsstand magazine as robbing him of material he really needs for his own thinking, research, and writing. Furthermore, such a journal provides an outlet for publications by black college faculty members; they are just as much subject to the "publish or perish" tradition as any white teacher, perhaps even more, for the black college has had to fight for recognition. As with the white journals, not all the contributions are equally important and some are insignificant. In view of the lack of study of black history and culture in the U.S.A., however, these scholarly journals sometimes are the only sources that can be consulted.

Howard University in Washington, D.C., has been an important source of such journals. The *Journal of Negro Education* is one of several Howard sponsors. It was begun in 1931 as "A Quarterly Review of Problems Incident to the Education of Negroes," by Charles H. Thompson, later dean of the graduate school. A typical journal of the American or British type in appearance, it carries articles by leading educators, black or white, and does not print advertising. Its circulation is 2,000.

An outwardly similar quarterly, the *Negro Educational Review,* "seeks to present articles and research reports," and carries book reviews as well. Advertisements of books by its editor-in-chief and managing editor were the only two in the issues examined, which emanate from Nashville, Tennessee. It carries analyses of educational problems.

Since 1952, the Central State University at Wilberforce, Ohio, has published the *Journal of Human Relations,* a quarterly offering scholarly articles on sociological and philosophical themes with an interdisciplinary approach: "The Homosexual," "Truth in Packaging," and "Cybernation and Human Values" are titles that show the range.

When W. E. B. Du Bois returned to Atlanta University to teach, after having made his imprint on American magazine journalism with the *Crisis* and other periodicals, he founded *Phylon.* When he left the university to go to New York, the combination scholarly and literary quarterly was edited by Dr. Ira D. A. Reid from 1944 to 1948 and by Dr. Mozell C. Hill, both heads of the sociology department at Atlanta. Often the motive power for these journals are such chairmen. Its current editor is Tilman C. Cothran, and *Phylon* still comes from the university. Subtitled "A Review of Race and Culture," it takes a more thoroughly scholarly approach than the purely literary and cultural affairs periodicals. A typical issue will carry several articles on black topics, such as "Negroes in the Armed Forces," book reviews, a short story, and a small amount of advertising. As do such intellectual publications as a rule, it has a small circulation, hovering around 2,000. It has not been accepted fully as an orthodox scholarly journal partly, no doubt, because of its mixed formula. A journal that concentrates on one subject, such as religion, education, or history, can make a solid place for itself as an authoritative medium. But one that publishes fiction, long suspect among scholars outside the foreign language and English departments, and also is hospitable to scholarly writings in any discipline is a nonconformist. Yet *Phylon* has endeared itself to many a black scholar and writer for giving him an outlet for his work.

Representative of the strictly orthodox journals is the *Journal of Negro History,* to which new attention was directed in the 1960's because of the intensified interest in the history of the race. And with it came heightened attention for the life of the man responsible for this major serious journal, Carter Goodwin Woodson. Long considered the foremost authority on the black society in America, Dr. Woodson founded the *Journal* in 1916. Published continuously since as a quarterly, it comes from the Association for the Study of Negro Life and History in Washington, and now has a circulation of 4,600. Intended for the advanced scholar, it has sought to carry out the Woodson view that the American black people have not been accorded their correct place in U.S. history. Traditional in format, it carries articles on such subjects as "The Canadian Negro," on various historical figures, including many not dealt with elsewhere, news of currently prominent black persons of historical importance, book reviews, and a small amount of advertising, about 5 per cent of the content. William M. Brewer was editor until his death in 1970.

Carter Woodson was a Virginian, born in 1875. He worked in the mines of West Virginia while attending high school, then went to Berea College. On completing the bachelor's degree work he taught and was principal of a black high school in Huntington, West Virginia. Later he became dean of the college of liberal arts at Howard University and at West Virginia State College. Woodson originated Negro History Week, wrote various books and monographs on black history, and founded the *Journal.* The annual history week is intended to popularize black history and correct earlier concepts. The black press in general assists by printing special columns and features, photographs of familiar black heroes, and editorials recalling the race's heritage.

A less elaborate publication than the *Journal* is the *Negro History Bulletin,* coming also from the association in Washington. It seeks to appeal to school pupils. Established in 1937, it is issued for eight months of the year in a more popular format than the *Journal,* carries illustrated historical and biographical articles, book reviews, news of association branches, and a little advertising. In 1969 its circulation was 8,070. In recent years its editor has been Charles H.

Wesley, successor to Woodson as association head, author of numerous historical works, and retired president of Central State.

Called an "interdisciplinary quarterly of the black world," *Black Academy Review* first was published in Buffalo, New York, in mid-1970, a neat, sixty-eight-page collection of six literary and historical articles and a book review. It is one of the enterprises of the Black Academy Press, Inc., primarily a publisher of books on black affairs and of black literature. Dr. S. Okechukwu Mezu, a Nigerian who teaches at the State University of Buffalo, both heads the firm and edits the magazine, a well-printed periodical of serious intent. Dr. Mezu, a poet and novelist educated at Georgetown and Johns Hopkins, directs the university's African Studies Department.

● THE TRADE JOURNALS

The black population of the U.S.A. has had little need for most of the magazines and newspapers usually lumped under the term trade, technical, or business publications. Having been mainly farm or industrial workers until recent years, and kept to menial jobs, they had little use for the technical content or the materials intended for business executives that one usually finds in these publications, which now are for the most part magazines and number about 2,700. But there have been exceptions. Where blacks have been able to go into businesses of their own, publishers have moved in with a service publication. And as black enterprise grows more will follow, although those activities that well-established white-owned publications cannot satisfy are the only ones likely to need their own publications. Over the years such papers and magazines have been launched. Few have survived; these have been mainly for two occupations: beauty shop operating and tavern and bar owning. The black newspaper press for a time had its own trade publication, but *PEP* went out when hard times came in the 1950's. The 1960's, however, gave impetus to several new publications.

Available in the 1970's is a handful that includes *Beauty Trade, Black Beauty, Pilot, New Negro Traveler and Conventioneer,* and *Black Business Digest.* Reported to be published are *Equal Opportunity, New Negro Business and Financial Journal, Journal of the National Technical Association, Project,* and *Contact.* The first two are intended for beauty salon operators. Their content is similar to that of white periodicals in the field—heavily illustrated articles on new hair styles, reports of beauticians' conventions, and features on individuals or establishments. Not as lush with advertising as their white counterparts, these magazines nevertheless sell more space than do many other black publications, except the national newspapers and a few consumer periodicals.

When he was a steward on a New York Central parlor car in

1944, Clarence M. Markham, Jr., began a magazine he called *Negro Traveler*. Once he had been a railroad news agency manager and thought a monthly concerned with the blacks working in transportation might help improve their status and morale. The publication was developed into a 75,000 controlled circulation monthly going to black travel agencies, offices planning conventions and conferences, and restaurants and taverns. It contains a high percentage of advertising from such firms as the Chrysler Corporation and Encyclopaedia Britannica, as well as from many motels, restaurants, and shops in black population centers. The editorial content provides coverage of large conventions, guides to hotels and restaurants, and listings of nationwide events. Of the business publications for blacks available, a magazine of this type should have a future others might not obtain, with some black Americans now in a better financial position to go on cruises, transatlantic plane trips, or journeys by car within the the U.S.A. The market for such a public has been neglected by white publications and only touched on by a few general circulation black publications, such as *Tuesday*. Byron E. Lewis, Jr., president of Uniworld Group, Inc., a black marketing, advertising, and public relations concern, told a travel conference in 1969 that $540,000,000 to $600,000,000 of the income of black Americans is spent on travel. Approximately half of this is spent by about 800,000 persons who attend at least one convention each year. Lewis estimated that if each spent $300, the expenditure on conventions for travel alone would reach $240,000,000.[15]

A quasi-trade or business publication and house organ is the *Pilot*, issued from Chicago six times a year by the National Insurance Association, a trade group of black insurance firms. It is sold, not going to members automatically, carries a small amount of paid advertising, and runs to sixteen pages an issue. News of people—deaths, new appointments, leading sellers among agents—dominates, but room is made for coverage of meetings, reprints of speeches, and reviews of pertinent books.

Equal Opportunity is a monthly for minority college students, published in New York by an interracial staff headed by Alfred Duckett, a black journalist and publicist, and John R. Miller III, white and a former Procter & Gamble sales manager. Launched in 1970, for use by colleges, by public and other libraries, and by minority community groups, its main aim, according to the publishing firm, is to bridge "the vital communication gap" between black students and corporations.

Another monthly reported to be helping black and other minority group members obtain employment information is *Contact*. Content includes facts about job opportunities among the magazine's advertisers. A controlled circulation of 50,000 is listed.

Late in 1969 plans were announced for *Black Enterprise*, "designed to advise and encourage the development of black entre-

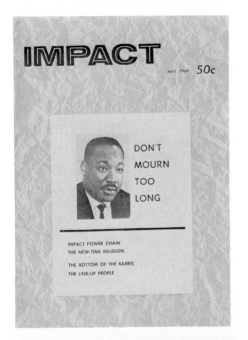

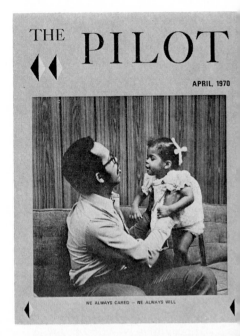

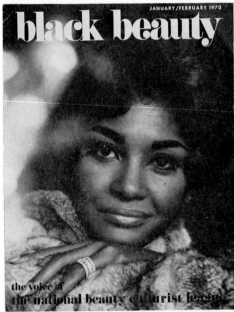

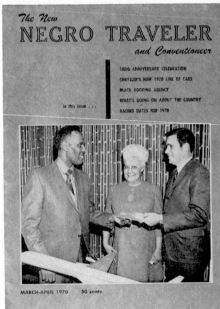

FIG. 8.2. Four specialized magazines from a variety of fields: **Impact** is for nondenominational, interdenominational, and separatist black churchmen; **Pilot** is for members of an insurance association; **Black Beauty** is a trade journal for hairdressers; **Negro Traveler** is one of the most widely circulated and oldest of specialized magazines.

preneurs," as publicity releases described it. The board of the magazine included Senator Edward W. Brooke; Georgia's black state representative, Julian Bond; and U.S. Congresswoman Shirley Chisholm. It first appeared in August, 1970, on a 100,000 controlled circulation basis, 45,000 going to black businessmen and the remainder to others who might be interested.

The other side of the coin of the business press is the labor press. It has taken black workers many years to be accepted by white labor unions; some still are not. They have few unions of their own. An outstanding organization has been that of the Sleeping Car Porters, of which the moving spirit for many years has been A. Philip Randolph, whose earlier career in journalism included coeditorship of an outspoken pro-labor magazine early in the century, the *Messenger*. He served for years as editor of the *Journal* of the porters' union, which had been preceded by the *Pullman Porters' Review*, which published fiction and other general material as well as news of members. A weekly *Negro Labor News* is on record as having been published since 1931 in Houston, Texas.

● INDUSTRIAL PUBLICATIONS

Often associated with the trade, business, and technical publications are the house organs, or, as their editors prefer they be called, the industrial or corporate publications. Printed for free distribution within a company for its staff and employes or outside the firm for its customers, dealers, and friends, these magazines, which the majority are, in the U.S.A. alone number about 10,000. This specialized journalism manifests itself in the black business world as well, particularly in that large area, insurance. Bearing such names as *Whetstone* and *Ulico*, these are internals for individual companies. Usually they are eight-by-ten inches in size, sixteen or twenty-four pages, use only spot color, and devote themselves to news of the business—coverage of meetings, personnel news, executive messages, speeches, and features on people. They carry only institutional advertising.

The *Ulico*, published quarterly by the Universal Life Insurance Company of Memphis, Tennessee, was begun in 1951. It is printed now on high quality paper. Its editor makes generous use of photographs, but runs no editorials. However, it does print copy on general black issues, which others tend to avoid.

George W. Lee, editor of the Atlanta Life Insurance Company's magazine, *Vision*, on the other hand, is free to editorialize on black affairs, perhaps because he is a vice president as well. Also a quarterly, *Vision*, begun in 1968, bears down heavily on material about people. It uses more color printing than is usually seen in these magazines.

Whetstone, a quarterly published since 1923 by the North Caro-

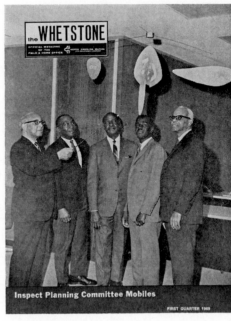

FIG. 8.3. Insurance companies are among the few black businesses that issue house publications (industrial magazines). **Whetstone** is from North Carolina Mutual; **Vision** is from Atlanta Life; the **Ulico** comes from Memphis, headquarters of Universal Life. Magazines of this type are usually quarterlies.

lina Mutual Life Insurance Company in Durham, combines news of the field staff and home office employes with articles on current black problems by prominent leaders, such as Floyd McKissick, Benjamin E. Mays, and Roy Wilkins, whose writings are available from syndicates.

Editors of these numerous but often little-appreciated newspapers and magazines, whether for black or white readers, generally have comparatively little professional journalism background or training; their experience more often is in advertising, public relations, or printing, if they have any communications background of any sort. The situation is changing as more journalism school graduates enter this specialized area and as more working journalists from the general field turn to house publications, trade magazines, and professional journals. One of the black editors with more than usual professional background is Murray J. Marvin, editor of *Whetstone,* for he was a reporter and art editor for several black weeklies and formerly edited the *Pilot,* the business magazine issued by the National Insurance Association. He also edits for the North Carolina company the *Hot Line,* a semi-monthly home office duplicated newsletter.

A few black firms have newsletters or small newspapers to serve as their house publications. Excelsior Empire Savings Bank in New York City began a small tabloid newspaper, the *News,* for its customers in 1967. Much like a small version of a commercial newspaper,

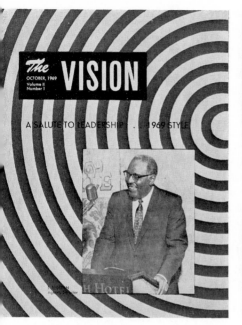

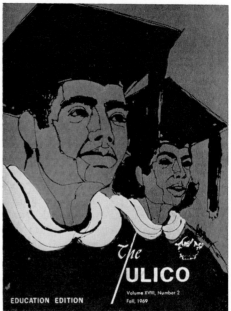

it publishes general and local features, an inquiring reporter-photographer column, and seasonal photographs, with far less exploitation of the bank than usually found in house publications.

Like many other similar small magazines and papers, those in this category suffer from lack of trained staff. Page after page carries pictures of stiffly posed figures; other pages are solid with speech copy. Yet they play a part in shaping public opinion about the institution that issues them, because the general press, even the black, has no room for such detailed copy.

Related to these papers and magazines is printed matter not ordinarily thought of as a form of journalism but rather of printing. These are the special publications, some regularly issued by companies for one or more of their publics. Included are annual reports, promotional leaflets, and special-purpose brochures. Often the editors and writers for the house magazine are called upon to produce such printed materials. The Golden State Mutual Life Insurance Company of Los Angeles, for instance, publishes the usual leaflet setting forth its annual report. But it engages in other printing as well. In connection with its fortieth anniversary—it was founded in 1925—its editorial people produced a twenty-page booklet containing reproductions of the permanent collection of paintings and sculpture by black artists exhibited in its lobby since 1949. For the same occasion, the company published a sixteen-page illustrated booklet describing the historical background portrayed in two murals in its office building.

These materials are public relations tools with some of the aims of the regularly issued external house publications.

● MAGAZINES ABOUT RELIGION

The black religious press comes almost entirely from the black organized churches. A few newsletters and a magazine, *Impact,* are issued by black churchmen from within the white denominational world or by black religious from black and white churches who have their own organization. White denominations, Catholic and Protestant, sponsor periodicals for blacks and even have black staffers producing them. But they are white in ownership and origin. Among the older of these latter are several mission magazines; *Josephite Harvest* of Baltimore and *Our Colored Missions* of New York City are two. Black Catholics are so few in the U.S.A. they perhaps could not support their own journal. The *Josephite Harvest* provides for a segment of Roman Catholicism, that affiliated with the Josephite Fathers, an order known as the Society of Saint Joseph of Sacred Heart. The magazine, at one time called the *Colored Harvest,* has a mission objective. "The Josephites are an American Society of priests and brothers who labor to bring the Gospel to all men and to work for the full incorporation of the Negro into the Church and into the society of man," reads a statement on its contents page. A bi-monthly, it is almost a picture magazine because of its heavy use of photographs supplemented by drawings. Articles describe interracial religious activities and the problems of black men and women who are the objective of the missionary activities. *Message,* a Seventh-Day Adventist magazine issued seven times a year, has somewhat similar objectives and content, but more variety in its fare, with room for poetry, editorials, and regular departments on topics this denomination is particularly interested in, such as health and food. Published by the church's house, Southern Publishing Association in Nashville, *Message* has 70,000 circulation and uses high quality printing, including color, possibly because the denomination is one of the most advanced of religious bodies in employing the printing press to further its cause. It is entirely nonfiction, for the policy of all Seventh-Day Adventist publications is not to print fiction.

What might be considered the genuinely black religious publications are those from the black denominations such as the National Baptist Convention, U.S.A., the National Baptist Convention of America, the African Methodist Episcopal Church Zion, and the African Methodist Episcopal Church. Like the press, the church has been a major influence among American black citizens. Its magazines and newspapers have given them a sense of security and hope. They have helped unite the people, and like other black media, have given them a sense of identity as well. When the churches turned to the printing presses in the nineteenth century the combination was powerful; because they could obtain subsidy for their journals the publications were among the longest lived.

One of the oldest extant black publications of any format is the *Star of Zion*, official paper of the A.M.E. Church Zion. Founded in 1867, it still is issued from Charlotte, North Carolina, with a circulation of about 4,500. This tabloid carries news of individual congregations, changes in personnel, general church notices, and reports on conventions and other meetings. It is published every Thursday.

Somewhat like it in appearance is the *A.M.E. Christian Recorder*, official organ of the A.M.E. denomination. Dr. B. J. Nolen, its editor, considers it "America's Oldest Negro Weekly Newspaper,"[16] although a 1970 copy carries in its first page folio line notice that it is volume 12, number 50. A *Christian Recorder* is listed by Mott, the leading historian of American journalism, as having existed from 1852 to 1931 in this denomination.[17] The present version is a weekly; in content it is like the *Star of Zion*; its circulation runs from 5,000 to 10,000. The African Methodist Episcopal Church also claims the oldest magazine issued by and for black people in America.[18] This is the *A.M.E. Church Review*, published in Tulsa, Oklahoma. A publication of that name from the denomination was founded in Philadelphia in 1884, with B. T. Tanner, at one time editor of the *Christian Recorder*, as its editor. Mott records that it ended in 1936,[19] yet a paper of that name is being published still. Also issued by this church are the *Journal of Religious Education, Women's Missionary Magazine*, and *Missionary Magazine*, the first from Nashville, the next from Lexington, Kentucky, and the last from Philadelphia.

Several religious journals have borne the title the *Christian Index*. The one which carried the name into black journalism was founded in 1867 and therefore is as old as the *Star of Zion*. It was begun by a black conference of the white Methodist Episcopal Church South and in 1870 became the official organ of what then was called the Colored Methodist Episcopal Church and today known as the Christian Methodist Episcopal Church, a black denomination. The nine-by-twelve-inch bi-weekly, edited by the Rev. John M. Exum in Memphis, has a circulation of 7,000 and contains news and articles similar to those in the other black church journals.

"The Negro Church is Dead," "Black Jews in America," and "The Pulpit and the Pill" are subjects to be found in issues of *Impact*, the monthly periodical issued by the black religious supporting the concept of a black church outside the framework of the existing black and white churches. Coming with the imprint of a Brooklyn publishing firm, *Impact* consists of sixteen pages of articles, poetry, departments for children and young people, and one or two pages of advertising. The expression of sharp militancy that might be expected is not present, but the editors insist that the black church and churchmen are important and potentially influential. It was begun in 1968.

Muhammad Speaks, the Black Muslim weekly newspaper, qualifies as a religious as well as a general black publication (see Chapter
5). The *New Day,* issued from Philadelphia since 1931, also a weekly
tabloid newspaper in format, contains largely magazine content. It
is the publication of the religious group founded by Father Devine,
the black leader who several decades ago gained a large following
among American blacks. It contains material chiefly about the activities of this group.

● **THE FRATERNAL PUBLICATIONS**

One of the more important national newspapers, the *Journal and
Guide* of Norfolk, Virginia, was created out of a fraternal organ (see
Chapter 4). Such fraternal groups—the Masons and Odd Fellows are
examples of one segment, college fraternities are another—have published journals for many years, a few going back to the nineteenth
century. At one time there was a *Fraternal Advocate* in Chicago that
served various orders as well as insurance and labor groups with news
of each other's doings.[20]

The *Pyramid,* begun in 1942, is the quarterly magazine serving
members of a freemason's group officially known as the Ancient
Egyptian Arabic Order Nobles Mystic Shrine of North and South
America and Its Jurisdictions. Newsmagazine size, it reports on the
order's activities and promotes its interests, such as the annual convention and trips abroad. Its 1969 circulation was 20,000.

Today each of the larger black college fraternal groups, four
fraternities and four sororities, has a publication of some kind, generally issued quarterly. They go to alumni and present members of
active chapters chiefly in the black colleges or to campuses where
segregation has created black fraternities and sororities.

● **COMMUNITY MAGAZINES**

Nearly all black community publications are in newspaper form.
Here and there one encounters a publisher who prefers the magazine
format, either to have something different to offer in a city where
black newspapers exist, or in a place where such newspapers have
usually failed. But it is an expensive formula and format, as the
experiences of some publishers in recent years indicate.

The Milwaukee periodical, *Echo,* and the one in Syracuse, New
York, *Around the Town,* were having financial troubles, at this writing, for lack of support from enough advertisers or angels. *Echo* has
depended for financing indirectly on the Milwaukee Inner City Arts
Council, which received its funds from the state for nearly three
years until October, 1969. The council maintained the Echo Writers'
Workshop, and three other arts groups; the magazine was related to

the workshop. The projects went on without funding. Late in 1969 came a temporary reprieve for *Echo* when the Milwaukee *Journal,* a major white daily, gave $1,000 to help the magazine and the workshop continue until "adequate state funding can be secured." The publication was edited by Mrs. Virginia Williams, who, about the time of the loss of funding, was appointed editor of publications by the Milwaukee school board, although she continued to edit the magazine. The magazine had some returns from advertising sales but not enough to meet all the costs of a monthly printed on high quality paper whose staff believed that the art work, short stories, and other content should be paid for; it was produced in the workshops conducted as part of the general project. Although *Echo* has taken no official editorial positions, its contributors often spoke out clearly for the freedoms they believed the black people deserved. The magazine, eight-by-ten inches in size and running often to forty-eight pages, sold for five dollars a year and appeared, comparatively, to have considerable advertising support, but its rate was low and the quantity was not enough.

Around the Town, published for Syracuse, was issued for about six months in 1969 and 1970, and had more of a local touch than *Echo* but was much like it physically. It was suspended, the publisher planning to revive it as an all-state magazine, a novel formula seeking to capitalize on the fact that New York has four cities with large black populations: New York, Buffalo, Rochester, and Syracuse. As a community periodical it contained more news and straight journalistic material than *Echo,* but was illustrated also with photographs. Some material was obtained with the aid of university journalism students and of townspeople. Cornelious Loftin, its publisher, said when he began the magazine that he hoped it would reflect the life of the black community. It was to give the black people of the area some identity, so that through it they would be motivated. But it was difficult to reach the audience, now formed into small groups as a result of urban renewal or dispersed to distant parts of the city and a few suburbs.

Community or city magazine stories out of Philadelphia, Dayton, Omaha, and St. Louis are more encouraging. Philadelphia, in fact, recently had two: *Pride* and *Philly Talk.* Their formula, as is that of St. Louis' *Proud,* is an echo of those used by some of the successful white city magazines of the 1960's: *San Diego, Philadelphia,* and *San Francisco.* A few decades ago the city magazine was a mouthpiece for the Chamber of Commerce and little more. The new-style version is independent, portrays conditions in the cities as they are without the tone of boosterism, and is well written, edited, illustrated, and printed.

Philadelphia's *Pride* was the best known of the black group. Far better produced than the Milwaukee and Syracuse periodicals, by 1970 it gave as its circulation 20,000 every other month. It was begun in 1966 and reported to have ceased in 1970.

Philly Talk, the other black magazine in Philadelphia, is some-

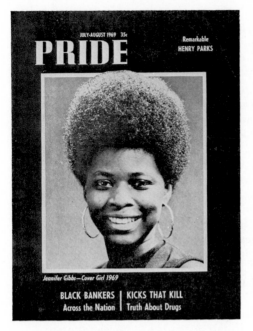

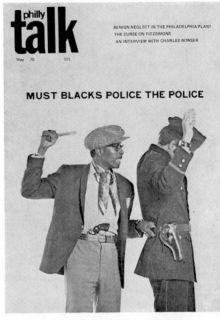

MUST BLACKS POLICE THE POLICE

FIG. 8.4. City or community maga-
zines, generally rising in popularity in
American journalism, are beginning to
appear for black residents. **Pride** and
Philly Talk were both published in
Philadelphia; **Echo** is for Milwaukee;
Around the Town was for Syracuse;
and **Proud** for St. Louis.

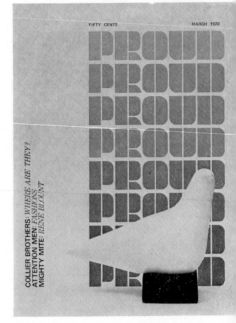

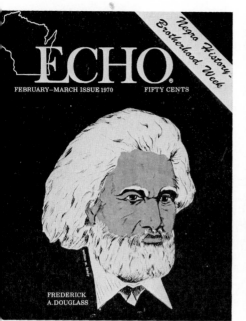

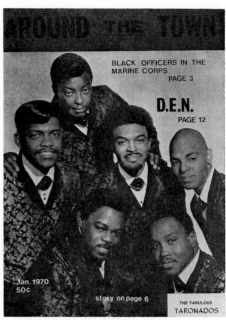

what more sophisticated than was *Pride* in content. Color is used on the covers and in a few spots inside. Satirical articles, feature pieces on social problems and on people, and departments on music and films give the magazine wide appeal. A monthly, newsmagazine size, it is well edited and printed. Begun in 1969, it reported a circulation of 32,000 in 1970, about half by subscription.

One of the oldest community magazines is *Everybody,* of Omaha begun in 1958. Issued every other month, it covers other cities. Today its newsmagazine-size pages shelter 50 per cent advertising. Editorial content is broad.

Dayton's *Rap* was begun in 1970 as a monthly; Rochester (N.Y.) has an even newer monthly, *About . . . Time,* seeking to give the city a publication totally devoted to black interests.

Magazines of this type can supplement the white newspapers as well as the black. As one staff member put it: "We feel there is much in the black community which has not been covered by the regular press in the past and are seeking to fill the void with a somewhat sophisticated and quality magazine. . . . in the past, the black press has tended to be somewhat slanted, amateurish, unsophisticated and militant. We feel this has had appeal for only one segment of the black population. . . . This seems to be a growing market, especially in light of the fact that more and more blacks are finally getting recognition in the professional areas and are moving up, proportionately, in the economic levels."[21]

This formula is being followed, as shown by the facing of local issues (an article describing the goings-on at the local Black Panther Party headquarters is an example), sophisticated writing, suitable illustrations, and the response of advertisers who include some major local firms.

It also is being followed in St. Louis, where *Proud* began in 1969. Like the others, it is a consumer magazine for a regional group of readers. Soon after its first issue came out in January, 1970, it began a promotion plan helpful to black newspapers and magazines alike: an in-service training program for young people; this group put out one issue, the Black Cultural Edition, in mid-1970. Running to forty pages a month, *Proud* carries articles on black history, local subjects such as the church and poverty ("Lead Poisoning in St. Louis"), musical groups, personalities, civic problems, food, sports, and fashion. Career opportunities for blacks are emphasized, a theme that appears in other community and regional magazines. *Proud* during 1970 had a circulation of about 15,000, of which 4,000 went to subscribers.

Urban West, a regional black magazine from San Francisco, has set a pace for attracting advertisers and within three years of its founding was planning to appeal to a national rather than only a West Coast audience. A bi-monthly, slick-paper periodical, it began in October, 1967, with considerable stress on fashion and making-it financially, with a Pacific coast emphasis. Gradually its base has broadened, however. Articles on urban renewal, the police mentality, music, and events in Africa began to appear. Its success with leading advertisers, if continued, will assure its entry into the consumer magazine class. Larger than most of the other city and regional magazines (nine-by-twelve inches), it uses color. By early 1970 it had a circulation of 21,000.

● OTHER SPECIALIZED PERIODICALS

Not all specialized black periodicals fit neatly into categories. Where, for example, shall the unusual *Negro Braille Magazine* be placed?

Unreadable by the sighted person of any race unless he knows how to decipher its surface of tiny raised dots impressed on heavy tan sheets, it draws from *Jet, Black World, Ebony,* and other black publications, and is a *Life*-size, seventy-eight-page quarterly. Naturally it is unillustrated. The only words for the sighted reader are in the combined flag and masthead on the cover. Advertising is not included. Published since 1952, it goes free to 400 persons. Not all readers are black and a number are on other continents. The unique magazine is the project of Mrs. E. R. Merrick, of Durham, North Carolina. Most of the years since its origin she also edited it, working alone. Its editorial work now is done by Mrs. R. E. Hackett. They give their services but other charges must be paid, such as production, which comes to $3,500 a year. It goes post free, being material for the blind. *Negro Braille* is financed by contributions from black organizations, individuals, and its editors.

Also somewhat unusual is *Golden Legacy,* a magazine of comic book format illustrating black history and issued from Hollis, New York. Unusual, also, is the way copies are distributed—by the Coca-Cola Company through its local bottlers, free to schools, churches, or other organizations. They are intended for educational use and obviously have the added value of building goodwill for the firm. Each issue is devoted to a different historical figure, such as Toussaint L'Ouverture and Harriet Tubman.

The world of black journalism, despite the wealth of publications whose history and characteristics preoccupy this book, has had few publications about itself. One of the most useful but least pretentious was the *Lincoln Journalism Newsletter,* begun in 1944 and lasting until 1957. It was duplicated, on business letter-size paper, and issued monthly, running from eight to twenty pages a time, with jaunty little cartoons to break up pages. Changes in publications, activities of editors, publishers, reporters, and other staff people were recorded; it called attention to new journalism books, courses, and other black journalism news, entered the controversies about the black press, and generally kept an eye on developments. During most of its life it was edited and largely written by Armistead S. Pride, chairman of the department of journalism at Lincoln University in Missouri. That university also for a time produced *PEP,* monthly organ of the National Newspaper Publishers Association, a pocket-size printed magazine containing news somewhat on the order of the *Newsletter* but supplemented with photographs. NNPA also at one time had *Dateline,* a quarterly. Both ceased when financial conditions became difficult in the 1950's.

Today no regularly issued publication serves black journalism as a whole, but a group of Californians working on publications in the San Francisco Bay area have brought out monthly since 1969, the *Ball and Chain Review.* It contains articles and cartoons relating the position of black journalists in the country now. Among titles in the early issues are "Plight and Promise of Black Journalism," "Press Parodies Propaganda" and "White Liberalism vs. A Black Reporter"; some contributions tackle more general matters, such as relations between white and black police officials.

Although most of *Ball and Chain Review* is devoted to blacks on white media, the black press receives some attention. One of the most important recent assessments of the press was the report of an interview with Hoyt Fuller, editor of *Black World,* in which he was adversely critical of the press, saying that the analysis of E. Franklin

Frazier, the black sociologist, is still valid and that the papers are not fulfilling their role.

The *Media Woman* is an annual magazine published by the National Association of Media Women, Inc.; the New York chapter also issues a quarterly newsletter.

Black Sports, a slick monthly begun in March, 1971, is of international scope. It is intended, according to its publisher, to reveal the the views of black athletes and provide them with a different image than they have possessed.   ●

9. WHAT IS IN THE BLACK PRESS?

BLACK PUBLICATIONS sit for their own portraits week by week and month by month merely by what they put in their columns. Here and there, in the first eight chapters of this book and in sections following this one, are indications of what is in the pages of the black newspapers and magazines of the U.S.A. A closer examination of their content, however, may give deeper understanding of the role of that press.

The more honest, courageous, and professionally competent the press the more nearly accurate the representation of its audience will be. Whether the black press of this time accurately reports the life style of the Afro-American is a question still without a scientific answer. Undoubtedly it mirrors the activities and interests of some of the people some of the time. But as with most segments of the American press, there is little depth to the portrayal. The newspapers, as usual, devote their space largely to the transient, fleeting news. They must do so, for the most part, for what happens periodically is the essence of journalism. Most of the magazines are specialized and therefore exist in compartments, meeting the needs of only portions of the black population.

Parochial as the press may be, it is much less so today than it was in the 1920's, when Frederick Detweiler devoted a chapter in his book to its content. He noted that much of the country correspondence began: "Please allow me space in your paper," an unprofessional touch no longer encountered. The folksy tone of much copy was an exaggeration of the informality of small newspaper journalism in general. "Our Eastern program was something rare," wrote the Pine City, Arkansas, correspondent of the Wichita (Kan.) *Negro Star* in 1921. Detweiler found editorials in most papers, large or small, a situation that still is true, but he made little attempt to evaluate those opinion essays and might have noted their wordiness if not their evasiveness, the latter a criticism all too easily made of many a black publication editorial today. High-sounding credos and platforms and slogans were common in the early 1920's; these have less prominence now, largely because a more sophisticated and cynical public finds it too easy to discover discrepancies between platforms and performances.

Columns, always popular in black journalism, were not so often political as they are today. The personal type, commenting on local activities, was common and has survived. Although poetry has little place today in the white newspaper and less than before in the white magazine, it was found in considerable quantities by Detweiler, and persists today in the black press. Fifty years ago, Detweiler said, it ranged from "humble attempts on local subjects to more ambitious verse." Much of it, whatever its range of subjects, was in the tone of this stanza from a contribution in the *Texas Freeman:*

> The Negro is a working race,
>   And so with circumstances
> Does try to reach some noted place;
>   In general he advances.[1]

Detweiler went into considerable detail describing the advertising content, finding many ads of the sort subject to adverse criticism since, preying upon the superstitions and fears of readers, but also a large amount, chiefly local, of legitimate enterprises in the communities.

Few national and international news events with a racial angle were given space either because few were occurring or were being reported by the press as a whole. Nor were readers of that day as alert to and actively concerned about social movements affecting the black society as they are today, for there was much less hope of solving their problems than now. But lodge, church, society, and sports news, and in the larger cities, music, theater, and other special subjects, were assigned generous regular space in the papers.

Since there was no important consumer magazine, the periodicals of the first quarter of this century were all specialized, Detweiler identifying 113, of which 82 were for schools. The rest were fraternal, music, religious, scholarly, or cause magazines except a few small ones with general content.[2] He found a number of favorite themes. One was ". . . an undercurrent of feeling that the race considers itself a part of America and yet has no voice in the American newspaper."[3] This complaint still exists, although some progress has been made in that the white paper or magazine now gives black Americans more place. Essentially, however, the white press leaves to the black papers and magazines the detailed coverage. Thus this theme still is present in the black press; admittedly it is a logical point for a press seeking to survive and strengthen its place.

Other themes noted by Detweiler were related largely to racial struggles; unfair laws, discriminatory acts of whites, such crimes against blacks as lynchings, and the positive achievements of blacks—new businesses begun, political offices gained, educational honors or progress made by individuals. Detweiler reveals the themes by citing mottoes of several papers of the time, most of them now gone. The Cleveland *Advocate* said it was "More than a Mere Race Paper, 'Tis a Voice that Asks for Justice."[4]

● TELLING IT LIKE IT IS

The modern black newspaper and magazine come much closer to living up to that popular slogan of modern America: "Tell it like it is," than did the publications of the past. Even the protest papers of the nineteenth century told only part of the story of the American black society of their day. They concerned themselves largely with the abuses of the black citizen. But most of the other interests and activities of readers were more or less untouched, partly because it was difficult to be fully journalistic and partly because it was not actually the *raison d'etre* of the publications.

But when the black press moved into the realm of business the "it" became more than racial injustice. Fuller reports on the ethnic group to which it was responsible became necessary. Steadily, therefore, the more effective papers and magazines have broadened their outlook. The survivors, from earlier in the century, have lasted because their owners and editors put so much into their pages.

Pride, in 1956, published a system of classifying the contents of black newspapers which still fits the press and can be expanded and adapted to more recent times.[5] First was what he called the characteristic Negro Story; it began with the Escaped Slave Story, then the Lynch Story, then the Protest Story aimed at jim crowism, and next the Integration Story. Since 1956 have been added the Black Power Story, the Separatism Story, and more recently the Black Revolution Story.

Next was the Achievement Story, now more common than then and at all times prime copy, mainly because blacks now have an opportunity for achievement more than in the past. The nature of the accomplishment has changed somewhat from 1956. Then it was achievement along the lines of white accomplishment—earning much money, being accepted by whites, having possessions and ease. Today it is achievement of a more socially conscious nature—leadership in power groups, in the arts, in the entertainment world, in social action.

Third in Pride's group was the Negro Angled Story: news of blacks taking part in white news events, but covering only the black participation. This type continues to appear.

Fourth was the Gossip Story: personal news of such great importance that it is put into the regular news columns—weddings and other social news beyond the routine. This story also has persisted.

To Pride's list now can be added the African Story. With the intensified interest in that continent in the past few years some American blacks have tried to identify themselves with the land of their forefathers, to the extent of wearing African garments, learning African languages, singing African music, learning African native dances, and visiting the continent, sometimes settling there permanently. News from Africa or reports of visits there by prominent or local blacks is copy to be found in both newspapers and magazines.

● THE KINDS OF CONTENT

Undoubtedly most editors and publishers would affirm that their readers look to the press to find out "what really went on" when a news story about blacks breaks, even though it may be covered by the white media. And unquestionably they must turn to their own press for details about the vast majority of events occurring in their ranks. Such information is the stuff of black journalism. Mrs. Elizabeth Murphy Moss, an officer of the *Afro-American* newspapers, tells the story of two young black men who one evening came to the paper's offices in Baltimore. Both were incensed.

"They told how the nurse in the emergency room [at Maryland General Hospital] refused to examine one of them. He had complained of a painful rash on his arm. The nurse had ordered him out of the hospital, had even called in a policeman with a K-9 dog to put the point across," she said.

Mrs. Moss, who was addressing a journalism educators' group after accepting an award to her paper for service to predominantly black communities, said that the paper sent its city editor and a photographer to the hospital. They also were treated with discourtesy.

"There was an implied threat of arrest if they did not leave the waiting room," she reported. But the young man was examined and given a prescription. And she believes that the presence of the paper brought about the change.

The *Afro-American* was not stopping there, however. It interviewed the hospital administrator, who promised to look into the situation in the emergency room. The next day the paper carried a story and an editorial about mistreatment of blacks by hospital personnel. Nothing about the incident appeared in the city's white papers.[6]

Mrs. Moss' account illustrates what some black papers contain as well as what some do by way of crusading. She also told the journalism educators of a survey by the Morgan State College news bureau which showed that the six dailies in Maryland, not including the two in Baltimore, "seldom, if ever . . . print news about black residents in the areas where they publish except for the sports pages." She also recounted various instances in which news was brought to the *Afro-American* that the white papers ignored, such as the death of a black Vietnam veteran killed in an accident not far from his home. He was to go back to the war scene the next week.

● ANGLING THE NEWS

As stated, much of the material in the black press is not found elsewhere. It consists of news stories of the dark-skinned citizens and their activities extending from society notes to encounters with the law and to political action. News features are personality sketches, interviews, historical accounts, biographies, human interest stories. The essay, the basic form of much content, is the editorial, and sometimes columns by individual writers, critical reviews of books, movies, recordings, and plays. Editorials usually are on subjects of concern to black readers: politics, government actions or plans, and white actions affecting black life.

The magazine short stories are conventional, plotted tales, with black, American middle class, Protestant characters (BAMPs instead of WASPs). The poems run the gamut of forms, are much more modern than the fiction, and are preponderantly about causes for which blacks fight today. Articles are wide in range, dealing with personal problems, racial issues, and instructions on how to perform some operation, such as repairing or building.

The typical content not found in the white press but common at least in the larger black publications includes special dispatches from Africa angled toward the interest in Africa of American readers. For these stories most papers depend upon publicity materials, feature services, or news agencies; a few have their own correspondents or accept material from free lancers. Of national scope is the news of activities of scores of black groups, most known only within the black world, such as the National Association of Fashion and Accessory Designers, the International Florists Association, the National Association of Negro Business and Professional Women's Clubs, and various religious denominations. A typical story was a report of a national meeting in Kansas City of four hundred black members of the United Methodist Church, a white denomination with a new subgroup of black members. Those in the subgroup questioned the value of the Christian church as it functions today and wanted changes. Their view was covered in detail.

On the local scene a story typical of the black press is that about the burning of a barber shop in Atlanta after a black barber received threatening letters. They began: "We don't see any reason you niggers should start wearing this long kinky hair down South. We're giving you 5 days to close this dam [*sic*] shop up. We're sick and tired of seeing you niggers downtown wearing this long kinky hair and it's coming from this very shop. . . ."[7]

A typical black magazine piece unlikely to be found in a white magazine is any one of these: an interview with only the black members of a mixed theatrical cast, a discussion of why black women resent black men dating white women, or a collection of soul food recipes.

Most dramatic is the difference in emphasis. In general news with a black angle much more detail is included. The news is played differently; it is on the angle. For instance, the St. Louis *Sentinel* put an eight-column streamer, two lines deep in 90-point type, on a story about Governor Lester Maddox of Georgia calling a certain black congressman a baboon and giving away ax handles in the House restaurant in Washington. It is unlikely that any white paper gave this story comparable play. It was big in other black weeklies as well. Similarly, the *Afro-American* devoted a full half-page, with six pictures, to the story about a model agency director who sued Time Inc., for three million dollars for ignoring her firm in a *Life* article about such black agencies and giving space, instead, to a white-owned one.

The story of the natural death of some accomplished or locally influential black receives far bigger play in the black publication than the white; furthermore, the deaths of blacks who were not extraordinary often receive no space in the white. As with so much other black news, the black publication is the only outlet for it, even black radio having limited news gathering resources and restricted time for news.

● BIASED NEWS

One tradition in American journalism to which black journalists usually have assented even though it is a white standard, at least in theory, is that of separation, so far as possible, of facts and opinions. The opinions are expected to remain in the editorials so the reader knows they are the paper's official voice. Or they are supposedly under the bylines of writers, assuring the readers that they are the writers' views and can be discounted or accepted from knowledge of the responsibility and reliability of the writers. In practice, however, there is considerable violation. *Considerable,* however, is a comparative. American publications are spotless in this matter when compared to those of many other nations. But when held up to an ideal situation they are far from being free of bias. The policy of a publication, the views and prejudices of editors and owners, or its poor organization can result in opinions straying off the editorial pages and out of signed columns into what is thought to be factual only: the news columns.

In the days when the black press was mainly a protest organ and not a commercial venture it had no pretense of objectivity in it. Virtually everything in the early paper was propaganda for a cause, a practice inherent in protest. Today, however, most of the black press is commercial and sets itself forth as fulfilling the traditional functions of newspapers and magazines: to bring readers facts and opinions, with a minimum of mixing. By its slogans and credos, the press has the agreement with its readers that it will be honest and keep facts and what someone thinks about them apart and recognizable for what each is.

Neither the black nor the white press succeeds. It perhaps is a matter of degree. The black press, particularly the newspaper, crusades more than does the white, having more to crusade for. Thus, having embarked on campaigns, it is likely that the fervor of campaigning will rub off on the presumably objective news stories. Journalists have several ways of breaking faith with the reader in this matter of attempting to tell the whole truth and nothing but the truth. One way is to use emotion-laden words in what supposedly is a straight news story and thus influence the reader. The black press has its practicers of the system. For instance, the Milwaukee *Courier* began a news story this way:

"Advanced methods of police methodology, seventh district style, saw a young Blackman handcuffed and thrown to the floor of a police wagon early Sunday morning following a speeding arrest." Late in the account appears this: "Milwaukee's finest, he said, graciously offered him a wet paper towel at the seventh district to wipe his bloodied nose."[8] The first eight words of the opening paragraph and use of *finest* and *graciously* later, in an anonymous story, are used by a reporter intending not to present facts only to the reader. There also was a conscious attempt to prejudice him. What is described is perhaps the way the reporter saw it but it is not necessarily telling it like it is—or was. If the events are as reported they can be described by witnesses or the victim quoted directly.

Such angled writing is to be expected in the ultra-militant publications, for they make no pretense of telling it like it is but only of telling it like the way they think it is (or want it to be or to be seen). Often it is the result of neophyte reporters and editors being given freedom to write as they wish without supervision of their copy before publication.

Not reporting the whole story or a story at all is the second way in which deliberately or innocently a publication controls or establishes opinion with facts. Leaving out what the owners or editors do not want publicized—or what the reporter or writer anticipates is not desired—is a common procedure in all journalism. Only the reader who has been on the inside of a story, perhaps himself played a part in the news event, can be aware of the omissions. More often, perhaps, the omissions occur because the staff is too small to report an event, especially if it is a complex happening reported by the white press. The black viewpoint on a major conflict within the black community or in the public schools of a large city is not easy for a community paper's staff to obtain. It takes several trained reporters to cover such a story, and since the basic facts usually are known already via the white media, including radio and television, it does not seem practical to neglect everything else, which might be necessary in covering the story fully. The existence of many factions within the racial community also increases the difficulties.

The third manner in which editors and publishers consciously or unconsciously try to influence the reader to their viewpoint is by the way they position and dress the news. Putting material on the first page is accepted as the way to tell the reader that the executives of the paper think it important or significant. It may or may not have high reader interest, but the editors want it to have.

Thus another Milwaukee black weekly, the tabloid *Greater Milwaukee Star,* put on its first page one week a story with a full-width headline reading, in inch-high letters: PASTOR HITS RACIST HEADLINES. It was a three-quarter column story about a local minister attacking the Milwaukee *Journal,* the large white daily, for using what he called "racist headlines." The whole account was largely the text of a letter the minister had sent to the *Journal,* but the reader was not told if the letter was printed. The *Journal,* it appears, had used a headline reading: YORTY DEFEATS NEGRO IN L.A. MAYOR RACE. The minister objected to the head because it pointed out the race of the mayor's unsuccessful opponent. Without arguing the point he made, a reader might wonder, however, if this out-of-town story was the major news of the week of interest to most black citizens of the area of Wisconsin covered by the paper, since they can read the white paper for themselves, and many do. Several stories inside the *Star* dealt with housing and other important subjects affecting the daily lives of Milwaukee's black citizens.

On the editorial page of the paper, furthermore, was another attack on the white daily. It would seem, then, that opposition to the white paper is a part of the *Star*'s policy.

● PUTTING IN WHAT SELLS

Newspapers and magazines that fail to publish what readers will read disappear. Their readers and advertisers decrease in number. Not even a subsidy can save any but the smallest. The black press realized this truism of publishing in the U.S.A., since it is a secondary press. The front page headline in a newspaper or the front-of-the-book articles or stories in a magazine are depended upon to pull in readers. Until recent years the streamers or banners on black papers dealt with crime. Now likely as not they are concerned just as often with some racial issue. A group of Syracuse University students noted that for twenty-five weeks the national edition of the Baltimore *Afro-American* gave its page one streamer to a crime story but that crime had little place elsewhere in the paper. Mrs. Elizabeth Murphy Moss explained why:

> What we do here is attempt to strike the best possible balance each week, without resorting to what we would agree to as sensationalism.
>
> This becomes a bit tougher and somewhat a mixed bag when you consider some of the factors which may not immediately be apparent in comparing a national paper and a local paper, particularly a daily publication.
>
> First, we are a second (or otherwise) paper. Second, some of the stories used which have crime appearances actually gain their prominence because of their civil rights context (examples: the one about white snipers using the gun of a police chief to fire on black protesters, and the one about South-Africa type arrests being used to arrest Mississippi students). The same is true of some of the crime appearance stories involving such groups as the Panthers and personalities like H. Rap Brown.
>
> It also would be useful, from our point of view, if your team considered that the AFRO considers it a responsibility to play up on front page as many civil or human rights stories as possible. When an editor leans heavily in one direction as a service, then it sometimes becomes necessary to lean in another direction to balance off the interests of the newspaper's readers.[10]

The *Afro-American* uses similar page one makeup every issue, two or three streamers and several spread heads. But few other black papers appear to have any such journalistic formula. With the majority one week the main heading is sensational; another week, if there is a streamer or banner line at all, it is on more or less routine news. Such formulaless editing tends to play the news with the emphasis it may deserve instead of forcing a story into a prominence it ought not be given, as in the instance of the story of a letter sent to a Milwaukee white paper.

● THE CREDO OF THE BLACK PRESS

Even if printing credos and platforms, as some black publications still do, were not a practice left over from an earlier day, when such statements were common, the policy would be worth noting because the aims of such statements are peculiar to this group of publications. Such documents are not comparable with those in any other press. The credos of some smaller papers appear in Chapter 6.

To be found in or near the editorial columns of the *Louisiana Weekly* of New Orleans, the *Weekly Bulletin* of Sarasota, Florida, and other papers is a statement resembling this:

The Negro Press believes that America can best lead the world from racial and national antagonism when it accords to every man regardless of his race, creed or color, his human and legal rights. Hating no man, fearing no man—the Negro Press strives to help every man in the firm belief that all men are hurt as long as anyone is held back.

The platform of the Chicago *Daily Defender,* under Robert S. Abbott, was longer in his time than it is today. The present-day statement offers seven points which are a substantial goal for any publication:

1. The obliteration of American race prejudice.
2. Racially unrestricted membership in all trade unions.
3. Equal employment opportunities in all jobs, public and private.
4. True representation in all United States police forces.
5. Complete cessation of all school segregation.
6. Establishment of open occupancy in all American housing.
7. Federal intervention to protect civil rights in all instances where civil rights compliance at the state level breaks down.

The *Afro-American* Newspaper chain carries on its editorial pages, above and below its name on the masthead, three statements. The first, from Martin Luther King, Jr.:

Let us not seek to satisfy our thirst for freedom by drinking from the cup of hate and bitterness.

The second, part of it a biblical paraphrase, was written by the late Carl Murphy, son of the founder, and declares:

May we let our light so shine that it will illuminate that which is good and beautiful, and magnify our Father which is in heaven. May we stand strong and firm against despair, falsehood, rudeness, hatred, pessimism and prejudice.

Perhaps the most famous *Afro-American* statement of policy was that written by its founder, John H. Murphy, in 1920, and reproduced regularly since in the chain. That credo says:

I measure a newspaper not in buildings, equipment and employees—those are trimmings.

A newspaper succeeds because its management believes in itself, in God and in the present generation. It must always ask itself—

Whether it has kept faith with the common people;

Whether it has no other goal except to see that their liberties are preserved and their future assured;

Whether it is fighting to get rid of slums, to provide jobs for everybody;

Whether it stays out of politics except to expose corruption and condemn injustice, race prejudice and the cowardice of compromise.

The AFRO-AMERICAN must become a bi-weekly, then a tri-weekly, and eventually, when advertising warrants, a daily.

It has always had a loyal constituency who believe it honest, decent and progressive. It is that kind of newspaper now and I hope it never changes.

The presence of such credos and platforms serves as a commitment of the paper to publish news and other information that will sustain the promises or aims of the platform. The *Defender*'s first goal, "The obliteration of American race prejudice," logically would mean recognition of the existence of black prejudice against whites or yellow peoples. Exposed as America's black population is to slogans—"More Power to the People," "Right On," and "Tell It Like It Is" are popular at this writing—publications of platforms serve, perhaps, as a rhetorical counterbalance.

● **HUMOR IN THE PRESS**

If this book gives the impression that the black press contains no relieving humor and no light touches it is a reflection principally of the newspapers; the magazines are considerably less sober. The papers overflow with news of racial conflict, columnar musings on the internal problems of the race, reports of activities, doleful editorials, and great quantities of promotion materials for entertainment and sports personalities or various business enterprises. The black newspaper is a clear denial of that stereotype of the American black citizen: always cheerful, singing no matter what his adversities or how badly he is rejected by others.

His press is not altogether long-faced, but it is close. It hardly has had reason to be other, but for the psychological effect perhaps it needs more balance. A little effort is made. Most newspapers have a few humorous comic strips or panel cartoons. Occasionally a columnist tries a quip; noted elsewhere is Louis E. Martin's character, Dr. S. O. Onabanjo, in the Sengstacke papers. One can read through scores of black papers from many parts of the nation and not once encounter what the newspaper business calls "a bright," i.e., a brief, human interest story, or a humorous incident in the news. Here and there some editor or publisher prints bits of wry wisdom. ("Be careful what you say in front of children, they are like blotters, they soak it all in and get it backwards" appeared in the San Francisco *Sun-Reporter*).

Black magazines do far better, having more time and being more of a target for free-lance writers. Cartoons do much to keep the balance: full pages, sometimes in color, as in *Soul! Illustrated,* share space with single panels and strips; an occasional piece of funny fiction appears in the community magazines. *Jet,* always breezy in its style, squeezes quips into some of its departments; *Essence* is giving space to entire satirically or ironically humorous articles.

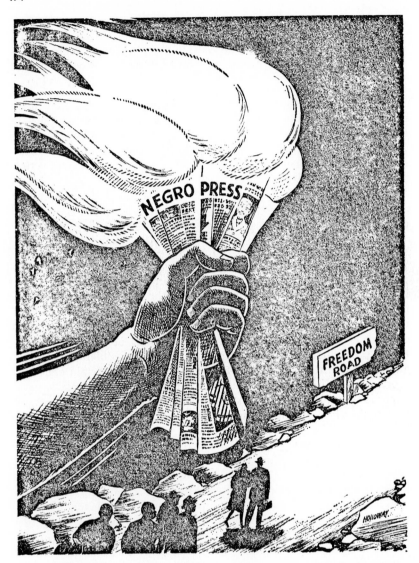

Lighting The Way To Freedom

FIG. 9.1. A typical Black Press Week cartoon.

One would not turn to either the black newspaper or the black magazine, however, for a dependable laugh. In these days the black man seems not to laugh much at himself or at others, for most of his humor is tinged with his social concerns.

WEE PALS By Morrie Turner

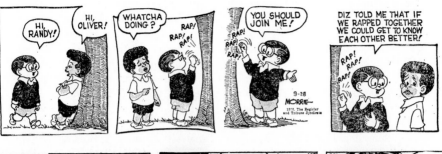

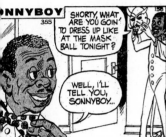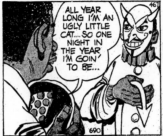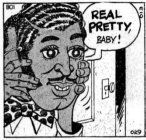

FIG. 9.2. "Wee Pals," drawn by Morrie Turner, a black artist, is syndicated to various black and white newspapers, and has characters of many races. "Sonnyboy," an unsigned strip carried in the **New Pittsburgh Courier**, is one of the few black-character comics being published in the black press. ("Sonnyboy" courtesy of Sengstacke Newspapers; "Wee Pals" courtesy of Register and Tribune Syndicate)

Turner's "Wee Pals." Examples of humor in the black press are coming strips and panel cartoons, some of which portray racially integrated characters but others black figures only. Both magazines and newspapers print such work by black artists; some also have found their way into the white press. One of the most successful is Morrie Turner's strip, "Wee Pals," which in 1970 was appearing in forty black or white papers. It goes beyond the usually integrated characters, for the small children who populate it include American Indians and Orientals as well. "The main purpose of 'Wee Pals' is to entertain," Turner has explained. "Then, I like to poke some gentle fun at adult black and white prejudices and misconceptions. Deep down is a signal to Americans that black and white children get along together famously until they learn about prejudices from adults." Then he went on to say that he tries to use his comic art to call attention to the good will in the world and how it might be applied to the adult society.[11]

Turner, who has won awards from the National Conference of Christians and Jews and the B'nai Brith Anti-Defamation League for his work, developed "Wee Pals" from an earlier strip, "Dinky Fellas." It was used by several large white and two black papers and then picked up by a national syndicate, an experience that white cartoonists also have had before their work gained wide attention. Lewis A. Little, president and general manager of the Register and Tribune Syndicate, points out that the strip was identical except for its name.

"Morrie and I merely decided to change the name to 'Wee Pals' when we started syndication in February, 1965. Before that he had been drawing the strip for four months for the Chicago *Daily Defender* and the Berkeley *Post*," he explained.[12]

Son of a Pullman car porter, Turner's serious cartooning began during World War II, when he was with the all-black 477th Bomber Group of the U.S. Army Air Force. He drew panels and strips for GI publications. After leaving service he worked eleven years as a clerk in Oakland, California, to support his family. Meanwhile, he free lanced his cartoons to *True, Argosy, Better Homes and Gardens, Extension,* and *Black World* magazines and the *Defender*. Impressed and inspired by Charles Schulz and his "Peanuts" strip, Turner at first had all black characters. He later included white, American Indian, and Oriental children. He was drawing it for the black weekly in Berkeley when Little spotted it. The "Wee Pals" strip has appeared in *Stars and Stripes,* the military paper. Turner reported a mainly negative response at first, some GI's thinking it anti-black and others having an anti-black reaction and demanding it be stopped. He attempts to make his social points and still be entertaining, a difficult combination. His own social philosophy, after much inner struggle, he arrived at following the assassination of Dr. King. It is belief in nonviolence.[13]

Surprisingly few black strips, that is, strips by blacks and about blacks, appear in the black press itself, probably because most cannot afford the cost of original work.[14] Among the few are "Sonny-boy" of the *New Pittsburgh Courier,* with numbers obscurely printed in several panels as an additional service to readers who want such gambling information. Atlanta *Voice* prints an untitled one, evidently syndicated, with black child characters. The rival weekly, Atlanta *Inquirer,* carries none, and the daily rival to them both, the *World,* has two white strips. The Chicago *Daily Defender,* in national edition, offers a full page of white strips. Its four-day local edition used to print another Morrie Turner strip, "Dogbert," with integrated child characters, but no longer does so. Turner's "Wee Pals" appears in the Baltimore *Afro-American*. The New York *Amsterdam News,* the largest commercial paper, carries no strips, nor do the important Norfolk *Journal and Guide,* Cleveland *Call and Post,* and Philadelphia *Tribune*. Numerous panel cartoons, humorous or serious, appear in *Muhammad Speaks,* but no weekly, continuous strips.

Ollie Harrington. The world of white journalism has had its Dave Breger, Bill Mauldin, and Herblock. The world of black journalism also has had cartoonists, some of them syndicated, who are popular, perhaps for different reasons. Breger reflected the views of the white rank and file soldier during World War II and the ordinary citizen in peacetime. Mauldin similarly drew wry cartoons about the thoughts of the man in the trenches or on the march and after the war pointed up in panels the ironies of current situations. Herbert L. Block, also a white artist, has been more concerned with the injustices suffered by America's black people than any other cartoonist who had access to large numbers of editorial pages in white publications, and sometimes bitterly limned their condition.

The black cartoonists are fewer in number, for if black journalism has barely been a living for many years, the career of a black cartoonist is even less promising, unless like the late E. Simms Campbell he manages to break into the big white magazine field, as Campbell did with *Esquire, Playboy,* and the *New Yorker.*

The one cartoonist that black readers know, if they are conscious of any who produce drawings for their papers, is Oliver "Ollie" Harrington, who labels his feature "Bootsie." The drawings, which appear in the *New Pittsburgh Courier,* portray some of the ironies of black life, but with a caustic humor. In one, for example, a little girl says to other black children playing outside a tenement: "I think I messed up in the civics class and ain't gonna git promoted this term. The teacher, Miss McCharles, been saying we be spreading freedom all over the world. Then I opens my big fat mouth and asked when it would git to Georgia and Florida . . . and Harlem!"

Harrington has recalled the origin of his popular feature. He temporarily, in 1936, was replacing the regular cartoonist of the New York *Amsterdam News,* receiving seven dollars a week for his work. "After awhile a rather well-fed but soulful character emerged and crept into each drawing." The atmosphere was provided by Harlem, where Harrington lived. The character was named "Bootsie" by Ted Poston, then city editor of the *Amsterdam News* and for many years thereafter a noted black reporter for the white New York *Post.*[15]

The cartoonist has gone far beyond the single-character drawing with his panels tackling subjects of the day. His cartoons are largely realistic but edged with caricature. A typical Harlem scene panel typifying his digs at whites shows scientists at dinner. The white scholars along the table are take-offs on the academic types to be seen among the full professors in the science departments. The bald chairman standing beside the elderly black visiting speaker says to him: "Doctor Jenkins, before you read us your paper on inter-stellar gravitational tensions in thermonuclear propulsion, would you sing us a spiritual?" His lime-flavored humor is not restricted to his drawings but also appears in his writing. Telling, for example, of restaurants

BOOTSIE
Ollie Harrington

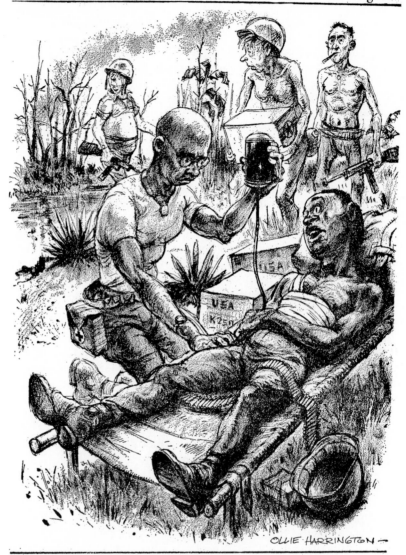

"Say Baby, you reckon they goin' to allow me to eat in one of their restaurants if I make it back to Mississippi?"

FIG. 9.3. Ollie Harrington, veteran cartoonist for the **New Pittsburgh Courier**, has made his "Bootsie" a black press institution. This one is typical of his ironic touch. (Courtesy of Sengstacke Newspapers)

in New York "where the greys wouldn't panic if a member appeared and ordered a meal," he adds: "But it would take a strong constitution to pass off the ground glass and other delicate spices they were apt to drop into that particular serving."[16]

Another cartoonist who has gained attention is Robert Brown, who signs his work "Buck" Brown. He has contributed a humorous panel drawing, "Fumbanks Tecumseh McShane" regularly to *Tuesday* since June, 1969, and also has appeared in *Esquire* and other national magazines. "Fumbanks" is a black who usually is in a humorous situation with his black employer; he is not bright and his boss despairs of him.

● WHAT IS NOT IN THE PRESS

The only nationally prominent black newspaper that shows an interest in other racial or religious minority groups is *Muhammad Speaks,* the organ of the Nation of Islam. Usually in black papers news of Mexicans, Arabs, Puerto Ricans, Cubans, Hindus, or American Indians appears only where there is a direct relationship, as in occurrences of anti-Semitism among New York blacks or when Puerto Rican and black youths unite in civic activities or politics. Here and there one finds references to American Indians.

With such notable exceptions as *Freedomways, Amistad,* and other limited circulation publications, black journals usually content themselves with editorials asking for cooperation between blacks and Jews in the efforts to bring about particular social reforms of common importance. Now and then one encounters a departure from this policy, as in 1963, when the New York *Amsterdam News* published a story to the effect that "Jews control New York City's top jobs." The article, based on a survey whose source was not disclosed, brought condemnation from Protestant and Jewish organizations. Fearful perhaps of handling material about other minorities as clumsily as the white press has handled news of themselves at times, black publishers move cautiously in the area.

Also not often in the black publication, especially the newspaper, is coverage of events that lack a racial angle. Since it is admitted to be a second paper, this is entirely logical; furthermore, it would be impossible for even the most financially substantial large black dailies and weeklies to duplicate—if it were necessary—what appears in the white papers in the same community, although in numerous American cities that are ill-served by one surviving paper or two under the same ownership it would be salutary if a black daily entered the scene and provided needed competition.

To the confirmed hater of blacks what is in their press is either frightening or ridiculous. He sees with fear the call in a few publications to a campaign to "kill the pigs" and stories in most others of the proud social and artistic accomplishments of some persons, daring to equate themselves with whites.

But to other outsiders, those nonblacks who are not beset with suspicion, discovering what is in the black press is an exciting experience. They turn the pages of a big national weekly crammed with news of the many activities and interests of black people or look at the increasingly successful consumer magazines, with their professional appearance, and are impressed. Another world opens before the reader who is not of it, when he has empathy for black America. ●

10. THE BLACK JOURNALIST TODAY

Stanley Roberts, while Washington Bureau chief for the Pittsburgh *Courier,* several times scored beats, but his best known exploit was in getting an interview with General Douglas MacArthur when all other reporters had failed. MacArthur had just returned to the U.S.A. from the Orient and was at the Waldorf-Astoria Hotel in New York City but refused to see newsmen. Roberts sent word to the general calling his attention to a situation overlooked by other reporters: some black papers were calling the general a supremacist and putting on him the blame for unjust treatment of blacks and for army segregation.

MacArthur called Roberts to his room and gave him a reply, denying the accusation and making a statement about black troops. "They didn't send me enough of them," he told Roberts. That led not only to a two-part article in the *Courier* but also to a piece about Roberts in both *Time* and the New York *Times.*[1]

This incident is an instance of a black reporter having an advantage over a white one in that he is more likely to be informed on the concerns of his particular ethnic group, and has a natural interest that white reporters are unlikely to possess. It is an argument for including black journalists on white staffs.

But the typical journalist working in the world of black journalism has gained little notice outside his own small circle. When *Time* published its informative special issue on April 6, 1970, called "Black America 1970" it devoted its Press section to the black journalist. Most of the four columns were about the place of blacks on white publications, news agency and broadcasting staffs, and restricted to seven newsmen then working for white-owned media. These were Carl T. Rowan, William Raspberry, Thomas A. Johnson, Lem Tucker, L. F. Palmer, Jr., William Drummond, and Ray Rogers. Black journalists on black-owned publications serving the black readers, however, received no attention beyond one sentence. The paragraph devoted to black publications merely recorded that the New York *Amsterdam News* is the largest paper, that the *Afro* chain then had

87,600 circulation and that *Muhammad Speaks* had 400,000 circulation. *Ebony, Jet* and *Negro Digest* were mentioned but *Tan* overlooked in the listing of Johnson publications. Thus would the general public as well as the uninformed black citizen gain the idea that the black press per se is of little consequence, with no black journalists of its own worth mention, and gain no idea of its size and extent.[2]

A few months before, the results of the work of two researchers, who had polled the NAACP's state conference and key branch presidents concerning black persons, were announced. They were asked whom they considered the ten most outstanding blacks, dead and living, and to say why they selected their first choice. Three among the first twenty-five of the living and two among the first twenty-five of the dead have had some identification with journalism. Roy Wilkins was ranked second, A. Philip Randolph fifth, and Adam Clayton Powell ninth in the first group. Among the deceased W. E. B. Du Bois was second on the list and Frederick Douglass third. It should be noted that no living practicing journalist was named in the first twenty-five, for Wilkins' journalism, all in the past except for his syndicated column, is not what made him known to the public so much as his work as secretary of the NAACP; Randolph has not been thought of as a journalist for many years, and Powell's journalism has not been full-time since the 1940's and he has written only sporadically since. But a few others beyond the first twenty-five among those who are dead were named as journalists, including Martin R. Delaney, who assisted Douglass; Samuel E. Cornish, co-founder of the first black newspaper in America; John B. Russwurm, his partner; William Monroe Trotter of the Boston *Guardian;* and T. T. Fortune of the *New York Age.* Carter Goodwin Woodson, founder of the *Journal of Negro History,* and Marcus Garvey also were on the list. Among the then living mentioned beyond the first twenty-five were John H. Johnson, head of *Ebony* and other magazines; Carl T. Rowan, Andrew T. Hatcher, and Louis E. Lomax.[3] The activities of most of these men are discussed in this and other chapters.

That black journalists deserve more than the short shrift they have been getting is evident from the records, sparse as they are, of their performance. They have scored their scoops on the war fronts as well as under more placid conditions, and often against handicaps white writers rarely experience, especially in those parts of the nation (but less so outside the U.S.A.) where they have not been admitted to certain hotels, clubs, and restaurants.[4] These obstacles are fewer today than ever before. But they still exist, as is known by black newsmen covering racial demonstrations and disorders who are mistaken for demonstrators and treated as protesters sometimes are treated.

The black journalists in the U.S.A. are reporters, writers, editors, and other journalistic staff members of black or white (or other minority) newspapers, magazines, news agencies, or in the journalistic end of broadcasting. They are not publishers, advertising people, or those in circulation or production, for these are identified with such other occupations as administration, management, selling, and printing, although they are closely enough related so that these services are dealt with briefly in this book.

The number of black journalists on white media is small, judging by the few clues we have thus far. Pride in 1968 published a figure of 175 blacks on white daily newspapers.[5] Columbia University, the same year, released results of a survey made jointly by the *Columbia Journalism Review* and the Anti-Defamation League of B'nai Brith. It showed that 4.1 per cent of all media workers were black. Replies were received from news publications and stations only; thus numerous general magazines were not included. About 44 per cent of the 388 units responded. Magazines handling news had hired the largest proportion of blacks, 5.1 per cent. Newspapers were next with 4.7 per cent; radio-TV last with 2.7.[6] A good many gaps in the survey may have skewed the results, since several major newspapers, one of the two national news agencies, and three news magazines refused to provide facts.

These surveys produced figures that undoubtedly are low, considering the omissions and the changes that have taken place since, for the push within the journalism and communications industries to obtain black talent and the increase in training recruits should have raised the percentages. The number still must be small, however, since there are about 1,780 white dailies and around 10,000 papers of other frequencies, and approximately 20,000 magazines of all kinds.

● BLACK JOB OR WHITE JOB?

Although the concern of this book is mainly with the journalists working on media issued by and for blacks, at this juncture it is appropriate to consider the merits of working for a black publication or a white one, from the viewpoint of the man or woman who might be attached to one or the other. A case can be made for each. Which one joins is perhaps less important than to go to journalism at all in preference for some other occupation.

Factors that the white-skinned journalist does not think of, for he need not, enter in this problem for the black journalist. Will he be assigned to cover black news only? Or write articles on black topics only? Will he be used as the house black, a victim of tokenism? Will he lose status with his soul friends, his family, by going to a white publication instead of a black, or vice versa? Does he feel guilty if he goes to a better-paying job on a white publication when he knows that black papers and magazines are seeking staff but usually cannot pay as well? Does he fear inability to keep up with the competition on a white publication staff? Are his chances of promotion on a white paper limited by his race? Will he, if he feels a change of mind after having first worked on a black magazine or radio station, be able to go to a white publication without loss of status or salary? Is the experience on a black medium inferior and professionally injurious? And perhaps the most important question of all: on which publication can he be of most service (if he wants to put it in such high-minded terms) to his race, to his country, to mankind?

These are among the many questions that arise. Often they can be settled only in individual instances by assessing the experiences of others, although what others have done is not an absolute guide. Luck, being on the right spot at the proper time, the ever-present "in" provided by friends, and changes in policies of publications in a rapidly altering racial situation all can be more important than is realized. The vocational problem of the black journalist simply is more acute than that of the white. The latter has many factors to weigh in making decisions about what kind of journalism to engage in, and even, in rare instances, whether the black press is perhaps the best place for him, considering his goals and ideals.

An examination of the careers of some black journalists should indicate what can be accomplished. Some have shown that the matter is not simply one of working on a black publication or a white one only but of working, at different times, on both. The decision is made out of necessity, perhaps; nothing else may be around to do.

When Virginia W. Williams, co-publisher and editor of *Echo,* the black community magazine in Milwaukee, wrote a special series of articles for the white Milwaukee *Journal* in 1969 while she was in Europe, she reported on what she had learned about race prejudice against blacks. Were these articles more effective in combatting prejudice or gaining understanding of blacks than they would have been had they appeared in *Echo,* read mainly by blacks and with an infinitely smaller circulation than the *Journal?* Or would they have been equally effective?

Easy answers to such questions do not exist, for only an expensive and elaborate research program would reveal them. But the black journalist must weigh such experiences, and, being within the black community, can perhaps guess at answers.

The condition of the black journalist on black media usually, as we have seen in the history of the publications, has been inferior to that of the white. His salary has been lower, his facilities not equal, his security little. The few black publications that provide pleasant working surroundings, job stability, and salaries at all commensurate with those of white offices are the exception. Walter White, at one time executive secretary of the NAACP, summarized the status of the black journalist at the time, 1948, when he wrote:

> In many ways the establishment and rise of the Negro press in America has been a miracle in journalism. Until quite recently no Negro could obtain employment as a reporter, editor, or craftsman on

any white daily newspaper or magazine. The Negro thereby had been denied the opportunity to learn the newspaper trade by working at it.[7]

He noted that a few blacks had been graduated from schools of journalism up to then and that more were taking courses as opportunities on both the black and white press increased. "But as a rule," he wrote, "the Negro newspaperman has had to establish his own practices and standards and the results have not always been uniformly good."

The situation improved in the two decades thereafter, the black journalist having been accepted, even sought after, in the offices of many white media and needed more than ever by his own press. More are attending schools and departments of journalism; others are being trained in short courses and workshops.

As in the past, some black journalists continue to work for the black papers and periodicals, either out of pride in blackness, a desire to see black journalism gain in influence, or because they merely feel more at home among blacks than among whites. Others go right to the white press, some from an unrelated occupation, others by shifting out of the black journalism sphere.

The Uncommon Backgrounds. Generalizations about the careers and backgrounds of the better-known black journalists are not easy to make. Some attended colleges; some preferred newspapers to magazines, some the reverse. Some chose the world of white journalism; others the black. Counting which did which is meaningless because studies to obtain such facts reliably have not been made, either of a representative group, if such there be, or the total of journalists. Both studies would be incomplete scientifically because the records of journalists are difficult to obtain; even some of recent years are unavailable, for the publications for which they worked often are not on file anywhere and office records of staffs have been lost in mergers, fires, and careless disposal.

A useful source is denied observers of the black press and black journalists: the autobiographies, biographies, and books of reminiscence so often written by white journalists, editors, publishers, and others connected with the communications industry. Such books are among the richest portions of the literature of American journalism, of vastly higher quality and importance than the hundreds of novels and volumes of verse about journalism published over the years which ordinarily constitute the body of strictly literary material about an occupation or profession. Yet of the many scores of such life stories few are substantially about black journalists. Ottley's on Robert S. Abbott, a half dozen about Frederick Douglass, three about W. E. B. Du Bois, two about Garvey, Gordon Parks' books, George S. Schuyler's autobiography, one on Trotter and the slight sketches in Penn on the journalists active in the black press during the nineteenth century constitute the extent of the source material in print form to this writing. Here and there are biographical articles, few of them in readily seen magazines and newspapers. This scarcity of information about these newsmen and magazinists makes all the more valuable what can be learned today about those of recent years and the present. For if one turns to the usual sources, such as biographical reference books, one finds little attention for journalists whose skin happens to be black.

● THE CAREERS OF BLACK JOURNALISTS

At the risk of seeming to offer an abridged Who's Who in Black Journalism, a volume that indeed would be useful, this section briefly tells the stories of a few black journalists who have gained public attention, often national awards, for their work. And, at a further risk, that of offending those omitted, or their families, it should be noted that this account makes no pretense of being a directory or catalog but seeks mainly to give the reader unfamiliar with these journalists an idea of their work and accomplishments. Women journalists are discussed later in the chapter.

Some of the men and women accounted for here have worked only for black media; these are emphasized, since their careers are more directly relevant to this book's scope than are the professional activities of those associated mainly with white publications and stations. But both are here. We begin with several who are no longer alive but who worked in a period beyond the years covered by the strictly historical chapters; they should not be passed over.

One of them was Allan Morrison, who died at fifty-one in 1968 while New York editor of *Ebony*. A Canadian, he had been the first black correspondent for the European edition of *Stars and Stripes*, the GI newspaper. After the war he edited the Harlem weekly, *People's Voice*, then joined the Johnson Publishing Company in 1947. He also did radio work while with *Ebony*.

Another *Ebony* staffer was a most versatile black journalist—Dan Burley, who died in 1963 when he was fifty-four. A Chicagoan originally, his first journalistic work was as a teen-ager with the Chicago *Defender*, and then, as either reporter or editor, he followed the tradition of the old-time tramp newspaperman who moved from publication to publication. His stops were at the New York *Amsterdam News*, of which he became managing editor; the *New York Age, Ebony, Jet, Tan*, an early version of *Muhammad Speaks*, and the *Crusader*. At his death he was publishing the *Owl* in Chicago. Burley had a variety of interests and talents. He not only was a skillful newsman and editor but also a composer of popular music, a critic, sports writer, and promoter of sports and entertainment events.

The War Correspondents. Stanley Roberts, who got the MacArthur story related earlier, was only one of numerous war and peacetime correspondents. Several dozen others served in the two world wars, the Korean War, and the Vietnam War. Their experiences in general were those of white writers entering the battle zones. Most lived to return to their home offices. One who did not was Albert L. Hinton, lost at sea in 1950 when a C-47 transport plane he boarded in Japan went down while he was on his way to cover the Korean War. Hinton was working for the Norfolk *Journal and Guide* but also filing to other papers in the National Newspaper Publishers Association pool. He had been with the *Journal and Guide* for twenty years. Others, some no longer alive, included Philip Dunbar, Roi Ottley, Fletcher Martin, John Jordan, Enoc P. Waters, Ollie Harrington, Francis Yancey, Ollie Stewart, Walter White, Art Carter, Lem Graves, L. Alex Wilson, and James Hicks.

Ollie Stewart still worked in 1970 as foreign correspondent for the *Afro-American,* writing stories with a racial angle from abroad, such as a report from Augsburg, Germany, relating how discrimination against black military personnel persists in the U.S. Army. Enoc Waters, now with the Health, Education and Welfare offices in Washington, wrote from overseas for the Chicago *Defender.* Thomas Sancton, a one-time editor of the *New Republic,* singled out Waters in a series about wartime race problems, saying, "By any standards, he is a first-rate reporter." Waters became a top *Defender* editor and then executive editor of the Associated Negro Press in the early 1960's; in the same period he was cited by Lincoln University in recognition of his service to journalism between 1932 and 1962.

Nunn and Rowan. A good many others gained attention during peacetime years, fighting another kind of battle. William G. Nunn, Sr., was on the Pittsburgh *Courier* staff for forty-four years, in the later years as managing editor. He left the staff in 1963. During his tenure the paper campaigned for integration of blacks in the military and in major league baseball. A son of the same name held his father's post on the *New Pittsburgh Courier* in 1970.

Carl T. Rowan is perhaps the best known of all present-day black reporters; he has had one of the most extraordinary careers among these journalists. It has included work not only as a newsman, columnist, magazine and book writer but also as a U.S. diplomat, military man, and government official. When he was nineteen he became a naval officer. This appointment took place during World War II, for he was born in Tennessee in 1925. Rowan was one of the first fifteen blacks in U.S. history to become an officer in the navy. After the war he attended the School of Journalism at the University of Minnesota; earlier he had studied at Tennessee State University, Washburn University, and Oberlin College, receiving a bachelor's degree from the latter. At Minnesota he earned a master's.

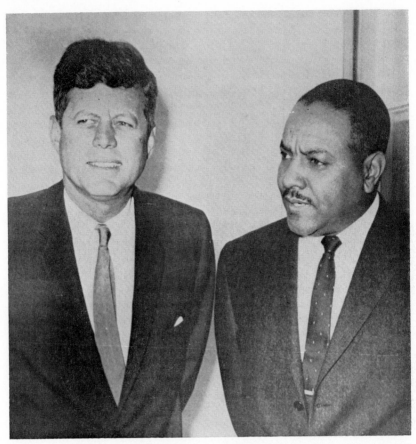

FIG. 10.1. Carl T. Rowan, Washington columnist and former U.S.
Ambassador to Finland and director of the USIA, with the late
President John F. Kennedy.

From study he went to the Minneapolis *Tribune* staff, at first as
a copy editor for that large white daily and then as a reporter and
foreign correspondent from 1950 to 1961. His series of articles on
conditions abroad and at home brought him to the attention of President John F. Kennedy, who in 1961 appointed him deputy assistant
secretary of state for public affairs and a member of the U.S. delegation to the United Nations. Two years later he was named U.S.
ambassador to Finland, for the liberal social attitudes of all the Scan-
dinavian countries usually have made them receptive to nonwhite
diplomats. While in that post he was the youngest U.S. envoy. The
next year President Lyndon B. Johnson recalled him; he then succeeded Edward R. Murrow as director of the U.S. Information Agency.
This appointment made him the first black to sit in the president's
cabinet sessions as well as those of the Security Council of the United
Nations.

Rowan left public service to become a daily Washington columnist writing for Publishers-Hall Syndicate. More than one hundred papers use his column, which deals with national and international affairs. At the same time he contributes to national magazines and to date has written four books. His honorary degrees and awards are more numerous than those of most other American journalists of any race.

The Alex Haley Story. One of the few writers, black or white, who has had a successful full-time career as a free lancer is Alex Haley, author with Malcolm X of the latter's autobiography. Haley was born in Ithaca, New York, while his father was a Cornell University graduate student. When his father taught later at southern colleges, which Haley also attended, he continued to move in academic circles. He then served in the U.S. Coast Guard for twenty years. There it was that he began free lancing, first to the original *Coronet* magazine, then to *Harper's, Atlantic,* the *Saturday Evening Post,* the *Reader's Digest,* and others. Before he left the Coast Guard in 1959, a rating of Chief Journalist had been created for him.

Haley then began to specialize in interview-writing, reporting on various black singers, political leaders, and athletes. He went on to take a law degree. Today his journalism is shared with writing nonfiction books and with lecturing. His most recent volume, *Before This Anger,* the story of an American black family traced back to its origins in Africa, is that of his own.

Wilkins, Holman, and Others. Roy Wilkins, the NAACP executive director, may not be thought of as a black journalist. Yet he has considerable practical experience in the profession and today writes a regular column appearing in dozens of papers. Wilkins' first journalism work was in college, while majoring in sociology at the University of Minnesota. He edited the *Minnesota Daily.* When he was graduated in 1923 he went to work for the Kansas City *Call,* a leading midwestern black weekly, eventually becoming managing editor. Even then he was a columnist, with one for the *Call* named "Talking It Over." He left black journalism to be assistant NAACP secretary in 1931. Three years later he added the editorship of the *Crisis* to his duties and kept it for fifteen years. His present syndicated column is "Along the Way" or simply "Roy Wilkins' Column" or "Roy Wilkins."

One of the earliest of the modern black journalists to join a white daily staff was Ben Holman. He was a 1952 graduate of the University of Kentucky when he became a Chicago *Daily News* reporter, but was drafted and spent two years in the army. He returned to the paper as a reporter. Once while on an assignment he disguised himself as a Black Muslim to write a series on that group.[8] He now is director of Community Relations Service of the Department of Justice and has counseled organizers of several regional conferences to bring together black and white journalists and publishers to consider race news coverage.

A successor to Wilkins as editor of the *Crisis,* James W. Ivy, has been on both black and white publication staffs. He joined the NAACP as an editorial assistant in 1943. Earlier he had been a Virginia high school and Hampton Institute teacher. Born at Danville, Virginia, he studied at Virginia Union University and New York University. Ivy left *Crisis* to serve as managing editor of *Common Sense,* a liberal white magazine of public affairs; his background for that post was his work in the late 1920's with the controversial black periodical, *Messenger,* as book review editor. When he returned to the NAACP magazine it was to be managing editor.

Another man who has been on both specialized and general publications is Roi Ottley, the biographer of Robert S. Abbott, founder of the Chicago *Defender.* After studying at the University of Michigan, St. Bonaventure University, and St. John's Law School, Ottley became a World War II correspondent for the unusual New York white paper *PM,* owned by Marshall Field. Its reporters signed their stories. Ottley also was on *Liberty* magazine, a onetime competitor for *Collier's* and other mass magazines. After the war he joined the Pittsburgh *Courier* as a special correspondent. While he was in Europe for the white publications he emphasized the roles of black people in both war and peace. He covered more than 30,000 miles and continued traveling when he went to the *Courier* staff. He already had published a highly successful book, his first, *New World A'Coming;* later he published *Black Odyssey, No Green Pastures,* and *The Lonely Warrior,* the Abbott biography.

Photojournalist-Editor-Cinema Producer. Certainly one of the most versatile of all U.S. journalists, regardless of race, is Gordon Parks. For he not only has been recognized as one of the best photographers and photojournalists of the country but he also is known as novelist, poet, cinema producer, movie writer and director, music composer, and most recently, magazine editor, and author.

Parks decided to become a photographer, he relates in an autobiographical book, *A Choice of Weapons,* when he stopped in at a Chicago movie house one day in 1937. Then he was a Pullman car waiter, newly impressed with the power of a picture after seeing many paintings at the Chicago Art Institute. At the theater he saw newsreel films of the Japanese bombing the U.S. gunboat, *Panay.* When the film was over, Norman Alley, the photographer who had taken the pictures, came on stage to talk about his experiences.

"I sat through another show," Parks recalled, "and even before I left the theatre I had made up my mind I was going to become a photographer." He was reminded by the pictures of those in magazines he had seen long before of poverty in the Southwest, taken by

Arthur Rothstein, Carl Mydans, Ben Shahn, and others working for Roy Stryker of the Farm Security Administration during the depression years of the early 1930's.

When his train run ended at Seattle, he relates, he immediately tried to buy a camera. He was appalled at the high cost of equipment. Finally he bought a second-hand one for $12.50, in a pawnshop. While shooting his first rolls of film he fell off a Puget Sound wharf and had to be pulled out. But the photographs were undamaged and so good, in fact, that the camera shop where he bought the film exhibited them. From then on he went everywhere experimenting with his new-found art as widely as his money would let him.

The St. Paul *Pioneer Press,* a large white daily in Minnesota (the other end of his run) printed some of his pictures; later the Minneapolis *Spokesman and Recorder,* a black weekly, ran Parks' work regularly on its front page, although neither paper paid him. But it put him into practical journalism, for he went to work as combination circulation manager and official photographer for the weekly, which bought him a press camera. But, Parks admits, he was not much of a salesman. Having to earn a living forced him back to railway work on the Chicago & North Western as a porter. He took pictures on the run between Chicago and the Twin Cities and continued his study of paintings in art galleries. "I read every book on art and photography I could afford," he later wrote.

When one day Bernard Hoffman, a *Life* cameraman, boarded his train, he questioned him for hours about the profession. By persistence, he got a chance to do fashion photography for an exclusive St. Paul store, nearly bobbled the assignment but came through with the needed films. After some delay because he had to move to Chicago; he soon was making a fair living with his camera there. At times he earned as much as $150 a day, a fabulous amount for the time, but there were some idle days. He continued to take fashion pictures and portraits of wealthy women, but he also spent some of his time exposing film in the Chicago ghetto districts; the photographs of people in those neighborhoods and living under similar conditions elsewhere have become his specialty since.

When Parks was awarded a year's Rosenwald Fellowship of $200 a month he decided to apply to the FSA, whose photographers earlier had so much impressed and inspired him. Under Stryker he was a trainee in Washington early in 1942, the World War II days having come. There he learned lessons not only in photography as an art but also about his reactions to race prejudice. The human compassion of the noted white photographers with whom he snapped pictures side by side kept him from being totally antagonistic toward whites. From the FSA he went to the Office of War Information staff and later to the Standard Oil Company of New Jersey.

Life's photo staff accepted Parks in 1949; he thus joined a cluster of some of the country's most famous photojournalists. He took many memorable pictures and series of photographs for the weekly until he became interested in book writing and motion picture making. His first book appeared in 1963, *The Learning Tree,* an autobiographical novel. Two years later came the partial autobiography, *A Choice of Weapons,* in which he explains not only his background but also his view that through his art he can fight the battle for his race better than by the use of more conventional weapons. Some of his poetry and color photographs appeared in 1968 in *A Poet and His Camera.* His writing, like his photography, is clear and realistic.

As the first U.S. black to produce and direct a full-length film for a major studio, Warner Brothers-Seven Arts, Parks in 1969 completed a cinema version of *The Learning Tree.* He also wrote the music, a symphony in three movements, although he never had music lessons. This experience led him to form his own motion picture producing firm. His most recent work in journalism was as editorial director of *Essence,* a sophisticated magazine for black women (see Chapter 7).

Why did Parks choose photojournalism, poetry, music, and cinema? His answer was quoted by *Jet* in 1969: "This leads me into bigotry and discrimination and all the indignities that black people have suffered here in the United States. And that leads me back to why I chose a camera. Why I have chosen the film. Why I have chosen poetry and music to fight these particular things. I think that these have been more effective than the more violent weapons such as the gun, the knife, the club or other weapons that you might use."

Parks' background was not what one might expect in so sensitive and artistic a writer and photographer. Born in 1912 in Kansas, he was the fifteenth child in his family. When his mother died fifteen years later he was sent to Minnesota to live in its slums, where he lived for fifteen years more, disappointed at not getting a college education but reading widely on his own and studying by himself the techniques of artists whose work was to be seen in nearby galleries and museums.

Conservative Spokesman. One black journalist who can be found in *Who's Who in America* is George S. Schuyler, long identified with the Pittsburgh *Courier.* Discussing the writing and writers in the black press, Thomas Sancton, writing in the *New Republic,* said that in his opinion Schuyler "is about the best."[9] This praise from a widely respected white newsman and liberal magazine editor may seem unusual, for Schuyler has espoused ultraconservative political and social views for much of his journalistic life and it has biased his work. Sancton wrote his opinion while Schuyler was moving from one social philosophy to another and may not, therefore, have realized the extent of the journalist's and columnist's eventual political change. It is not, however, that Schuyler has been so ardent a conservative; it is that his viewpoint has warped so much of his work. It would have had the same effect had he held to directly opposite be-

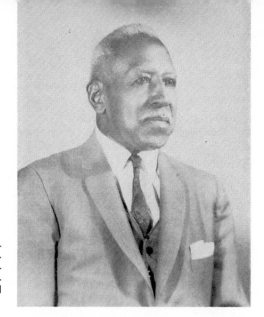

FIG. 10.2. George S. Schuyler, for many years a Pittsburgh **Courier** editor and writter, member of staffs of various black magazines, and author.

liefs, such as he had in youth, and strained everything he saw through them.

A Rhode Islander born in 1895, Schuyler has been a journalist since he was twenty-eight. He was assistant editor, then managing editor, of the *Messenger,* the gadfly magazine then considered radical, edited by A. Philip Randolph and Chandler Owen. He edited *National News* briefly in 1932, then went to the NAACP's publicity department. From 1937 to 1944 he was business manager of the *Crisis.* In the latter year he left for a long tenure at the Pittsburgh *Courier* (1944 to 1964). On the *Courier* he was a special correspondent in South Africa, the West Indies, French West Africa, and the Dominican Republic. At the same time he edited *National News* for a year and worked for the white press as a special correspondent in Liberia for the New York *Evening Post.* In 1953 he became a columnist, writing regularly until 1962. In 1960 he also began work as a foreign correspondent once more, this time for the North American Newspaper Alliance, a white syndicate, in Nigeria, Portugal, and East Africa, meanwhile doing other writing for NANA.

So energetic and prolific a writer as Schuyler has turned to books and articles as outlets for his work. He is author of three volumes, two of them novels, and has contributed to numerous magazines, the articles tracing the changes in his views over the years. In early days he wrote for *Nation, Plain Talk, Common Ground, World Tomorrow,* and *Americas,* all white, and what can be called liberal publications. He did not neglect the black press, for his byline also was in *Opportunity, Negro Digest,* and *Crisis.* But in the past few decades his work has appeared, when in magazines, in the rightist periodicals, socially and politically: *Freeman, National Review, Human Events,* and *American Opinion,* the latter the John Birch Society magazine. All are white.

In 1953 he was cited by Lincoln University for his performance in journalism. Fifteen years later he had come to represent ultra-reactionaryism to the militants among the nation's blacks. He documented his position in a straight-forward autobiography, *Black and Conservative.* Whatever one thinks about his social outlook, his writing style and use of irony and wit in making his points mark him as outstanding among black editorialists. Sancton called him "a clear and vivid writer," adding: "Sometimes he writes with a mordant sarcasm, but he does not let it unbalance the order of his ideas. And he hammers what seems to me the soundest line of all: that the Negroes' natural friend, and natural ally, is the white worker, and that the two should strive for a unity of purpose in the labor movement."[10] From this comment it is obvious that Sancton was writing in the early 1940's, when white labor was identified with the hardships the black society still has not overcome.

During Marcus Garvey's day Schuyler was skeptical about the man who has been called the black Moses, chiefly because he sought to lead the black man out of his misery with various somewhat grandiose plans. When Garvey founded a new church body, the African Orthodox Church, and wrote that God was black, Schuyler commented: "Last summer Marcus accused the Deity of being a Negro. No wonder the luck went against him!"[11]

Schuyler, less productive as the 1970's began, nevertheless was still in view. *American Opinion* at that time carried a picture of him on its cover and a tribute to his social philosophy inside.

The Black Sportswriters. A. S. (Doc) Young, himself one of the most widely known black sportswriters, told the stories of some other sports journalists of the black press world in *Ebony* in 1970. Young observed that editors often are overworked because they lack staff assistance. Frequently writers only are tolerated by their white colleagues, and they are bypassed by prominent black athletes on stories and book manuscripts, since the stars tend to take their material to white writers and publishers. Moonlighting often is necessary for the sports, journalist, Young notes, and cites the experience of Brad Pye, Jr., sports editor of the Los Angeles *Sentinel.* To get the income he needs to support his family, Pye must be sports editor, sports publicist, scout, sportscaster, and a member of the Los Angeles Recreation and Parks Department.

Among the sports journalists of the past he mentions Frank A. (Fay) Young (no relative), who for many years was sports editor of the Chicago *Defender.* He considers Young the dean of them all and father of the sports section in the black newspaper. Others singled out are Bill Nunn, Sr., Bill Nunn, Jr., Wendell Smith, and Chester L. Washington, all of the Pittsburgh *Courier;* Eric (Ric) Roberts, of the Atlanta *Daily World,* and Abie Robinson, sports editor of the *California Eagle* and the Los Angeles *Sentinel.*

First Black TV Newsman. Faced with competition the white journalist does not have to confront, the black newsman or magazinist has found that versatility or intense specialization is an asset. A number of the journalists mentioned so far in this chapter have possessed one quality or the other. The late Louis E. Lomax, who broke a precedent when he became the first black newsman on television, was another who had various talents. A Georgian, born in 1922, he came of a family of teachers and writers. At Augusta's Paine College he began his journalism by becoming editor of the *Paineite,* the college paper. His first professional journalism was with the Baltimore *Afro-American.* He continued his formal education by attending American University in Washington for graduate work. This study led to a faculty post at Georgia State College in Savannah, where he taught philosophy. He did further graduate work at Yale.

Lomax returned to journalism as a staff writer for the Chicago *American,* now called *Chicago Today,* a large white daily. It was in 1958 that he went into television, at WNTA-TV, New York, and was the first black newsman for what was then a fairly new medium. He continued writing by contributing articles to such major magazines as *Harper's, Nation,* and *New Republic.* Three years later he published his first book, *The Reluctant African.* It brought him the Anisfield Wolf-*Saturday Review* Award for 1961. He also wrote *To Kill a Black Man, When the Word is Given, The Black Revolt,* and *Thailand.* His television work was writing and producing as well as handling news. With Mike Wallace he wrote and produced a program called "The Hate That Hate Produced." He also was associate producer of a prizewinning documentary, "Walk in My Shoes," seen on American Broadcasting Company stations. At his death in 1970 in an automobile accident he was professor of humanities and social sciences at Hofstra University.

The Washington Scene. Louis R. Lautier broke into the news himself in 1947 when he became the center of a case in which, because of his race, he was refused admission to the Congressional Press Gallery in Washington, an area for reporters covering Congress. This and other media galleries are operated under rules adopted by the standing committee of correspondents whose members are elected by the newsmen. Reporters whose credentials have not been approved by the committee cannot sit in the gallery. Lautier was turned down ostensibly on grounds other than race but fought the case out and was recognized. The National Press Club, which for years has occupied two floors at the top of the National Press Building in the national capital, also held out against admitting not only black journalists but women applicants as well. Lautier gained admission in 1955; the stricture against women was dropped in 1970. It was the restrictive attitude which led to formation of the Capital Press Club by black journalists working in Washington. Both men and women of any race are accepted.

Lautier worked for the National Newspaper Publishers Association in the days when it ran a news service for its member papers; he also was on the staff of the Atlanta *Daily World*. He won a Willkie Award for Journalism as a result of his successful fight to gain admission to the press gallery.

As will have been noted by now, most black journalists who have attained home degree of public recognition had accumulated journalism experience before attaining their topmost positions. But Charles Sumner Stone, Jr., better known as Chuck Stone, appears not to have had any such preliminary preparation. Yet, before he was forty, he had been the top editor of three major national black newspapers: *New York Age,* the Washington edition of the *Afro-American,* and the Chicago *Daily Defender.* During his ten years in black news work Stone won two awards and then moved on to organization and government committee public information activity.

A St. Louisian, born there in 1924, Stone went to New England for his first college degree and then to the Midwest for his second. From Wesleyan University he received an A.B. in 1948; from the University of Chicago a master of arts degree in sociology two years later. From 1956 to 1958 he was employed by CARE, the first year in India, Egypt, and Gaza and the next as an educational consultant in the U.S. In 1958 he went to *Age* as editor; in 1960 moved to the Washington paper; in another three years to the Chicago daily. He won a first prize from the National Newspaper Publishers Association for the best column of 1960 and was named for an Outstanding Newsman of the Year award the next year.

Stone left journalism for the tangential field of public information, becoming executive assistant for the committee of education and labor of the U.S. Congress, public information director and vice chairman of the National Conference on Black Power, and a member of the steering committee of the Black United Front, Washington. In early 1970 he became director of educational opportunity projects, Educational Testing Service, Princeton, New Jersey. During 1969–70 he appeared every few weeks on NBC's television program, "Today," as a commentator on racial problems. He withdrew from the program in 1970, saying that he was unable to communicate with "white America" and reported receiving antagonistic mail.[12] Stone is author of three books, *Tell It Like It Is* and *Black Political Power in America,* both non-fiction, and a novel, *King Strut,* published in 1970.

Also active in government service has been William Gordon, a senior officer of the USIA in Washington, who has as one of his duties the writing of a weekly column on civil rights for distribution to media of communication in other countries and to the Department of State's agencies abroad. Since the citizens of other nations, especially those with nonwhite populations, watch the racial events in the U.S.A. closely, Gordon is in a vital and sensitive position.

His journalistic experience before joining USIA was extensive.

His first work came in 1947, after he had received his A.B. from LeMoyne College. He was a copy boy at New York *PM,* the adless daily. He became an editorial clerk there before serving for a few months late in 1948 as a special assignments reporter for the New York *Star,* another white paper that tried to stay in New York after *PM* failed. During most of 1949 he was city editor of the Newark (N.J.) *Herald News,* but moved from there to the Atlanta *Daily World,* the great training ground so many black journalists have used. During nearly a decade there he was associate and then managing editor. During 1958–59 Gordon was an Ogden Reid International Journalism Fellow in Africa, remaining on that continent for five years more, leaving then for government service, at first as branch public affairs officer in Enugu, Nigeria, and then chief information officer at Lagos in the same country. He was assigned to Sweden in 1964 as director of USIS in Stockholm for two years. He did graduate work at Columbia and New York Universities, in 1949 receiving a master's degree in economics, the subject of his undergraduate major. In 1952–53 he was a Nieman Fellow at Harvard. Gordon served, in 1969–70, as Kemper Knapp visiting professor in the School of Journalism at the University of Wisconsin, a post for which he also had preparation, since he had taught journalism and other subjects at Morris Brown College and Cannon Theological Seminary in Atlanta while on the black daily there.

Clarke, Scholarly Journalist. An entirely different experience has been that of John Henrik Clarke, whose journalism has been combined with historical scholarship despite early lack of formal education. He has been identified with five black publications. Born in 1915 in Union Springs, Alabama, he grew up in the textile mill city of Columbus, Georgia, one of nine children. His boyhood is a familiar one of being in poverty, learning to read sooner than others in the family, and being expected to accomplish much. Even at grammar school he was interested in history and was an eager reader of books, magazines, and newspapers. During his two-faceted career he has contributed short stories to many U.S. and foreign publications. Creative writing attracted him early; he went to New York in 1933 to study at the League of American Writers School and at Columbia University. He also became interested in the writing of poetry and has contributed verse as well as articles and criticism to numerous publications. Some of his tales have been on the "distinction" list in *Best American Short Stories,* an annual compilation.

Clarke's publication connections include being co-founder and fiction editor of *Harlem Quarterly,* book review editor of the *Negro History Bulletin,* and associate editor of *Freedomways,* his present principal journalism activity. He has been a feature writer, also, for the Pittsburgh *Courier* and the Ghana *Evening News.* His articles have appeared in numerous other black periodicals.

Like most scholarly journalists, he has had a hand in book writing and editing, largely the latter, editing several volumes of black literature, such as *American Negro Short Stories* and *Tales from Harlem,* as well as books on Harlem or leading black figures, including Malcolm X, Garvey, and Du Bois.

He now teaches at several institutions as a lecturer on history. He also is on the Urban Leadership training program faculty. His devotion to black history, in which he has had classes at Hunter, Cornell, and Columbia, began when he was told that the black people had no history. One day he saw an essay by Arthur H. Schomburg about the black man's past. He sought out Schomburg, who now is best known for the branch of the New York Public Library in Harlem bearing his name which is a center for study of black history and culture. Clarke was told to "study the history of your oppressor" and to understand the history of his people.

Probably Clarke is known most widely for his work in the somewhat controversial 108-part television series, "Black Heritage, A History of Afro-Americans," shown on the Columbia Broadcasting System network in 1968. He coordinated it and was a member of the committee that developed the program and gave some of the lectures. Subsequently he began editing a twenty-volume illustrated work based on the series.

Other Types of Experience. Two other men illustrate other types of experience, Henry Lee Moon and George M. Daniels. Moon, now director of public relations for the NAACP and editor of its magazine, *Crisis,* had a labor union connection before he went to the association. He was assistant to the director of the political action committee of the Congress of Industrial Organizations. Moon also is among the journalism school-trained black journalists. His bachelor of arts degree was earned at Howard. The next year, 1923–24, he attended Ohio State and received a bachelor's degree in journalism as well. Seventeen years later he took courses in public relations and public administration at American University.

In the meantime he was a journalist, from 1926 to 1931 as editor of the Tuskegee *Messenger* and assistant to the press relations secretary of Tuskegee Institute. Then he went to the staffs of the Cleveland *Call,* Cleveland *Herald,* and the New York *Amsterdam News,* all black weeklies. He also covered the organizing meeting of the World Federation of Trade Unions in London in 1945 for the Chicago *Defender.* His experience also includes six years, 1938–44, as regional racial relations adviser with the Federal Public Housing Authority. More recently he was for six years a member of the board of directors of the Joint Queensview Housing Enterprise and for another period on the boards of the United Housing Foundation and the National Housing Conference. Moon has done considerable magazine writing, having contributed articles to *Nation, New Republic, Saturday Review,*

New Leader, Phylon, Opportunity, and *Crisis* as well as to the New York *Times,* New York *Post,* and the London *Tribune.*

Public relations has lured black journalists just as it has white. The road to such work for George M. Daniels, director of interpretive services of the United Methodist Church's Board of Missions in New York, led through editorial positions on a black news agency, a black daily, a black fraternal magazine, and two white religious magazines. A Drake University and Columbia University graduate, with journalism degrees from each, Daniels soon after graduation from the Des Moines institution became a rewrite man and foreign news editor for the Associated Negro Press, a wire service. He went from there, in 1954, to the Chicago *Daily Defender.* There he was awarded the Chicago Newspaper Guild's Page One Award for "outstanding performance in the field of journalism." He left black journalism to do editorial work in Chicago for *Together* and *Christian Advocate,* two large magazines published by the white denomination, the United Methodist Church. This work led to a move to New York to his present post. In addition for three years he edited the *Sphinx,* the magazine of Alpha Phi Alpha fraternity.

Two books have come from his deep interest and personal experiences in Africa: *The Church in New Nations* and *Southern Africa: A Time for Change.* In 1962 and 1965 he visited that continent and has been in nine of the countries.

***The Johnson* Ménage.** Because of their prestige, the higher salaries that may be paid, or for less realistic and tangible reasons, certain publications attract more of the talented journalists than others. The New York *Times* and the *New Yorker* magazine have done so in the world of white journalism. *Ebony* magazine has gained that reputation in black journalism. Some writers and editors came to it via its companion magazines, *Jet, Black World,* and *Tan* as well as those no longer issued, *Hue* and *Ebony International.* All are or were owned by the Johnson Publishing Company in Chicago.

Alex Poinsett, an *Ebony* senior staff editor, has specialized in education writing. He won a trophy and a $1,000 cash award in the second annual Penney-Missouri magazine competition for his article, "Ghetto Schools, An Educational Wasteland." He won another for his education writing in 1963. A journalism graduate of the University of Illinois in 1952, he remained another year to earn his master's degree in philosophy, and then did graduate work in library science at the University of Chicago. He went to the Johnson firm in 1954.

Another award winner in the Johnson *ménage* is Simeon Booker, a Washington reporter since 1949. Now head of the *Ebony-Jet* bureau in the nation's capital, he also has done national radio and television broadcasts on racial problems and is a commentator for the Washington TV-radio group. Booker, who came from Youngstown, Ohio, attended Virginia Union University and was a Nieman Fellow. Like

Poinsett, he won a Wendell Willkie award for an educational series.

Booker has worked for the Cleveland *Call and Post* as well as the large white Washington *Post,* where he was its first black reporter. He is author of several books. In *Black Man's America* he discusses the black press as well as other black institutions. In *Susie King Taylor* he tells the story of a black nurse. His viewpoint can be gauged by an incident that occurred in 1969 while he was chief of the bureau in Washington. He was invited by the Mayor's Human Relations Commission to speak at its annual dinner in his home town of Youngstown. But when he was asked to avoid any mention of the city administration and the mayor he left the banquet hall without speaking because he objected to what he considered censorship.[13]

Black photographers and photojournalists who have received recognition for their work are few. One, Moneta Sleet, Jr., brought the Johnson publications a Pulitzer Prize in 1969 with his picture of Mrs. Martin Luther King, Jr., and her daughter Bernice, taken at Dr. King's funeral. A staff photographer for *Ebony* since 1955, he had worked behind the camera for five years before that for *Our World,* another black consumer magazine. A Kentuckian, Sleet was born in Owensboro in 1926. He studied at Kentucky State College; after graduation he attended the School of Modern Photography, New York. He also received a master's degree in journalism from New York University and has taught photography at Maryland State College.

Photography has not led many black journalists into the field of journalism but it was a factor for Herbert Nipson, managing editor of *Ebony* since 1963. He was a cameraman for the *Daily Iowan* in Iowa City and a writer-photographer stringer for the Cedar Rapids *Gazette* before going to *Ebony* in 1949. Nipson came from North Carolina, born in 1916 in Asheville. When two years old he was taken to Clearfield, Pennsylvania. He went to high school there and then on to Penn State University, receiving a journalism degree in 1940. While there he wrote for the *Penn State Collegian* and two literary publications. After graduation he joined the staff of the *Brown American* magazine in Philadelphia, first as assistant editor and then editor. After military service from 1941 to 1946 he took a master's in fine arts at the University of Iowa. Once on the *Ebony* staff, in 1949, he went on to become co-managing editor in 1951 and managing editor twelve years later.

One of the most scholarly of the Johnson staffers is Lerone Bennett, Jr., associated with the firm since 1953. He is author of a half-dozen books, the contents of some widely read because they first ran as *Ebony* articles; several are being used in black studies programs at various colleges and universities. He has become a recognized historian of black America.

Bennett's study of and writings on black history have not been free of controversy. In 1968 *Ebony* carried an article which startled readers: "Was Abraham Lincoln a White Supremacist?" He concluded that the president had been one, and cited the researches of white scholars as well as his own investigation in support of the view. His books include *Before the Mayflower,* tracing the history of blacks in America from 1619 to 1966; *Black Power U.S.A.,* describing the Reconstruction period, a time in history when blacks had considerable power. Several other volumes are on contemporary social problems; another is a biography of Martin Luther King, Jr. Born in 1928 in Clarksdale, Mississippi, and a graduate in economics from Morehouse College, he went into full-time journalism from college. At Morehouse he edited the *Maroon Tiger.* As a teen-ager he had worked on the black papers in Jackson, including the *Mississippi Enterprise.* Like several other Johnson editorial people he is a one-time reporter for the Atlanta *Daily World.* Beginning as a reporter, he had become city editor by 1953. In that year he undertook his first work at the Chicago magazine company, as an *Ebony* associate editor. In 1958 he became senior editor.

Poinsett, Booker, and Bennett are among the writers and editors on the Johnson magazine staffs who have received considerable public recognition. Other, younger men and women have had less spectacular success with their work but should not be overlooked. A dozen other names could be added, for these publications have been published since the 1940's and 1950's. Other present or recent staff members who have played important parts within the organization are Robert E. Johnson, not related to the owner, executive editor of *Jet;* Hans J. Massaquoit, assistant managing editor of *Ebony;* Hoyt W. Fuller, managing editor of *Black World,* and Phyllis Garland, *Ebony* New York editor.

Robert Johnson's original intention was to become a lawyer, but journalism interfered with his plan. An Alabamian by birth, he gave journalism a start in his life before the law had an opportunity by being editor of *Trail Blazer,* the Westfield High School paper in Birmingham. This work threw him into association with the paper's faculty adviser, a history teacher who also was managing editor of the Birmingham *World,* a black weekly. That led to two jobs, as cub reporter and salesman. When Johnson attended Morehouse College, still planning a law career, like Bennett he edited the *Maroon Tiger.* He added editing of the yearbook, *The Torch.* World War II and the navy interrupted his college work but not his journalism, for in the service he was assigned to be a reporter for the *Masthead,* a San Francisco naval base weekly. He was ordered to do this work because the paper's editor had published an anti-black joke and it was thought that giving him the black news beat would allay the criticism that had resulted from printing the joke. In the year he was on the naval paper Johnson went from reporter to managing editor. The law career was as far away as ever, but not forgotten.

Next the Twelfth Naval District Press Association selected Johnson to be a war correspondent. He interviewed sailors for stories to be sent to their hometown press, going to the Hawaiian Islands,

Okinawa, and the Philippines on these assignments. His naval journalism experience covered more than three years. When he was discharged in 1946 he attempted to continue his law plans. But he still lacked two undergraduate college years, so he returned to Morehouse, was graduated in 1948 and went, not to law, but back to journalism by joining the Atlanta *Daily World* staff, covering the standard beats. From reporting sports, police, and courts he became city editor in a year. The law definitely had lost out by 1951, when he took a leave of absence to work on a master's in journalism at the School of Journalism at Syracuse University. After a year, master's in news editorial work safely in hand, he returned to the *World*. While in Atlanta he added free lance writing to his interests.

Among the publications that took his articles was *Jet,* the small-format newsmagazine of the Johnson firm. One day he had an offer of full-time there, but refused it. Eventually, however, he agreed and became an associate editor in 1953, and successively assistant managing editor, managing editor, and then executive editor, his present title. He told an interviewer in 1970 that he has no regrets about having chosen journalism over the law, although he still takes an evening law course in Chicago occasionally.[14]

Specialized Journalists. Not all black journalists work only for consumer newspapers and magazines and broadcasting stations. A few are to be found on the staffs of trade and technical journals and those numerous but often forgotten examples of specialized journalism, the house organs or industrial publications. The nature and number of such publications as members of the black journalism corps are obscure (see Chapter 8). The stories of a few of their staff members have come to light, however.

In the world of the business press is a group of about 2,700 newspapers and magazines, mainly in the latter format, which cover more than business but generally are linked with the type of publication identified with merchandising, professions, institutions, and techniques. Almost all are white-owned. H. Lance Barclay is in this aspect of journalism, connected with the Reuben H. Donnelley Corporation of New York. He became director of special projects of the magazine division of the firm, in 1970, after having been district manager of *Textile Services Management* magazine and before that business manager of two international magazines also issued by the firm, a position which took him overseas to attend conferences and on other business missions. He also was responsible for an industry market letter. A graduate of Franklin and Marshall College and of Columbia University, he has been working for a Ph.D. at New York University in the field of American urban history and urban problems. Barclay has been a consultant to *Scholastic* magazines, publisher of many periodicals and books for youth, on its American Negro History Project.

Among the few editors of publications in another area of business journalism—house organs, or as their editors prefer to call them, corporate or industrial publications—is a veteran black journalist, George W. Lee, editor of *Vision,* the internal or employee magazine of the Atlanta Life Insurance Company. Although lacking in editorial experience when he became responsible for the magazine, one typical of the approximately 10,000 publications of this type in the U.S.A., he has engaged in other activities that involve different writing problems, particularly the production of books. A Mississippian born on a farm early in this century, Lee received a bachelor's degree from Alcorn College. He then went into the insurance business as an agent, going on to a district managership and his present post in the executive offices, for he also is a vice-president of the firm. Like many another house publication editor, he knew far more about the field of insurance than he did about that of journalism. He is author of three books. One, *Beale Street,* grew out of his friendship with W. C. Handy, of jazz music fame. His editorials in *Vision* are concerned with general problems of the black race, in contrast to the mainly company or personnel news on other pages.

And Many, Many More. Among other black journalists known within the profession is Layhmond Robinson, who has been with the New York *Times* as a reporter and WABC-TV, New York, as a correspondent, in public relations work for the National Urban League, and in 1970 was named chief information officer of the New York City hospital system.

Lestre H. Brownlee, a Chicago *Defender* staffer after he left the Medill School of Journalism at Northwestern University in suburban Evanston, Illinois, at first was a reporter and rewrite man. He then joined *Ebony* as associate editor of that monthly, also published in Chicago. He left to become the first black reporter for the Chicago *Daily News,* then returned to his old paper, the *Defender,* to work in its advertising and public relations department, moving from there in the late 1960's to WLS-TV, a Chicago station, as a newsman. Thus he has done newspaper, magazine, and broadcasting work.

Martin D. Richardson, who was connected with various papers, at one time was managing editor of the Boston *Chronicle* but worked mainly on the black Cleveland *Call and Post.* William I. Gibson has held top posts on the *Afro-American,* including managing editorship of the Washington edition. The late Clifford Wesley Mackay was with both the country's black dailies. On the Chicago *Daily Defender* he was theatrical editor; on the Atlanta *Daily World,* managing editor. He also was editor-in-chief of the *Afro-American.* Another *World* man, Stanley Scott, a member of the family that owns the paper, left it because he wanted to cover more than the black community. For a while he was with the NAACP, but then became a reporter for WINS, New York, where he covered other than black assignments. He was one of the first black reporters with United Press International, to which he went from his family's paper. In 1970 Scott won the Russworm Award of the National Urban League for "sustained excellence in interpreting, analyzing and reporting of the news" and his "use of the immense power of the press in advocating equality for all in the best American traditions."

Other prominent journalists include Moses J. Newson, executive editor of the Baltimore *Afro-American;* Claude Lewis, formerly of *Newsweek* and the New York *Herald Tribune* and later an NBC commentator; Jesse H. Walker, executive editor, New York *Amsterdam News;* Thomas A. Johnson, New York *Times* reporter; William Worthy, controversial *Afro-American* foreign correspondent and a Nieman Fellow at Harvard; Louis E. Martin, editor-in-chief, Sengstacke Newspapers; Ted Poston, once on the New York *Amsterdam News,* but long with the New York *Post;* John Pittman, writer and editor for both black and white papers; Rudolph A. Pyatt, Jr., Washington correspondent, Charleston (S.C.) *News* and *Courier;* Ernest Dunbar, senior editor, *Look;* William J. Raspberry, Washington *Post* columnist; Lutrelle F. Palmer, Chicago *Daily News* reporter and columnist; and Fletcher Martin, city editor of the Louisville *Defender,* and war correspondent.

Some from the past who worked mainly on white publications were Orrin Evans, of the Philadelphia *Record* as well as the *Philadelphia Tribune,* the first a white paper and now defunct, the second still one of the major black papers; Horace Cayton and Joseph Bibb, both of the Chicago *Sun-Times* when it was only the Chicago *Sun;* Edgar T. Rouzzeau, of the now departed great New York daily, the *Herald Tribune;* George Anthony Moore, the Cleveland *Press;* Earl Brown, *Life* magazine staff man and later active in New York City political life; Frank Harriott, of New York *PM;* Eugene Gordon, New York *Daily Worker;* and Michael Carter, Brooklyn *Daily Eagle.*

● TODAY'S WOMEN JOURNALISTS

This report on the black journalists discusses women in a separate section because the relatively few who have been productive writers and editors would be lost in the accounts of the men. Although in black journalism there is somewhat less tendency to give men the job advantages than exists in white newspaper and magazine work, women nevertheless are a small minority. The reasons do not necessarily include sex discrimination. Black women, even more so than black men, have had little chance to obtain journalism training. Opportunities leading to major positions are claimed by men, as in white journalism, because traditionally the male is the family head and financially responsible. Work on black publications, especially newspapers, is more difficult than on white, since the black paper does not have the entrée accorded the white, as a rule. If black journalism is more nearly a man's job than white journalism, women make less progress in it. Nor have many women been interested in journalism as a life work; they too have heard of the long hours and low salaries.

But the romantic view that some persons have ink instead of blood in their veins exists for black journalism as well, with the result that some women have made a reputation for themselves in this occupation. And in recent years, women's place has become a little larger, with the increase in consumer and specialized black magazines, although the greatest area of growth has been on the white publications. By this time it is clear that the situation is better for the black woman journalist.

Until now only a few have had much opportunity to make their skills and views felt. Chapter 2 presents what Penn, the recorder of nineteenth century black journalism and journalists, had to say about black women journalists. In what follows some of the better-known twentieth century women are accounted for.

The title "International Editor" is an unusual one in U.S. journalism. Its meaning is not exactly clear, but it is the designation for one of the widely known black journalists of either sex, Miss Era Bell Thompson, a member of the Johnson firm. She occupies this position at *Ebony* and for some years has lived up to one sense of it by being international in her movements, particularly in journeys to and from Africa.

The senior member of the staff aside from the company's founder, John H. Johnson, Miss Thompson has been connected with these publications since 1947. She began as an editor of the first periodical, *Black World* (then *Negro Digest*) and went on to executive positions at *Ebony*. An Iowan born in Des Moines, she spent two years at the University of North Dakota, and then completed her bachelor's degree at Morningside College in 1933. During 1938–40 she did graduate work at the Medill School of Journalism, Northwestern University. Before putting her journalistic training to work she was a senior interviewer for the U.S. and Illinois employment services. She then was given a general assignment as an associate editor at Johnson's. After her stint with *Negro Digest* she was named co-managing editor of *Ebony,* holding that post from 1951 to 1964. Her world traveling increased in the latter year, when she was made international editor.

Although Miss Thompson has gone to all continents as a writer, she naturally has concentrated on Africa. From there she has written articles on such subjects as the progress of the new black republics and about safaris of black hunters. She has not been welcome in South Africa, once spending a night in jail awaiting deportation. On a second attempt to enter that country of belief in apartheid she was denied a visa. Like several other Johnson staffers she writes books. *American Daughter,* an autobiographical work, was written before she went into journalism and sheds no light on her writing career. She speaks frequently before women's groups, black and white, and is active in various religious, social, and cultural organizations.

Another women journalist identified with a prominent publishing firm is Mrs. Elizabeth Murphy Moss, of the *Afro-American* newspapers. Mrs. Moss, who has been a war correspondent as well as managing editor of the Baltimore paper, is now vice-president, treasurer, and editorial supervisor of the publishing firm, of which her family has long been the owner. She is one of several black women in executive positions on newspapers; in most instances the others are officers who have succeeded their husbands as owners, managers, treasurers, and secretaries when they were made widows.

Up to early 1970 Miss Ethel L. Payne, Washington correspondent of the Sengstacke Newspapers, was the only black newswoman to be assigned to cover the Vietnam War. She spent ten weeks there in 1966–67, writing about the activities of black servicemen from Da Nang to the Mekong Delta. She also sent dispatches from Hong Kong, Korea, Thailand, and Japan. In 1970 she was one in a group of journalists who accompanied the U.S. Secretary of State on an Asian tour. War, however, has not been Miss Payne's only assignment. She has covered a wide variety of other stories. Her regular beat includes the White House, Capitol Hill, the District of Columbia, and various government agencies. A Chicagoan and like Miss Thompson a onetime Northwestern journalism student, Miss Payne was one of a group of thirty-five reporters who in 1957 went with then Vice-President and Mrs. Richard M. Nixon to various African and European nations. Earlier she had covered the Asian-African conference at Bandung, Indonesia. She also was sent by her papers to write about the Nigerian civil war in 1969 and the World Council of Churches assembly at Uppsala, Sweden, in 1968.

Miss Payne also has had experience in government posts. She has been a consultant to the Special Security Administration and visited twenty-two cities for the Medical Alert Program. As a staff member of the AFL-CIO Committee on Political Education in Washington she wrote for and edited its bi-weekly, *Notes from COPE*. She has worked as well for the Democratic Party in Texas and for the national party's Conference of Women. She has won numerous awards for her work, twice being given the Newsmen's Newsman Award of the Capital Press Club, of which she became president in 1970.

Describing how she entered journalism in the first place she has said: "My career in journalism began by accident. While I was working in Japan as an Army Service Club hostess, I put down my impressions of life under the Occupation . . . those jottings found their way into the Chicago *Defender* and caused an earthquake in the high command. But for the intervention of Thurgood Marshall, who happened to be in the country on a court martial case, I would

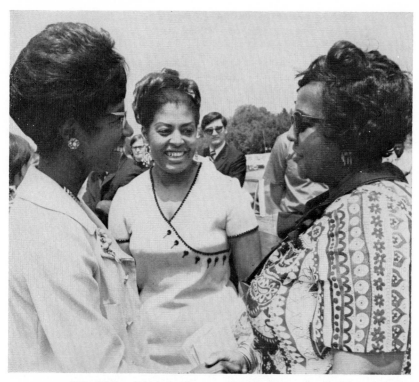

FIG. 10.3. Ethel L. Payne, Washington correspondent of the
Sengstacke Newspapers (right) with Representative Shirley Chisholm (left). Miss Payne has had numerous awards for her work.

have been cashiered and sent home in chains for allegedly upsetting
the morale of the troops. Six months later, I left under my own power
and joined the staff of the *Defender,* where I have remained off and on
for the past 19 years."[15]

On Smaller Publications. Because their publications are recent and
small, two other black women journalists with like aims and interests
have not become widely known. They represent the personnel of
small newspapers and magazines. One is Mrs. Barbara Winters,
editor of the *Star,* a weekly newspaper published in New Haven,
Connecticut, and the other is Miss Virginia W. Williams, co-publisher of *Echo,* a local magazine in Milwaukee. Mrs. Winters was
editor of her college paper at Bennett, in North Carolina, and then
became a staff member at the Hamden (Conn.) *Chronicle,* a weekly.
In early 1969 she took over the editorship of the *Star,* which had
begun as a newsletter the year before but had become a printed,
tabloid newspaper called the *Crow* until 1971.

Miss Williams, originally from Birmingham, Alabama, received
a degree in elementary education at Alabama State Teachers College.

Later she did graduate work in education, English, and journalism at Marquette University, Milwaukee. Her study of creative writing led her in 1966 to establish with a friend a monthly community magazine and a writers' workshop, all as part of a federally supported community project. In Milwaukee she also works as an editor for a city agency.

Two others represent the few women who have taught journalism. Mrs. Thelma Thurston Gorham and Miss Consuelo Young both were at one time on the Lincoln University department of journalism faculty. Mrs. Gorham edited *Step-Up,* a magazine for black businessmen, is a writer on black journalism, and now on the staff of *New Lady* magazine as a senior editor. She also has been managing editor of the Tulsa (Okla.) *Eagle.* She received her master's degree in journalism from the University of Minnesota in 1941, writing on "Negro Newsmen and Practices of Pressure Groups in the Middle West."

Miss Young, whose master's degree in journalism came from Northwestern in 1943, served in India on assignment from the U.S. State Department and in other posts. She also has made special studies of black journalism in the U.S.A. and written about it.

Other black women have served on publications and broadcasting staffs. Mrs. Dorothy Gilliam, formerly of the Washington *Post* and then at WTTG, Washington, also teaches a course on black journalism history at American University, one of the first of its kind. Lena Rivers Smith has been on the staff of the Pittsburgh *Courier,* Kansas City *Call,* and with the *Informer* chain, where she was once managing editor, in Houston. Miss Lucile H. Bluford, managing editor of the *Call,* was cited in 1961 by Lincoln University for her work, by then amounting to a quarter of a century, as a reporter and editor for that weekly. It was her suit against the University of Missouri, recounted elsewhere in this book, that led to establishment of Lincoln's journalism department.

Mrs. Walter Stoval, who writes for the New York *Times* under her maiden name, Charlayne Hunter, in addition to being a byliner for that daily has twice made national news herself. In 1961 she was the first black woman to be admitted to the University of Georgia and one of the first two black persons accepted there. A campus riot greeted the two new students when they arrived at the Athens institution. She was graduated in 1963. For many years women journalists have been denied membership in Sigma Delta Chi, professional journalism society. In 1969 the doors were opened to them. Miss Hunter was the first woman admitted to the Georgia chapter and thought to be one of the first two women accepted by this large national group.

Many black newspapers and a few magazines have on their staffs women writers and editors. Scores are society, women's interest, and religious editors or columnists, few of them working at it full time, however. Among the more familiar names are those of Betty Granger Reid of the New York *Amsterdam News,* Theresa Fambro Hooks of the Chicago *Daily Defender,* Nancy L. Giddens, Philadelphia *Tribune,* and Toki Schalk Johnson of the Pittsburgh *Courier*. The larger papers have as many as a half-dozen women contributing special depart- ments—society, food, religion, fashions, entertainment, and gossip— in every issue.

Women staffers on magazines, as in other periodicals, have risen to places of control in some instances. Much of the work in the editorial departments of the four consumer magazines published by Good at Fort Worth is done by women staff members. Edna K. Turner is editor of *Sepia;* she also is managing editor of *Jive* and *Hep,* and co-managing editor of *Bronze Thrills.* Eunice J. Wilson serves as man- aging editor of *Sepia,* is co-managing editor of *Bronze Thrills* with Mrs. Turner, and associate editor of *Jive* and *Hep.* Miss Leoma Wheat heads the art department of all four.

● WHITES IN BLACK JOURNALISM

A look at black journalism in the U.S.A. should not fail to note that a few whites have worked for black newspapers and magazines. It is a two-way street, although most of the traffic has been one way. The motivations of those whites who have gone to black publications are not always clear; few have explained their reasoning. It is not unwarranted to assume that some certainly have done so out of ideal- ism, hoping to assist the race in its fight for just treatment. A few active in this sort of journalistic switch or crossover are noted here.

Ward Caille, for twenty years on the Chicago *Daily News* staff, left that paper when he was night editor to become managing editor of the Chicago *Defender*. Ben Burns was among the early managing editors of *Ebony* (see Chapter 7) remaining until his somewhat sensa- tional policies appeared to be losing subscribers. Earl Conrad, a New York newspaperman who went to the *Defender* also, served voluntarily, it has been said. He headed its New York bureau. He wrote fre- quently as well for major magazines and published a number of books about black life, including *Jim Crow America,* which attracted wide attention in the later 1940's.

A few black newspapers and magazines today carry the work of other white journalists, but usually as outside contributors. With the growing desire of blacks not to be dependent upon whites if avoidable, and the clear opposition of certain militants toward any reliance whatsoever upon "the man" or the "honkies," employment of whites is largely clerical or in highly specialized positions which few blacks are as yet trained to fill.

● PRESS ORGANIZATIONS

The black journalists have few organizations of their own. Some belong to the various white-dominated groups, such as the one large labor union, the American Newspaper Guild, or to comparable organizations in the broadcasting field. An increasing number are joining Sigma Delta Chi and Theta Sigma Phi, national journalism honoraries, either through college chapters or professional units in the larger cities. They are affiliating also with various associations, also dominantly white, existing in a few specialties, such as the Religious Public Relations Association, the Associated Church Press, and the Religion Newswriters Association.

Four black journalists' groups were united in 1970 into the National Association of Black Media Workers as an outcome of the case of Earl Caldwell, a black correspondent for the New York *Times* in San Francisco who refused to testify before a grand jury investigating the Black Panther Party. These included Black Perspective, of New York, which earlier had rallied to Caldwell by hiring a lawyer to help defend him and had affirmed its position on the integrity and freedom of the black reporter; the Black Journalists of the San Francisco Bay Area, publisher of the *Ball and Chain Review,* one of the few publications on the black press, and similar groups in Chicago and Nashville. NABMW, beginning with fifty members, decided to accept both print and broadcast personnel.[16]

In a message "to the Black Community from Black Journalists" Black Perspective had said:

> We will not be used as spies, informants or undercover agents by anybody.
> We will protect our confidential sources, using every means at our disposal.
> We strongly object to attempts by law enforcement agencies to exploit our blackness.[17]

Among the signers were mainly staffers of white New York publications, broadcasting stations, news services, and book firms, but writers for *Essence, Jet,* and *Ebony* magazines and the *Amsterdam News* and New York *Courier* also were in the list. The *Times* supported Caldwell by hiring a constitutional lawyer to represent him and advising him to refuse to appear with his notes.

Another organization is the Afro-American Employes Association of the New York *Times.* The organization at the *Times* was founded by the black employes there "to protect their interest, welfare and security." It charged the New York paper with "a white racist attitude towards black workers," saying that the paper employs about 6,000 persons, of whom about 450 are from minority groups and that most are service workers and office and clerical help in lower level jobs.[18]

In Washington, black journalists of both sexes, rejected for many years by white organizations, formed their own Capital Press Club in 1944. Black women communicators have an organization of their own, somewhat like Theta Sigma Phi, which has had many black girls as members but is a dominantly white honorary society, or the white National Federation of Press Women. It is the National Association of Media Women, Inc., begun in 1966. Its present membership is between 150 and 300 in chapters meeting in Los Angeles, New York, Detroit, and Philadelphia. Its aims are to provide members with an opportunity to exchange ideas and experiences, to hold research seminars to find solutions to mutual problems, and to enlist young women in mass communication careers. For a time it published the *Media Woman*, a slick paper magazine. It came out several times a year and now is an annual. Eleven women originated the group, headed by Mrs. Rhea Callaway, formerly woman's editor of the *New York Age* and now manager of the Brooklyn edition of the New York *Amsterdam News*. She was the first president.

● WIDENING OPPORTUNITIES

The black journalist today stands nearer the edge of wider acceptance and opportunity than at any time in American journalistic history. The situation is favorable largely by comparison, for he had little acceptance of any sort until recent years. His own publications were too poor economically to sustain him. The white ones had no interest in him, even repelling him. For whomever he worked he might face humiliation and obstructionism. Jules Witcover, a white Washington correspondent, tells of the experience of a black member of the press corps there, working for a large black weekly who related an experience of his earlier days. He was covering a racial trial in the South. He had to go to the courthouse a day ahead of time, finding places where he would be allowed to eat, park a car, and telephone his story back to his paper. On the day of the trial he got up early and put an out-of-order sign on a phone booth so he'd have one to use.

"Then, after the morning session, I ran out and called in my story," he told another Washington reporter. It worked the first day, but on the second the operator said: "Aren't you the nigger boy who called yesterday? You just put that phone down." He protested but had to go to another phone.[19]

Training and education also no doubt played a part in the rejection of the black journalist and now are more than ever important in his new possibilities for service to his people and to himself. Under today's conditions there is less reason for lack of either to be used in refusing him an opportunity to practice the profession of journalism. ●

11. TRAINING AND EDUCATION

WHEN Miss Lucile H. Bluford, managing editor of the Kansas City *Call*, accepted a citation of merit for outstanding performance in journalism in 1961, she responded with this observation:

> Today, there is no limit for the graduate with ability and good training. The journalism graduate of today can aspire not only to positions of responsibility on one of the 142 Negro weeklies in the country—many of which are badly in need of competent editorial department personnel—but there are opportunities on metropolitan dailies, on the slick magazines, and in government and industry which were unheard of a few years ago.[1]

Miss Bluford could repeat her words today with great assurance that she is correct. Publishers of black newspapers and magazines complain of the difficulties of finding staff. John H. Sengstacke, president of the largest black journalistic empire, considers that he runs a journalism school himself, he prepares so many young men and women for the occupation, some of them going to other publications. And William O. Walker, editor and publisher of the Cleveland *Call and Post*, pointed out in 1970 that the white media, seeking at least to give token employment, have raided black newspapers for reporters and printers. The desperation about lack of staff sometimes expresses itself in incidents such as one that occurred early the same year when ten black students from Morgan State College visited Baltimore and Pittsburgh newspaper and television offices as part of a journalism course. At the Pittsburgh *Courier*, reported *Editor & Publisher*, a student was offered a job after being shown the office.[2] Several of the author's black journalism students, on visits to black publication offices as well as white to gather facts for class use, have been offered jobs on the spot, all in editorial positions.

In the decade since Miss Bluford first spoke her words in Jefferson City at Lincoln University, the efforts to train and educate black journalists have increased many times over. The problem today is not only to provide training but also to arouse interest in journalism as an occupation.

At the beginning of the 1960's a small number of students studied journalism in the white as well as black institutions. Scholarships and special training programs were few. This is not to say that the programs now available are sufficient in value or number, but they are far in advance of what existed only a few years ago.

Two principal methods are bringing more minority group people into journalism. One offers short courses and workshops for quick imparting of skills, usually but not always elementary. The other makes it easier for such persons to obtain a university journalism education, not by lowering standards but by providing practical help. Variations on these plans exist, including combining them, but in the long run the aim is the same: to train adult men and women or youths who have certain skills and know how to follow specific procedures and to help young persons, especially in getting a general education which includes a certain amount of professional training. The latter offers studies intended to help develop the mind and insure that students acquire knowledge beyond the area for which they are being prepared.

The goals of both training and education programs are broader than the vocational.[3] Other intentions are to enable blacks (as well as members of other ethnic groups) to fit into the economic structure, to be able to compete with the dominant group, to realize their ambitions, to use their talents, to drain off their dissatisfactions with society by giving them a stake in it, to obtain their cooperation in correcting the evils about which they complain, to obtain needed personnel for publishing houses, and, as one major plan explains it, ". . . to challenge and confront the racism so often apparent in many American newspapers, especially Southern newspapers."

● EXAMPLES OF TRAINING PLANS

The activities concerned purely with training vary in length and content. One of the most ambitious is the Frederick Douglass Fellowship Program launched in early 1969 by the *Afro-American* newspapers and the Virginia Council on Human Relations. Financed by a $123,000 grant from the Ford Foundation, it was open to fifteen young, would-be journalists. The scholarship winners were recruited from such disparate areas as colleges, prisons, the military services, VISTA volunteers, and returned Peace Corps members. Three hundred and fifty-five persons applied; fifteen were accepted and given a year's stipend of $4,200. All but one were black. They ranged in age from eighteen to thirty-nine, and six were women. Ten came from the South. After the program began one left to be married. Under direction of a former newspaperman and teacher, Frank T. Adams,

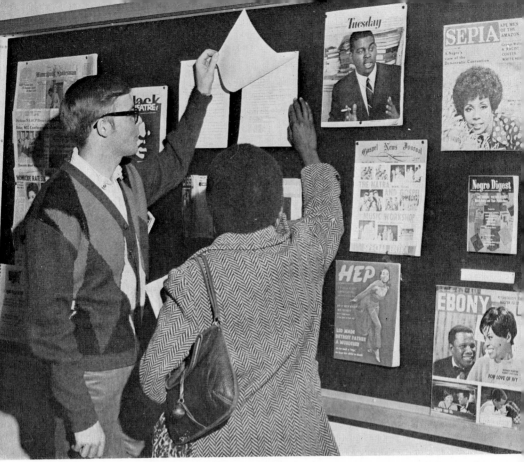

FIG. 11.1. Black newspapers and magazines on exhibit in the Newhouse Communications Center tie in with the course, "The Black Press," taught at the School of Journalism, Syracuse University. (S.U. News Bureau photo)

Jr., with William Worthy, a prominent newsman, as director of instruction, the program proceeded according to a plan worked out between Adams and Raymond H. Boone, editor of the Richmond edition of the *Afro-American*. After a three-month orientation session in Richmond, the Fellows spent six weeks in Washington observing methods of government coverage and five weeks in Baltimore headquarters of the *Afro-American* papers learning production, advertising, editing, and management techniques.

The remaining half-year was used for independent study projects in journalism. Jobs were guaranteed to successful trainees by several white papers, including the Atlanta *Constitution*, Greensboro *Daily News*, Norfolk *Star-Ledger*, the Norfolk *Virginian Pilot* as well as by the one black sponsor, the *Afro-American*. Other agencies were expected to aid in placement as well.[4]

A shorter but more varied program was begun at Columbia University in 1968. Also Ford-sponsored, it received $250,000 and was able to assist more persons than the Douglass plan. Offered in the summer only, for eight weeks, it provided less thorough training for twenty minority group members interested in careers in print and broadcast journalism.

One hundred and twenty-five applied in 1969. Twenty-two of those accepted had no previous journalism experience. Their ages ranged from twenty-one to forty-one; thirty-one were blacks and twenty-five were men. Two-thirds of the students were sponsored by ten broadcasting stations and ten daily newspapers. Tuition and room and board costs were provided free, cost-of-living stipends and family allowances based on need also were assured. Eighteen of the students were married. All who wished to work on the media were placed. Professor Fred W. Friendly, formerly a president of CBS and the Edward R. Morrow professor of journalism at Columbia's School of Journalism, directed this program on a volunteer basis for several years. He was aided by various regular and special faculty members.[5]

Discussing the 1970 program with a news service feature writer, Friendly observed that the program is "trying to find people who ought to be journalists regardless of their education or current occupations. . . . Too few blacks, Puerto Ricans or members of other minority groups understand this. I wish they would ask themselves, 'Who is in a better position to influence America—another black lawyer, or a black Walter Cronkite?' "[6]

Thirty-seven members of minority groups, all but six of them black, completed the 1970 program and all were placed. Thirteen went to newspapers and twenty-four to broadcasting stations, all of them white media, and including mainly large publications and stations.

Most of the schemes have been intended to produce more editorial personnel for the various media. But some also are aimed at increasing the available pool of advertising talent. A plan similar in some ways to those so far described was carried out in 1969 in New York City for black persons interested in training for timebuying. Twelve advertising agencies and the International Radio and Television Society combined efforts for this program. It was a free twelve-week course, with classes from 6 to 8 P.M. once a week, administered by leading media men of six agencies. The twenty-seven students, all in their twenties and thirties, who completed the work were hired as assistant buyers at varying salaries, with prospects of becoming buyers at $10,000, head buyers at from $15,000 to $17,000 and eventually supervisors at $20,000 or higher. The cooperating agencies included such large white ones as N.W. Ayer & Son, Inc., Cunningham & Walsh, Foote, Cone & Belding, and Young & Rubicam. Agency executives taught spot broadcasting, media planning, buying, the language of buying, reading of basic references and other documents, and additional practical aspects.[7]

Other training programs in the advertising, marketing, and pub-

lic relations fields have been arranged through the American Association of Advertising Agencies as well as by individual agencies in
both New York and Chicago; the latter city began such a program
in 1968.

One of the most practical and realistic training schemes centers
on a New York weekly tabloid, *Manhattan Tribune*. First issued in
1968, the paper covers the news of Harlem and the West Side
neighborhoods and is aimed at black and Puerto Rican readers. One
purpose is to provide a training ground for reporters for these two
minority groups (see Chapter 6). Some of the neophyte newsmen
cover small stories in the Harlem area; others, as they absorb more
experience and training, are assigned to investigative stories. They
work under the guidance of professionals, both blacks and whites.
Trainees do not receive salaries and are screened before being
accepted.[8]

Other plans have been functioning at the San Francisco *Examiner*
and Long Island *Newsday*, both white dailies. Blacks have been included in the award of scholarships to young people through a plan
financed by eight newspapers or newspaper groups and a press club
in a six-week summer journalism camp at the University of Kansas.
A program of training ten youths, described as "hard-core jobless," as
copyboys by the New York *Times* under a $34,000 Federal grant, and
an after-school weekday journalism workshop for Detroit area senior
high teen-agers, coordinated by the Downtown YWCA, are two more
plans. At least a dozen more seminars and short courses similar to
these were reported between 1968 and 1970.

The San Francisco *Examiner* program provides thirteen-week,
on-the-job training internships at the paper, a large daily, for reporters
and photographers from minority groups; the Newsmen's Job Re-
ferral Committee in the same city, which seeks out the names of
minority group people and sends them to communications media
in Northern California, helps recruit people for the *Examiner* program, established a weekly news-writing class at San Francisco City
College, and conducts seminars at the San Francisco Press Club. Another California program is in Los Angeles, where workshops have
been held for several years. The participants, meeting Saturdays,
work at the University of Southern California. Stressed are reporting
and editing, which are taught to low-income students, both youth
and adult.[9]

In the Midwest are the Ohio University Urban Journalism
Workshops, sponsored by seven white papers in Ohio, an industrial
firm, Ohio University, and The Newspaper Fund, a project of the
Wall Street Journal.[10] Baylor University, the University of Kansas,
and San Fernando Valley State College in California also have offered
such training.

Certain white special centers also are offering training and further experience in journalism to black applicants. Although orig-

inally not intended to give special aid to black young people, the Washington Journalism Center in the national capital has granted forty fellowships each year to applicants, half of them to black applicants. The Fellows with journalism experience attend seminars with members of Congress, government officials in other posts, Washington journalists, and representatives of private organizations. Those lacking experience are assigned to publications suitable to their special interests for an internship but also share in some seminars. Each Fellow receives a $2,000 grant to cover living expenses. The sixteen-week program is financed largely by the Ford Foundation.[11]

From various national organizations or individual newspaper and magazine publishing companies have come additional types of aid. The American Newspaper Publishers Association for several years has made grants to black college students interested in journalism careers. During 1968–69 a total of twenty-six students attended eighteen universities under this arrangement; forty-five black journalism students, in 1970–71, were placed in twenty-eight accredited journalism schools and departments. The fund serving as the source was organized after the association received a contribution of $100,000 from the Robert R. McCormick Charitable Trust of the Chicago *Tribune*. Another $135,000 was pledged by a group of white dailies and newspaper chains. In addition, the Frank E. Gannett Foundation gave five scholarships; the winners work part-time on the two Gannett dailies in Rochester, New York.[12]

The American Newspaper Guild, an AFL-CIO union of below-executive level employes of print and broadcast media, in 1970 began including in its contracts a clause concerning job-training programs for members of minority groups "to assure equal opportunities for job advancement."[13]

Beyond these opportunities are scores of other journalism scholarships or nonjournalism grants that may be applied for short-term study and are not intended necessarily for any particular racial group. Thus considerably more money is available to black students than ever before. But few of the grants are fully adequate to the needs of people in the lower economic levels, who sometimes come with insufficient clothing and without the basic supplies needed.

● HIGH SCHOOL LEVEL WORKSHOPS

At the college or older age level the plans generally are from one to four or six months, or even a year in length, with classroom work as well as field trips and seminars. At the high school level the plans run more toward workshops of a few weeks, with emphasis on rapid learning of a few basic techniques. In the past few years workshops for high schoolers were offered by several universities and in at least five communities. Four grew out of a plan stemming from The Newspaper Fund. Called Urban Journalism Workshops, they were held in summer, 1969, for example, in Washington, Detroit, Plainfield, New Jersey and Athens, Ohio. As explained by a report, the workshops were "designed to identify ghetto high school students with talent and provide them with fundamental training in the field." Credit was given for the work. The Newspaper Fund, local papers, and, in three instances, journalism schools cooperated in sponsoring the one- to four-week sessions. The goals were stated to be:

> (1) To instill in the students an understanding of the need for improving communicative skills; (2) To publish a student-written and student-edited workshop newspaper; (3) To expose students to the opportunities, challenges and disadvantages of journalism careers; and (4) To explain the role of the newspaper and its responsibility to the community it serves.[14]

Under direction of experienced teachers of high school journalism the aims were achieved, according to reports made after the sessions. Smartly prepared newspapers, produced by young people, were issued. The students reacted much as do high schoolers who attend the conventional summer press conferences conducted for many years in various parts of the country by Temple, Columbia, Syracuse, Northwestern, and many other universities. They enjoyed the companionship and the chance to learn new skills.

In 1970 the Fund's program was expanded. Originally it was begun in 1958 to attract young people in high school to the news profession; twelve years later it doubled its plan of steering minority students toward journalism as a career. Several hundred took part that summer. Since the Fund was set up it has spent more than $2,500,000 on the plan.

● JOURNALISM EDUCATION

As differentiated from training in crash programs or other plans separated from general education, journalism education is not new even for members of minority groups; in the North, black students have been studying journalism since such education began more than half a century ago. With one exception, however, virtually all such degree-courses are in white institutions. Separate courses, in English or other departments, are taught in a number of black colleges and universities, some going back to the 1930's. But lack of interest in journalism as a profession, high tuition costs, inadequate background preparation in many instances, and unavailability of jobs when candidates finished their degree work kept enrollments of black students low. While a little higher today, they still are out of balance with white enrollments numerically even in proportion to the total population and certainly are far short of what the profession could absorb. Attempts to remove these obstacles to bringing more blacks into journalism are being made but far too slowly to solve the immediate problem of adjusting the black student to the white press world or attracting him to work on the black press.

Educators Work for Change. The Association for Education in Journalism in 1968 appointed a special committee to perform "the task of ascertaining, stimulating, and coordinating the activities of AEJ members in bringing more blacks and other minority group members into our pipeline," explained Dr. Lionel C. Barrow, Jr., committee chairman. His Ad Hoc Coordinating Committee on Minority Group Education set four goals for AEJ. It included seeking five hundred scholarships for minority group members for the 1969–70 academic year; establishing cooperative relationships with more black colleges and junior and community colleges to help them establish communication courses on their own campuses; getting pledges from local media that they will hire minority group members and establish internships for them, and "The incorporation by all schools and departments of mass communication of material on the role of minority groups in America and on the portrayal of that role by the media into existing or new courses."[15]

Although the committee was unable to accomplish these goals in as short a time as it had hoped, it did, judging from its survey of what is being done, discover there were some accomplishments and plans. Financial support of one degree or another was available specifically, it learned, for at least 250 black students and undoubtedly more than that number because at least twenty-three plans were listed as being "for minority students," and surely would include some black young people. The report also noted that financial assistance then was obtainable for attending short courses or workshops for from 166 to 184 black high school students, eighty-two to eighty-seven black community residents, plus the number of blacks that would come under the label *minority*. Such support, the report observed, ranges in scope from textbooks to $9,800 a year.

Professor William R. Stroud, committee secretary, was somewhat disappointed by the report, believing that many more scholarships, workshops, and other of the aids desired by the committee should be forthcoming. The committee nevertheless made further recommendations for the future, including recruiting of black and white students on a national scale; supplementation by the schools of journalism of their present texts and courses so that they "present an unbiased view of the role of black and other minority groups in America"; indicating "the manner in which minority groups have been or are being portrayed in the mass media"; and helping to "prepare students for work in urban areas." A related recommendation was for AEJ to establish or designate a library to collect materials to be used in fulfilling these purposes.[16] In 1970 the committee became permanent, named Division of Minorities and Communication.

Performance of the Schools. Slow as the progress appears to be, a number of journalism schools are attempting to educate members of the minority groups by giving them a sound general education along with training in use of basic journalistic techniques. Some provide them with the opportunity to prepare for specialties at the same time. These possibilities are in addition to the scholarships, short courses, workshops, conferences, and the other programs already described. E. Franklin Frazier, the black sociologist, wrote as long ago as 1955 that "Negro journalists have been recruited on the whole from the inferior, segregated Negro schools, and their outlook has been restricted by the social and mental isolation of the Negro world."[17] But white journalism schools, until recent years, were only on suffrance in both the journalistic and the academic worlds and even today still must defend in some quarters their need for more financial support and equal treatment with other studies. They are among the minority groups of educational institutions, not segregated but certainly discriminated against. And if the school or department (more likely only two or three courses) exists in a black college it is a minority group within such a group.

Whatever the cause, little was taught about black journalism and relatively few black journalists were educated for life and the profession in either black or white college journalism courses, although more of the effective practitioners had such schooling than may generally be realized. And the white press, despite the occasional hiring of a black reporter (rarely a black editor or other executive) was actually blameworthy, doing little either to cover the black community or give blacks journalistic experience and responsibility.

Two 1968 studies reported by Dr. Edward J. Trayes, of Temple University's School of Communications and Theater, bear on the acceptance of blacks in both classrooms and offices of newspapers and magazines. One study indicated that the percentage of black news executives, deskmen, reporters, and photographers on newspapers in large cities was extremely low. The other study showed that the enrollment of black students was even lower. Of 6,418 juniors and seniors majoring in news-editorial or photojournalism at eighty-three colleges and universities, less than 2 per cent were black. About half the schools had no blacks in their degree sequences.[18] Professor Trayes, reporting on an early 1970 survey, found that the proportion of black news-editorial and photojournalism majors—junior and senior undergraduates—had increased more than 50 per cent during the preceding year but that the extremely low level of black enrollment persisted in most undergraduate programs. More than 40 per cent of the schools studied had no black undergraduate news-editorial or photojournalism majors, he learned.

Simeon Booker, Washington bureau chief for *Ebony* and *Jet*, said that he often had wondered "why the major journalism schools refuse to recognize the Negro press and do not attempt to improve its quality, as is done among white newspapers and magazines."[19] Some attempts have been and are being made, but there is a fallacy in his assumption about the schools' attempts to improve the white press. They have helped better it largely in technical matters: writing, layout, desk techniques, marketing. Few have been critical of the white press' coverage, of its ethical standards. Instead they have served, on the whole, as handmaidens, preparing young journalists to serve just as uncritically on it and rarely calling the newspapers and magazines to task for their faults, and virtually never for their neglect of the black world's news and for their unfair treatment of blacks when they did make news. Usually it was only crime or sports involving blacks that found a place in the pages. Contented or indifferent as the schools were about the white press' handling of racial news, the schools hardly would be interested in the black press, although they might have been had they not over the years been so understaffed. As the eighth decade of the century begins, however, there are signs of discontent among some journalism educators as well as students with the handmaiden attitude or the view that the function of the journalism school is to train staff members for publications and stations.

The Black Press Attitude. Nor, for that matter, has the black press, any more than the black college, until recently done much to promote journalism education. In a recent 144-page tabloid-size vocational supplement published by a major black newspaper, the only mention of journalism education or training, a line in a one-half page advertisement taken by Lincoln University and a story about its journalism department running a bit over a column, was hardly in proportion to the space for other vocations.

During most of American journalistic history it has been the practice of some journalists to scoff at journalism education; it is a commonplace experience for a reporter's or editor's son to be discouraged from entering his father's profession, being told it is only an area of low pay, hard work, and little other reward. The press has done little to cover its own news, under the excuse that the general public is uninterested in the internal affairs of journalism, an excuse that might also free the press from the necessity of dealing with what is going on within the profession that not always is pleasant. A casualty of this policy has been journalism education, which rarely is mentioned.

When the black press has printed stories about itself they have been confined to obituaries of editors and publishers, brief reports of annual conventions, boasts of honors received by owners and publishers, and other self-exploitation. Negro Newspaper Week and other such promotions have said little about the need for more and better staff by black publications or urged young people to consider journalism as an occupation. The white press has been similarly neglectful. At that, it is only some of the larger firms concerned enough about their future personnel who send recruiters to schools of journalism. Some recruiters are on the watch for able young nonwhites. With few whites inclined to work on black publications and not many black students enrolled, it would not be practical for even the larger black firms to send emissaries in search of talent, although one or two scouts might be so assigned by the National Newspaper Publishers Association in behalf of the newspapers and magazines who belong to it.

The Education Available. Journalism education is available to the black man or woman who wants it in the environment supposedly most familiar to him: the black college. About seven hundred were studying mass communications in one or more black college courses, a 1968 study by the United Negro College Fund indicated.[20] Around 30,000, the vast majority of them whites, did so in the 145 white institutions having degree programs covering bachelor's, master's, and doctor's. The Negro College study, made for the AEJ, did not confine its investigations to journalism education but covered as well what it called mass communications areas. These were general mass communication, journalism, mass media, radio-TV, advertising, and communicology. The research department did not make clear the differences between these areas or define communicology. The findings indicate the attention seventy-four accredited four-year b'ack colleges give the areas; they represent 90 per cent of the eighty-five such institutions in the U.S.A.

Five—Hampton Institute, Lincoln University (Missouri), Norfolk State College, Shaw University, and Texas Southern University— were found to have mass communications departments, with four offering a major in one or more of the sub-areas. A sixth, Bishop College, offered a major without a department by cooperation with white Southern Methodist University. An additional three offered minors, and thirty-three more offered one or more courses.

When narrowed down to journalism it was learned that Hampton, Lincoln, and Texas Southern had departments in the field, to which should be added departmentless Bishop. Minors are offered also by Grambling College, Howard University, Norfolk State, and Xavier University (cooperating with Tulane University). Thirty-one more offered one or more individual courses. Four hundred students were in journalism courses, by far the largest in any one area. Hampton and Shaw both reported radio-TV departments and offered majors as well as minors; Lincoln also offered a minor. A half-dozen more offered one or more courses in this area, in which there were twenty-nine students. No advertising departments or majors were uncovered. One institution, Lincoln, offered a minor and seven others scheduled one or more courses. Nevertheless, there were eighty-seven in advertising classes.

Among journalism educators exists the view that this specialized education should be left to the institutions staffed and equipped to provide it. The teachers and administrators holding that opinion—frequently at the big state and private institutions—discourage the development of many small programs, believing that like law, medicine, forestry, and other professional specialties journalism training and education cannot be conducted properly in the usual small liberal arts college. But their attitude does not consider the geographical and financial problems of the black student.

Perhaps in response to the idea of offering such education on a broad scale, two black universities recently announced ambitious programs. Howard University in Washington, D.C., in 1969 made preliminary plans for a school of communications and since then has been refining them. It will merge existing programs in film-making, journalism, advertising, television production, speech and information sciences. Clark University, a unit in the Atlanta University Center, in 1970 announced a plan to establish "a wide variety of programs in all areas of mass communication." The university by then had obtained a $1,500,000 grant from the Board of Missions of the United Methodist Church to begin such work. Journalists, teachers of mass communication subjects, and film and broadcasting officials were brought together to discuss the plan.[21]

The Lincoln Program. The Lincoln University program at Jefferson City, Missouri (another Lincoln, in Pennsylvania, offers a little journalism) which was begun in 1942, has pointed to what the black colleges might do. The instruction came into being when Miss Lucile H. Bluford wished to enter the noted school of journalism at the University of Missouri and was denied admission because of her race. She eventually completed her work at Lincoln. Today the curriculum is similar to that at many white colleges of about the same size; Lincoln has about 1,900 total enrollment, with a separate department of journalism. Three-fourths of the work of journalism students is in liberal arts courses; the rest is news-editorial or advertising and management, a plan designed to give the student a sound basic education plus the specialty. Work on the campus newspaper, the *Clarion,* is required for two of the four years.

Attention to black journalism, as explained by the department chairman, Armistead Scott Pride, "is fused into courses in news editing, history of journalism, introduction to mass communications, newspaper management, writing for publication, and the seminar in mass communications problems. . . . In the history course I devote three lectures to the Negro Press and snap at it here and there throughout the course."[22] Students tour black publishing plants and are assigned projects using the university's collection of black press material. "Thus," Pride also notes, "in spite of the absence of a separate course in Negro publications, the students are exposed to the field and become aware of the role of the Negro journalist in various ways."

Many Lincoln graduates have gone to the black weekly papers, at least at first. Later they may go into editorial positions on white dailies, in federal offices, or on to either black or white magazine staffs. "They have, or have been, the top editors at the major, as well as smaller, black papers (Chicago *Defender*, Baltimore *Afro-American*, Atlanta *Daily World*, St. Louis *Argus*); they work on the dailies (Chicago *Daily News*, Washington *Post*, San Francisco *Examiner*, etc.)," Pride reported in 1970.

Awards are made annually to black journalists for their accomplishments and to newspapers and magazines contributing to racial understanding and national unity. Lincoln also is an important repository for microfilms of black newspapers of historical importance; it receives about a third of the black publications.

A change is occurring at Lincoln, Pride reported in 1970. "Since 1955, when universities in the South and elsewhere began beckoning to black students, those interested in journalism study have tended to study near their homes; consequently, Lincoln's black student enrollment in journalism has declined while the white student enrollment has increased," he pointed out. "In some years since 1955 there have been no black graduates, only white graduates. Schools like Temple, Columbia, and a number of others are making a firm effort to recruit black students in journalism. Even University of South Carolina is making a bid. Half a dozen years should bring the total black student enrollment to a respectable figure. If not, the whole problem of black interest in journalism will deserve more concentrated study."[23]

● BLACK JOURNALISM IN WHITE COLLEGES

At no black institution, it appears, is any extraordinary attention given to black journalism as such. Pride's lectures about it probably are the extent of the attention anywhere, although no doubt in discussions of the influence of the media, regardless of color, its impact is talked about in sociology and public affairs classes. More intensive study of the black press apparently has been left to white institutions; none did much about it until recently but several now are giving it its due. A few have taken the initiative with complete courses (not programs or sequences and nothing leading to a separate degree, as in Afro-American studies; as yet black journalism resources are not great enough for a series of courses in depth). These include American, Syracuse, Michigan, Iowa State, Kansas State, Houston, University of California at Berkeley, Humboldt State College, California State at Hayward, and San Jose State. Several others plan such courses, although most of these will be about treatment of mi-

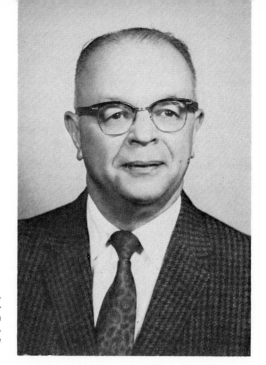

FIG. 11.2. Dr. Armistead S. Pride, chairman of the Journalism Department at Lincoln University, Jefferson City, Mo., and a leading scholar of the black press.

nority news by the mass media, reporting ghetto news, or interracial reporting.

Two of the courses directly concerned with black journalism are those at American University in Washington, D.C., and at Syracuse University, in Syracuse, New York. Their nature indicates the lines college and university schools of journalism can follow. That at American, begun in 1968, is on the "History and Evolution of the Afro-American Press and the Afro-American in the Mass Media" and is taught by Mrs. Dorothy Gilliam, who has been a black staff member of the white Washington *Post,* a major daily, and now is in broadcasting. The course, which may have been the first ever offered dealing with the history of black journalism, begins with 1827 and goes to the present, ending with the related topic, "The Negro and the Mass Media." Syracuse's course, begun also in 1968, includes such history but its major attention is to the contemporary black press and such auxiliaries and competitors as the news services, broadcasting, advertising, circulation, and production, covering most of the chapter topics of this book. The teacher is white (at present the author of this book), so black journalists are brought in as guest lecturers as are white specialists in black journalism. As at Lincoln, and doubtless at many other schools of journalism, information about the black press has for years come into certain other Syracuse courses.

Discussed at the outset of this book was the validity of the concept of a black press. In this chapter, as part of the examination of the training and education of the black journalist, there should be inquiry of the validity of teaching black press courses, for in some quarters these have been questioned as unnecessary. "Journalism is journalism, whatever the color," sometimes is heard. The more militant blacks attack black history courses in general as being taught only in the perspective of white history. It is true that if the events of white history are the only guideposts such a course is artificial and unrealistic. Related to this charge is another: that black subjects when taught by whites cannot be taught adequately because whites do not have—and cannot ever have—the understanding of the black experience and point of view that only black persons possess. It is conceivable, however, that an informed white teacher, a professional in two fields, education and journalism, can impart facts and ideas and can direct analysis of such facts and ideas perhaps more successfully than a black teacher who brings an inner understanding of certain aspects but may lack expertise as an educator. Furthermore, so few persons are available to teach courses in black journalism that the educational world will have to rely on both white and black instructors.

Black studies courses are thought to be an attempt to be popular, especially when taught by whites.[24] White colleges and universities are charged with trying to do what now is wanted, just to placate sign-toting, protesting students, after having neglected black subjects for years. Perhaps these accusations are deserved on some campuses. One might ask, however, at least in the instance of a course on black journalism, whether proposals to teach about that journalism, if made in the past, would have been considered seriously. It is doubtful that they would have been accepted. And perhaps they could not have been in the mood of the time. To begin with, to have done so in the 1940's and 1950's would have been damned as discriminatory, as downright segregationist. It was not so long ago that college admissions offices refused to issue figures about the number of black students accepted or enrolled because they had abandoned taking racial counts. Also, there was not the possibility of support for such courses equal to the small amount existing in the years since 1968, when the first was begun. The climate of opinion was not warm enough, any more than it was at one time for classes in religious journalism, science journalism, or other specialties.

So long as separation thrives, black journalism courses will be useful. And when it is discovered that the subject contains considerable substance it will continue to be taught, since black journalism has a rich content and a great potential for study, particularly if broadened to include the African background and influence upon that continent.

● A TEACHER OF JOURNALISM

Because the teaching of journalism has been so restricted in black colleges and universities and in white-run institutions of higher

learning, they have had no money in the first instance and no interest in the second in hiring black instructors for their journalism programs. A black teacher of this subject in a white college is a rare
being. Of those in black colleges the great majority spend nine-tenths
of their time on duties other than classroom work, usually as directors
of public relations. The reasons for the lack are clear, aside from the
prejudice or indifference of white institutions. Salaries in black colleges have been low, journalism instruction only a fringe activity, experienced and degree-laden black journalists have been uninterested
in such teaching as a vocation, as well as few in number. And today,
with the greater chance for a profitable and enjoyable career in white
journalism, there is even less likelihood of obtaining their help.

One black teacher, although he had comparatively little practical experience in journalism, has for years been outstanding if not
entirely alone in the teaching profession. This pioneer is Armistead
Pride, of the Lincoln University mentioned earlier. He has been dean
or chairman of its work in journalism education since 1944. A Wash-
ingtonian born in 1906, Pride also is unusual in that he has the full
list of academic degrees: an A.B. from the University of Michigan, an
A.M. from the University of Chicago, an M.S. from Northwestern's
Medill School of Journalism, and a Ph.D. from the English department
of the same university with a journalism subject dissertation.

Pride's journalistic background is less impressive than his education, but some of the other widely known teachers of the subject have
had little practical experience, as for example the internationally
noted teacher, administrator, and historian, Frank Luther Mott, one
of whose histories in journalism won a Pulitzer Prize. Pride was city
editor of the Lamar (Colo.) *Daily News,* in 1933 and 1934, and at the
same time area correspondent for the Associated Press. Earlier, for
two years, he was an editor in the department of forms and reproduction of the Massachusetts Geodetic Survey. But the rest is teaching.
At first it was English for several years in Southern colleges and at
Lincoln, where he was an assistant professor of that subject in 1937,
moving into journalism fully in 1942. In two years he was acting
director of the school of journalism, becoming director the next year,
dean and full professor in 1947, and remaining as chairman when
journalism was put on a departmental instead of a school basis.

During several leaves of absence he has made an international
impact. He served as a Fulbright lecturer at Cairo University, as well
as at American University, in Egypt. Another year he was at the University of Rome; later at Chungang University in Seoul, Korea. In
1969–70 he was a visiting professor at Temple University.

His major contribution to black journalism in America, aside
from educating dozens of students over the years, has been by exploring the history of the black newspaper. His doctoral dissertation at
Northwestern was an invaluable record and historical account of these
papers from the first in 1827 to 1950, when the dissertation was com-

pleted. This thorough and careful study is far more than a checklist, for the history in general and that of individual publications are discussed and analyzed.

In addition, Pride has contributed articles on aspects of black journalism to the *Nation, Editor & Publisher, Journalism Quarterly,* the *Quill, Gazette,* and other professional journals. He has been active in the American Society of Journalism School Administrators, a constituent part of the Association for Education in Journalism, and directly with the AEJ as well. His bibliography of the black press for the latter's Ad Hoc Coordinating Committee is the most comprehensive thus far issued. He launched the *Lincoln Journalism Newsletter* in 1944, maintaining it as a continuous record of events in black journalism for more than a dozen years.

● EVALUATING THE PROGRAMS

A member of the Columbia University Graduate School of Journalism faculty who developed the print journalism portion of the training program there, described earlier in this chapter, has examined the ways being used to solve the problem of obtaining more "black and brown faces," as he put it, into journalism classrooms and newsrooms. Writing in a journalism periodical, Professor Melvin Melcher in part evaluated the existing programs; he was adversely critical of some.

"Many training programs for black and Spanish-speaking men and women," he wrote, "prepare them to go out and look for jobs rather than to progress in jobs guaranteed them on successful completion of the program."[25] He also noted that several plans broke down under the often well-founded suspicion that those who took part would face the usual barriers of job-getting. He said he believed that the plan of attaching minority group students to working newsmen does not succeed because the regular staff people are too busy and are not necessarily competent teachers. The newcomers learn only the way it is done at one office, may which or may not be the best.

"No one proposes," he wrote, "that quickie medical licenses be given, despite the shortage of doctors. Yet programs are being financed that would place in sensitive posts men and women whose training disposes them only to repeat the errors of the media." Nor is the journalism school approach the solution, either, Melcher wrote. Its courses are irrelevant to the minority groups. Practice courses do not cover the ghetto, for instance. Lack of balance in the staff, such as no black and Spanish-speaking journalism teachers, and of money with which to recruit are additional handicaps to the schools. Melcher makes the point that it is vital that such teachers be at the front of the room because they have a perspective others do not possess. He saw the need for money to finance the journalism education of minority group members as enormous and that journalism schools are not prepared to meet it. Scholarships must be large, since students come without money. Therefore he proposed a program of all-cost national fellowships and a coordination of present efforts, under a journalism education council.

Professor Melcher's points are important. Some schools of journalism eager to be of help with special programs have been unable to assist because their own administrations cannot finance the plans. Nor has there been success in obtaining outside funding. But the danger in his view about schools of journalism is that their past performance and potential will be downgraded and their effectiveness impaired. So many of the more accomplished black journalists, as recounted in earlier chapters, are products of journalism education, that it might be simpler and wiser to supplement the schools' work rather than imply that it is not a satisfactory source of a solution to the staff problem.[26] Journalism programs may be unworkable with students right out of a black community if no special preparatory work is done to ease them into the technical work. An institution that can offer a substantial program of terminal preparation should be able to set up advance schooling as well. It also should be remembered that the black American is developing into a middle class member of society and that the traditional college education and training will be increasingly within his reach, despite costs, because of the steady increase in financial aid to students and the greater possibilities of part-time work. Yet the person thinking of applying for some program noted here might well check it against Professor Melcher's views. ●

12. PUBLISHERS AND THEIR PROBLEMS

IDEALISTIC BLACK JOURNALISTS are torn between the opportunities offered in the white and the black worlds of journalism. They see, on the one hand, the higher salaries in white organizations, the prestige connected with certain publications, and the chances for future accomplishment, especially in these days when blackness alone offers an entrée to some positions.

Another point of view exists, however. The black press, in the opinion of many, is "beautiful," and deserves the loyalty of the people it is published to serve. Because it is not getting such fealty, publishers of newspapers are confronted with numerous problems. They face all the dilemmas confronted by other racial groups of publishers and certain ones especially their own. To delve into the problems common to all journalism would call for many more chapters; discussion of these is found in the comparatively richer literature of white journalism.[1] Today most newspaper and magazine proprietors hold their aching heads while they face rising costs of equipment replacement, delivery, supplies, staff salaries, maintenance, taxes, and rents. Staff turnover, changes in the national economy, consumer reaction, competition with other papers and magazines and with the nonprint media, the need to diversify operations, and labor unrest inside and outside the industry, all bedevil the black publisher. About the only problem not acute is that of unionization. The labor movement is weak in the black press because the vast majority of publications would have to go out of business if their owners attempted to meet union contracts on wages and other provisions. The black magazines, like most periodicals, come into contact with unions only through their hired printers or distribution firms, for unlike the newspapers, they usually do not own their own equipment.

At least a half-dozen special problems, or angles of general ones peculiar to this ethnic journalism, confront owners and publishers of the black press. They are staffing, the philosophical and political battles going on in the black society, the broader interests of the enlarging black population or market, as the businessmen call it, the methods of reaching well-educated blacks, the temptation to pander for the sake of advertising, the threat of new competition, and the dilemma presented by such ideological conflicts as racial and cultural ill-feeling between blacks and other ethnic groups.

● LOSS OF STAFF

The beckoning finger of opportunity, part of a hand holding far higher salary checks than most of the black press can afford, comes not only from the offices of the relatively few affluent black publishers. A look at the biographies of the black journalists in Chapter 10 shows that a large number went either from small black publications to the larger ones or left black journalism for white entirely. The "come join us" invitations now arrive more often and strongly than ever before from advertising agencies, public relations firms, broadcasting companies, and the public relations, advertising, promotion and other divisions of white industries and professional groups.

What annoys the publishers and other black executives is that this increased raiding of their staffs may or may not be on merit. It is done, in some instances they suspect, to put some black faces into the office. Robert E. Johnson, executive editor of *Jet*, observed during a Sigma Delta Chi Headline Club discussion in Chicago in 1969 that the white publications cannot truthfully allege that they have been unable to get black journalists, because they have been there all the time. Some black students were graduated from schools of journalism in the 1950's and 1960's but few were given opportunities on white publications. The white employers now realize that and are seeking to make up for lost time, a boon to the employe but a headache to the black publisher. This staff raiding undercuts the possibilities of building reasonably permanent staffs on the black publications. Also irritating black owners is the fact that although financial conditions are improving for a few of them, enabling them to do somewhat better with salaries than before, they have not yet become competitive, by any means.

John H. Johnson, editor and publisher of *Ebony, Jet,* and other magazines, hearing about an agreement made by the owners of the German magazine, *Der Stern,* with its editors to give them greater freedom, observed that his company had given its editors more freedom for a long time as an effort to keep them.

"Not only have we been working for their independence and freedom," he said, "we've also been working for their happiness, we are forced to give editors what they want in an effort to keep them. As a matter of fact, I have a little sign on my desk . . . 'What should I do today to insure that my editors will be happy and contented and will not leave me?' " He added that "we also have to think about the wives. So we occasionally arrange for an editor to take his wife on a trip overseas, to Africa or to Asia, and when he thinks about leaving, she tells him, 'Oh, remember that nice trip we took, dear,' and this tends to discourage them." He mentioned also that the company reminds single girls just out of journalism school that the Johnson magazines have many single men on their staffs.[2]

But no other company equals the Johnson firm in affluence. The typical black newspaper or periodical publishing house can offer no such inducements, must less hard cash equal to that of white firms of only moderate size. Small community papers, which are the bulk of the black press and could offer opportunities in different regions, employ few people, single or married, and barely can afford to send them to the state capital, much less Asia or Africa.

Journalists traditionally are among society's thoughtful citizens and for years were considered the rebels in society, although today they seem to have been outdistanced by people of all ages and colors who follow programs which mean peaceful or violent revolution against the established order. Although lagging as social critics, black as well as white journalists continue to be skeptical about much that occurs. Increasingly, some are not content with any job, even if it does include Asian or African trips or an opportunity to meet a future mate. These writers and reporters want meaningful work which contributes to the solution of social problems facing the nation or humanity as a whole. The pursuit of personal affluence may be the goal of many journalists or would-be journalists but by no means all. Some uncounted number is standing off, critical of the status quo, seeking ways to have its part in eliminating or correcting what is wrong.

One of the author's black journalism students had opportunities to work on either a large white newsmagazine or on one of the largest black newspapers. The dilemma about which to choose plagued her for months. She realized that her ultimate goal might be a deciding factor. She was torn between her loyalty to her race and a desire to be a success in the white world. This conflict is acknowledged by most of the black students with whom the writer has been in touch during many years of teaching. Those who seized the biggest dollar sign, whatever its source, were few.

This particular student, in her college years as an undergraduate and then a graduate student, had been a girl of comfortable family giving little thought to her race; in fact, she was inclined at first to ignore it. But the drive of many of her black friends—and white ones as well, for some whites can be blacker than blacks—towards pride in her race led her to change her personality. She let her hair grow naturally and gave up trying to make her skin lighter. She had no difficulty being proud of black novelists, poets, painters, athletes, and statesmen. Black, to be sure, was beautiful. Black music was beautiful. "Why wasn't the black press beautiful, in the same way?" she was asked.

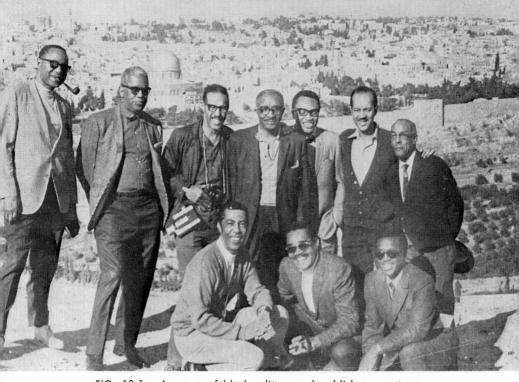

FIG. 12.1. A group of black editors and publishers went on a fact-finding tour of Israel in 1969, under sponsorship of the National Newspaper Publishers Association and other groups. Standing **(left to right)** are John H. Sengstacke, president of Sengstacke Newspapers; Dick Edwards, New York **Amsterdam News**; John Murphy III, president of Afro-American Newspapers; Howard Woods, St. Louis **Sentinel**; Dale Shields, New York disc jockey; Kenyon Burke of the Anti-Defamation League, one of the sponsors; John Bogle, **Philadelphia Tribune.** In the foreground are Thomas Picou, Chicago **Daily Defender**; Garth Reeves, Miami **Times**; and Robert E. Johnson, **Jet** magazine. (**Daily Defender** photo)

She persuaded herself that perhaps the black press was, and took editorial work on a major periodical. Her salary was adequate and the working conditions satisfactory. But the idea of meeting single men meant little to her. She had traveled abroad before joining the staff, so that benefit—which was offered to almost no woman, anyway, she reported—was less important to her than it might have been otherwise. What she missed was a direct confrontation of the social issues whose solution she believed so important to the welfare of the black people. After a time she resigned to go to work for a white publication concerned with social problems, not a radical journal but one bringing a scientific approach and as a whole concerned about human beings.

Motivated black journalists such as this young woman want from publishers a more candid attitude. If publishers are to appeal to them to become staff members there must be some compensation for the low comparative salaries, the lack of the usual benefits, such as severance pay, insurance, sharp definition of duties, expanding vacation periods with pay, and retirement plans, often not available in black offices. That compensation might well be a purpose beyond commerce. The freedom fighter dormant in many a black journalistic breast is not unduly upset by inferior working conditions and lack of benefits if the warrior for the right is single and in good health and convinced that by joining the staff of a black publication he can accomplish something for the betterment of the race. If it means only a way to bring money to a few or encouraging black readers to be concerned only about their personal pleasures, black journalism will not command the respect and assistance of these idealists.

"Negro publishers are apt to be primarily businessmen whose interest in race welfare is secondary to their interest in selling newspapers," Thomas Sancton, an astute white observer of the black press, wrote in the World War II years. He goes on to describe one that he knew then, as a "patronage politician, a political reactionary, and an anti-Semite. . . . He was exactly like the majority of white publishers."[3] A quarter of a century has passed since that was printed. Both black and white publishers are less commercial and far more socially conscious than they used to be, pressed to those positions by the forces of events and public opinion. It must be remembered, however, that no business operation which must sell its product and rent its space to advertisers can be so quixotic as to put race welfare first even in this day of social ferment unless some other source of revenue is available. And the business operations are so complex and hedged with so many problems such as those already noted that little time and energy are left to do much else but keep the publication from sinking into the graveyard of black publications. The publisher may have to battle for survival in the marketplace, but his employes usually know what is dearest to his heart.

● THE PHILOSOPHICAL BATTLES

From the publisher's point of view, especially if he attempts to stand off from the scene either to keep from entanglement with any faction or because he respects the long-held view of American journalists that the press is a watchdog, not a partisan, the various philosophies of social change are confusing. And some are a threat to him and the owners of the publication.

Like his fellow white publishers, the black entrepreneur is subject to the many pressures of change; he now feels them sharply. Lerone Bennett, Jr., *Ebony*'s senior editor and an historian of Afro-Americanism, told a conference on "The Media and The Cities" in Chicago in 1968 that "The black revolution is a total revolution, and every institution in the black community is bending to the winds of change. Black media are becoming more militant, more black. . . . There is a new tide of black consciousness in the black community. Black readers are more assertive, more demanding, more militant. They are demanding more information about themselves and their struggle. As a result, new media are springing up across the country, and established media are expanding their formats to satisfy new demands."[4]

So the publisher raises questions. Is his audience actually more militant? No doubt only a portion, but how large a segment? And what is militancy? Is the reader in a small southern city just as militant as one in a far western community or that of Harlem or Bedford-Stuyvesant, that other restless part of New York? How militant must he be to retain the respect of his readers and, not so incidentally, the patronage by them of his advertisers? And how much militancy will his advertisers stand for? One month he receives this anonymous letter:

> I am not renewing my subscription because I believe that your magazine has become too militant. I am not renewing because I believe that you now cater to the vocal minority which does not abide by our democratic traditions.
>
> Your magazine began to lose favor with me after an editorial a few months ago in which you advocated that all blacks get together and vote as a bloc, and vote only for the candidate who says he will do most for this segment of our population. . . . I think that your proposal . . . could lead to the worst form of divisiveness and demagoguery that this present generation has yet witnessed. Also, getting back to general attitudes, has the word "Negro" gone out of favor? You don't seem to use it anymore. I don't think that's right, either.[5]

Later comes another signed letter, reading:

> I have just finished reading the letter by the "Former Subscriber" . . . I am going to keep on subscribing to your magazine if nobody does, because I am proud of it. I'm not a militant; I am just concerned about my race. I take every issue of Ebony to school and show my classmates that black is not only beautiful, but very interesting and educational as well. I am proud to be black and you've made me even prouder.[6]

Can the publisher judge by the number of letters how his readers react? Probably not. Shall he make a reader interest survey? If he can afford it, he does, but it may be necessary to conduct more than one and even if a series is completed there is no certainty that it portrays his readers' reactions, for the climate of opinion is changing rapidly.

The general effect of the current social and political philosophies as a white observer sees them among the American black people is examined in Chapter 15. Special attention is given to one, black power, because it is of deep concern to the press as a whole. Here, however, we look at aspects of the social ferment particularly relevant to what in the publishing business is called the front office: the owner's or publisher's sanctum. Atop the problems of many years' standing, such as persuading a firm to advance credit for purchase of new printing equipment, comes that of having to contend with a boycott of local merchants, some of them users of space in his paper. If militant actionists, with entire justification because of overcharging or refusal to employ blacks, conduct such a boycott the publisher is in the middle. He can oppose the action, but if he does he is suspected of protecting his profits. He can report it and remain neutral; he then is called an Uncle Tom and blamed for not helping the brothers and sisters in their campaign for justice. Or he can side with the actionists and earn the enmity of his advertisers and a section of his readership. Earlier in this book is the record of the occasional personal attack on publisher or editor. Burning crosses on lawns have been among the milder methods used, not by the black readers but by the white enemies of a militant press.

The upsetting social theories of the day touch more than the advertising department. How is the publication to treat, in coverage and editorial comment, the actions and utterances of the Eldridge Cleavers, Robert Williams', Rap Browns, and Stokely Carmichaels? Shall they be reported straight? What is "straight"? With or without pictures? On page one? On the cover? How important is the street corner speech of an unknown man or woman who gains a quick following in a crisis situation, perhaps resorting to demagoguery to get it? Some publishers have a solution. Most of those attending the 1968 convention of the National Newspaper Publishers Association were of the opinion that the mission of the black press is "to preach law and order while attempting to understand the militants and translate their demands into meaningful objectives."[7]

In recent years that policy is what has been followed by scores of newspapers and most of the few magazines that possess discernible editorial policies. That statement naturally does not hold for the angry publications, such as *Muhammad Speaks* and the *Black Panther*. But for the bulk of the regular, noncause press, it does and earns in return the contempt of the strongly protesting papers but the applause of the moderates.

The black publisher also is acutely conscious of his geographical location. If his paper (and it is the newspaper owner who experiences this more than the magazine owner, whose periodical usually is national and more remote from the local citizen) may be in the North, where the press can afford to be much more militant about stories of police brutality occurring in the South or Middle West. But, as Lomax observed, the northern press "cannot expose sharp business practices and loan-shark dealings that keep the masses of Negroes in perpetual debt."[8] Unless, he might have added, it is completely detached from the business system, as in the long run even the militant papers find it impossible to be.

Bound firmly by his economic ties, the publisher is affected even by the presence of types of white newspapers in his community.

St. Louis, known for two major white papers, the outstandingly liberal *Post-Dispatch*, and the relatively conservative *Globe-Democrat*, is the home of the St. Louis *Sentinel*, a crusading weekly. The Washington edition of the Baltimore *Afro-American* similarly has no trouble keeping up with the liberalism of the white *Post* and the comparative liberalism of the conservative rival, the *Star*. The *Afro*, however, would be a radical sheet in Jackson, Mississippi, where the black *Advocate* on some issues reflects the conservatism of the community.

Although some black publications rely on general statements to encourage their readers to get on with the business of righting the wrongs against them, only the outrightly militant believers in the efficacy of violence are willing to tell readers to use "whatever means necessary." The dominant black press wants a revolution of sorts but is not sure of just what kind. It is fairly well united in urging its achievement by legal means, whatever the revolt's goal.

● FAVORING THE ADVERTISER

Although it is not by any means exclusively a practice of black publishers, they are particularly vulnerable to the temptation to favor their advertisers and have been since the press was founded, purely because advertising space has been so difficult to sell. All publications are so accustomed to doing something extra for advertisers that the practice is overlooked or condoned. Travel, automobile, and real estate pages in even the largest white papers, with few exceptions, set no example for the black publisher, for they are laden with free advertising. The degree to which such special favors go is great in any journalism. But a publication that runs laudatory articles about its advertisers, sometimes in columns adjoining the paid space, is hardly being subtle. If its editorial policies are generally namby-pamby or nonexistent, it seems reasonable to assume that the owner has no intention of telling the whole truth, as his masthead slogan may declare, because it is not expected of him to bite the hand that signs the checks to pay for his space. Or, it may be that it simply is inexpedient for him to do anything but ignore what it is pleasanter to ignore: the questionable methods of a political boss or the prejudiced hiring policies of an industry or store or bank that advertises. It is difficult to know what a publication omits without living in the community it serves, but there are clues from towns and cities with competing black papers.

● GRATIFYING THE READER

Closely related to that practice of letting, or having to allow, the advertiser call the tune is that of giving the reader solely what he wants. Oft-debated by the press as a whole, both newspapers and magazines face the decision. All publications, to some extent, give the public what it wants, but it is a question of how much and which of the public's wants are gratified, and which public is being catered to. The readers of *Muhammad Speaks,* for example, have a deep interest in the spread of their beliefs and in the righting of wrongs practiced against blacks in general and certain ones in particular. If a reader is against racial intermarriage, as is the Black Muslim group officially, he is pleased to see that the editor has included news or views concerning that policy. If the majority of the publication's readers follow that philosophy the editor is giving his readers what they want. Yet he may consider himself an independent editor, beholden only to the organization's officers. That same editorial staff does not, as do some of the white/black underground papers like the Berkeley *Tribe,* condone acceptance of lubricious advertising or print articles laden with obscene words; it is likely that a considerable number of readers would enjoy such material. A line has been drawn, after all. Copy encouraging superstition, news stories furthering rumor, or fiction pandering to the desire of some readers for vicarious sexual thrills, all published for the sake of selling the publication, are giving the public—a portion of the public, in any case—what it wants at the expense, perhaps, of the public's moral fibre or sense of fair play toward others.

Black publishers learned long ago that the practice of giving the public what it wants without much concern for its effect upon the public sells papers or magazines; in the long run the policy is not enough to produce papers that influence public opinion on major social issues, as has been shown by the history of the Chicago *Defender,* in black journalism, and the Hearst chain, in white journalism. There always will be some audience for the sensational; if the level of education of readers is not yet such as will make them demand a higher quality of content giving them the better quality can be a failure. When Mr. and Mrs. V. P. Bourne-Vanneck, the English couple, took over the black weekly, the *New York Age,* in 1949, they found they could not succeed with the paper with their policy of omitting sensational copy. They observed: "A lot of people preach progress, integration, and the need for a new clean newspaper in Harlem . . . but did you know that some of these same people do everything possible to hinder and crush our 'new' paper with malicious lies and rumors?" The Bourne-Vannecks were reported, along with other investors, to have lost considerable sums by the time the Chicago *Defender* took over the paper in 1952.[9]

As with playing favorites among advertisers by cutting rates or running free plugs for them, the practice of pandering to a certain element among readers still goes on in the black press. It has been much criticized (see Chapter 16). Some weeklies fill their first pages with crime stories, others play as the main story of the week a crime report in which blacks are the major figures. Crime sells papers. The publisher is faced with the questions: Does such treatment overemphasize it? Does it develop an inordinate interest in such happenings? Does it further the concept that the black is naturally criminal? Does it not really become an easy way to obtain a big front-page story rather than do more difficult and controversial reporting of what is happening in the black community in the way of social action or social progress?

● REACHING THE EDUCATED

A friend of the author who is among the scores who have supplied information for this book one day out of curiosity asked a young black woman, at one time a secretary in a white magazine office, which of the black papers of the city she reads. "Never read them," she told him. Faithfully, however, she reads both the large white dailies. The author asked a black retired official of a racially mixed peace organization her opinion of the black press. She had heard of and glanced at a few papers and magazines. But all her life (she was middle-aged), she insisted, she never had read any of them, always the white press. She had grown up in a fairly well-to-do part of the Midwest and her family had no interest in black news. There was no special interest in blackness for its own sake; on the contrary, they all worked for racial integration. The black press, apparently, simply kept blackness alive and in their opinion to the detriment of all society.

The black publisher therefore welcomes the new interest in Africa and its culture, the attempt to rewrite the U.S. history books to show what part black people had in the story of the country's development, the efforts to tell their story fully in books devoted to black history. What can he do, however, to reach the well-educated blacks who lack this pride of race, who do not care about the columns of personal news, the accomplishments of individual blacks who are total strangers to them, the goings on in the black colleges and among black sportsmen, and much else that fills the pages of black newspapers and magazines? If the publisher's paper is not even a second one to such readers, what hope has he of gaining them as his own?

The magazine publisher, rather than the newspaper publisher, can hope to reach the black intellectuals, but whether it will pay him to do so is another matter. He can offer erudite articles, and literary and art work rather than the straight news which perforce is largely what appears in newspapers. For while the educated black may be indifferent to the community life he often is concerned about the social problems or the cultural progress of his people. And with the new interest in separatism the publication that gratifies such interests will gain and hold readers. Now is the day for publications named

Freedomways, Black World, Amistad, Black Scholar and *Phylon*. For the black intellectual, like the same being of white skin, has little respect for most newspapers, whatever their origin. The dailies and weeklies are by the nature of their hasty production forced to be somewhat unscholarly and incomplete and to be written and edited by persons who are not specialists in the interests of the intellectuals: the arts and literature, science and sociological and philosophical ideas, revolutionary politics.

● THE NEW COMPETITION

In an attempt to encourage black enterprise, the Ford Foundation in 1969 granted $70,000 to a predominantly black publishing firm so it could restart a black women's magazine, *New Lady*. Another $70,000 was provided the firm, Mecco Enterprises, Inc., in Hayward, California, by seven Pacific Coast banks. Staffers of *McCall's*, the huge magazine for women in general, agreed to give *New Lady* technical assistance. Later the founders and staff of *Essence*, another magazine for black women, also received financial aid from business sources and technical help from executives of prominent magazines and advertising agencies (see Chapter 7).

The foundation explained the plan a little more in detail, saying that *New Lady* was to be "the first nationally circulated family service publication serving black women. The magazine hopes to develop a strongly ethnic identity among Negro women as well as serve as a training ground for black editorial and managerial personnel."[10] Commenting on this development before a magazine conference, John H. Johnson, owner of *Ebony* and other magazines, including *Tan*, directed at black women, said:

"Your presiding officer was saying something about the fact that *Ebony* and our publications were still trying to bridge the gap between races and that perhaps the militants wanted to remove that. I also think that some of the liberal whites are trying to do the same thing. As a case in point [here he restated the *New Lady* plan]. So I want you to know that, in rebuttal, I'm looking for a struggling white publisher who needs money and technical assistance so he can give some competition in the white field."[11]

Such new competition for black publications comes on top of the long-standing editorial and advertising opposition from white newspapers, magazines, and broadcasting companies, now emphasized because they are more hospitable to news, articles, pictures, and even fiction about blacks. That the publishers are troubled by it was indicated as long ago as 1956. That year at their annual NNPA convention "It was agreed that Negro newspapers . . . would do well to follow the course of national news magazines and attempt to review, analyze and present such news in further detail than the dailies do."[12]

● THE TENDEREST SUBJECT

Picking their way between the various types of militants and radicals is a difficult enough problem for these essentially moderate or conservative publishers. Those rebels with laudable aims but unlaudable methods must be distinguished from those with methods as well as aims that may be called anything but laudable.

More ticklish or tender than any of the black social and political programs is the subject of anti-Semitism in the black society. Not a recent development, as is known from the subjection of blacks to attacks by a Jewish editor in New York in the early history of the black press, it is perhaps now more of a problem because of recent events. Aggravating it are the setting up of the nation of Israel, with the Arab-Israeli warring, and the fights in black neighborhoods between black and Jewish groups, the blacks asserting their resentment for what they call overcharging by store owners and the Jews resenting what they consider lack of appreciation for their services and their patience. Bad blood also arose in some cities between Jewish white members of labor unions which will not admit blacks or who work for employers unable or unwilling to hire blacks. The blacks resented the whites' fear of loss of jobs.

Some of this feeling reached the black press world in 1967 when two prominent blacks resigned from the advisory board of *Liberator* magazine in protest against publication of articles they considered anti-Semitic. The protesters were James Baldwin, the author, and Ossie Davis, the playwright and actor. Their resignations came about because of a series of articles by Eddie Ellis, a Harlem writer. Called "Semitism in the Black Ghetto," they described alleged exploitation by merchants and landlords, charging that Zionists dominated black colleges and organizations and manipulated the civil rights movement.[13]

But such views rarely surface in any large black publication; when they do they are reported guardedly, for the publishers or their editors seem to realize the dangers of sensationalizing or fanning the latent animosity. One important paper, however, takes a definite position on the Arab-Israeli War: *Muhammad Speaks,* which has a substantial circulation in Chicago, New York, and other large cities with big Jewish and black populations. In one issue alone stories appeared under these headlines:

16,000 ARABS IN ISRAELI JAILS

Middle East Report—
ARAB LEADERS: NO OIL FOR U.S.A.

Champions of Freedom?
ZIONISTS SILENCE ISRAELIS WHO DO NOT SUPPORT WHITE RACIST ZIONISM

ARAB VALOR: ISRAELI REPRESSION

U.S.-Israel-Portugal-W. Germany-South Africa—
BIRDS OF FEATHER PLAN ARSENAL IN AFRICA

In addition there appeared a three-column photograph of Senator Jacob Javits with cutlines reading: "Jewish U.S. Senator from New York grins as he discusses the Arab-Israeli situation with Shah Reza Pahlevi of Iran." Iran is referred to as "a neo-colony of the U.S."[14]

All these accounts, to be expected in a Muslim publication with a deep interest in Africa, with one exception ran from one to two columns in length. They are credited to Jordan and Tel Aviv; the latter is a Liberation News Service dispatch; others are not clear as to origin, although one has the byline, Ali Baghdadis. The *Black Panther* unquestionably supports the efforts of Arab guerrillas.

Other controversial events are handled with caution by the regular commercial publications if not in the cause papers and magazines. And they are thus handled because they also are tender topics: attacks on the clergy, on such folk heroes as Adam Clayton Powell, Jr., or on popular entertainers; articles or editorials praising accomplishments of the Castro government, reporting in any favorable way on North Vietnam, the Viet Cong, North Korea, or other countries aligned with either Soviet Russia or mainland China. The problem of treating such news and views is settled, by and large, either by ignoring it or taking the safer position of consistently unfavorable presentation.

● THE UNITED PUBLISHERS

Perhaps the problems would be more numerous or even more unsolvable if the nation's black publishers, at least of the larger newspapers and several magazines, were not organized. The black magazines in general are so diversified, being concerned largely with specialties and using a wide variety of formats and formulas, that it would be difficult for them to unite, just as it has been in the white magazine industry, where only the relatively small number of consumer magazines and a minority of the business and religious periodicals have their own organizations.

The newspaper publishers' group grew out of a meeting called in 1943 by Walter White and the NAACP, of which he then was executive secretary. The editors of twenty-four of the largest papers, with an aggregate circulation of three million a week at that time, came together to discuss attacks upon the black press from both black and white critics. The charges were that some papers oversensationalized news, particularly of racial discrimination. The acceptance of doubtful advertising such as that for love potions, dream books, and good luck charms also had been frowned upon. Out of the sessions came the Negro Newspaper Publishers Association, with John H. Sengstacke as the first president. White reported that moderation of the treatment of news followed. The objectionable advertising was dropped, he wrote.[15] Some of it, however, has been resumed since (see Chapter 13).

The group, which later changed its name to National Newspaper Publishers Association, is similar in function to the large white organization, American Newspaper Publishers Association, and to numerous state bodies of white published weeklies and dailies. It promotes its particular phase of U.S. journalism, using the Negro Press Week annually to call attention to the black press. This event is its best known effort at developing a favorable public opinion, but it also has rallied aid for publications or individuals it deems unjustly brought before the law. One such was an editor and publisher in the South indicted in connection with stories written about a young black man electrocuted following conviction on a charge of attacking a sixteen-year-old white girl. The editor had not published the girl's name but was indicted under a code statute which prohibits such publication. The paper had printed an interview with the convicted man who alleged that the girl had cooperated.[16]

Other NNPA activities are less dramatic. The president may meet with the members; generally he or some other public officials say something appropriate, such as praising the papers for championing minority rights or being vital sources of information to their readers. At one time NNPA had a national news service to provide news and feature copy for papers published by its members (see Chapter 14). It also has undertaken market studies.

Just how seriously NNPA's efforts are taken by its public is difficult to say. Certainly intervention in cases of misapplication of the law win respect for the press and its publishers' organization. The articles lauding the past editors or the present performance of the press probably get little attention. The newspaper business itself, white or not, never has fascinated the customers, who presumably are more interested in the results than in what goes on behind the scenes, although they need not be sheltered so thoroughly as they usually are in the press' pages.

Now NNPA has about seventy members, almost all newspaper firms, whose buyers number around 1.5 million. The organization has served to give the publishers and editors a chance to discuss ways to deal with some of the problems faced in common by the nonwhite newspapers. ●

13. THE BUSINESS OPERATIONS

KINZER AND SAGARIN, in *The Negro in American Business,* insist that the black press cannot be judged as a business as can other enterprises run by members of that race. "For primarily," they write, "the success of the press is not measured by its financial statements, its ratio of advertising to editorial space, but rather by its influence over its readers, and by its ability to plead their cause and express their hopes."[1]

Although the black newspaper and magazine should not be downgraded because it has not, throughout its history or to any great extent now, set any records as an investment and should indeed be taken seriously as a factor in public opinion about black America and as an influence upon that population, it nevertheless must seek to operate like an efficient business if it is to survive. In its existence the black press as a whole has had comparatively little opportunity to fall back upon resources that would supplement advertising and circulation income. Even returns from running a job printing plant along with the publication of a newspaper or magazine have often not been sufficient. Church, lodge, and college papers have had supporting capital, but never as lushly as have the periodicals of some of the large white denominations or giant universities. Black society's political and social groups have not been in a position to finance in any substantial way publications intended for the general consumer. The press, therefore, has had to depend upon its ability to function as a business institution, particularly in the past half-century. This necessity accounts for the great mortality among the publications since the first was issued in 1827 and the hand-to-mouth existence of many that did not survive more than a few years.

Government, which in recent years has helped many other types of business directly through the Minority Small Business Investment Company and other programs, has not been welcome in American journalistic operations during this century, usually for fear of attempts at political control. The black press has been like any other in this respect, but the word *directly* must be emphasized. Distribution of government advertising money has kept many a white newspaper alive, especially in a county seat town, via the official advertising. Black publications have not been so favored.

And if any publishing ventures could have benefited from financial assistance it is the black newspapers and magazines. Since their beginning about a century and a half ago, with some exceptions they have been undercapitalized, underequipped, and understaffed. And many remain so. Kenneth O. Wilson, a vice president of the *Afro-American* newspapers, speaking at a panel of six black executives of black publications or members of the staffs of large white firms, said that of the 150-odd black owned and operated newspapers . . . there are probably only about sixteen who are doing well.[2]

Yet this picture is different only in degree from a large segment of the white newspaper press. Numerically the bulk of both the black and white presses is made up of weeklies and a few issued twice or three times a week, a few out every other week. Two of the approximately 250–75 black papers (Wilson apparently was using the Ayer figure available at the time) are dailies; about 1,780 of the 12,000 white papers are dailies. For many years the white weeklies had financial troubles similar to those of the black papers, although not so severe or general. The great decrease in their number, from about 16,000 in the first part of the century to around 10,000 today, occurred because the financially feeble ones simply lost with the rise in cost of operations.

In recent years the black press, particularly the middle-sized and large daily and the consumer magazine, has gained a measure of comparative business stability, but only a measure. What improvement has occurred has taken place largely in the last quarter of a century, reflecting the gradual rise in purchasing power of a segment of the black society and a greater rise of literacy among black workers. It also is evidence of the greater business opportunities of the owners.

The differences between the business operations of the black and white presses are few. Their managers are in the same positions of finding ways to keep publishing. They attend the same workshops or at least the same kind, if they are able to stand the cost of travel and enrollment; they use the same guidebooks; they are quick to appreciate cost savings through new mechanical devices although they can afford few of these inventions. Even the physical quarters are much alike: unpretentious, crowded, and looking a little rundown in many instances. If one wants to understand the inside operations of black publications, one can see them described and explained in the usual books and periodicals devoted to the world of publishing. The equipment is much the same. The black paper's may be somewhat outdated, but it printed, in all likelihood, a white paper once, before it was sold at secondhand. Except quantitatively and in some matters qualitatively, the two use the same organizational plans and the same procedures. Black publishers, even if they wished, have no other choice. Presses are made for any user, as are typewriters, file cabinets, and cameras. The equipment is color blind.

The differences are in the race of the owners and most of the staffs, the subject matter of the publications, the number of publications, and some of the particular problems facing those who own and operate this black business. Differences in quantity or number of publications and the quality of their product are serious, but not as much as they used to be. Through the years many black publications have been shoestring operations. Their owners have had no choice but to use ancient equipment or to depend upon white printing establishments. They had little access to trained personnel, the more skilled a worker became the more likely he would be enticed by the higher wages and better working conditions of white firms or the few more affluent black ones.

As is traditional with small publications, weekly newspapers especially, publishing a newspaper still is not enough. The press would stand idle six of the seven days. Thus job printing is undertaken—handbills, stationery, posters, leaflets, letters, wedding invitations, business cards, and the like.

Although the basic business operations of a black publication follow in general the lines of any other, several special aspects of advertising, circulation, and production should be realized by persons seeking to understand black journalism. These three areas undergird the business operations of a publishing firm. Other operations, less essential, as well as several services and competitors, are discussed in the next chapter.

● **ADVERTISING**

Functionally, advertising in the black journalism world is no different from that in any other. In both it is intended to provide revenue to the owners, to perform a service to readers by informing them of the availability of products and services, and to aid producers and service institutions to reach their markets. In scope, this advertising is like all other. It is national, regional, or local; it is display or classified. Space is sold in the usual ways: agents represent the papers and magazines or the publications' own salesmen sell it.

Two primary differences exist, however. They are in the slant, appeal, or content of copy and in the volume obtained. Both are changing.

Adverse critics of the black press for years have commented unfavorably on certain types of advertising to be found in it. At one time even the publishers themselves agreed to avoid it, but it continues in some papers. These types were for aphrodisiacs, patent medicines, clairvoyants' services, lucky charms and other appeals to superstition, and skin lighteners. The appeal to superstition, to fakery in religion, and to preoccupation with sex still can be found in some of the most prestigious papers. Nothing today is as extreme, perhaps, as the patent medicine ad found by Detweiler in the Chicago *Defender* of July 9, 1921, which read:

> IF YOU SUFFER FROM
> Malaria, Chills and Fever, Loss of Na-
> ture, Catarrh, Dropsy, Ulcer, Prickly
> Heat, Tired Sleepy Feeling, Headache,
> Pain in Neck, Sides, Shoulders, Back
> or Hips; Sick Stomach, Kidney and
> Bladder Trouble, Female Diseases and
> Women's Troubles, Bad Colds, La-
> Grippe, Stomach Ulcers, Fever; Mean,
> Tired Feeling, by all means take a
> bottle of Aztec Kidney and Liver Med-
> icine. It has made hundreds well and
> strong again.[3]

More popular today are such small ads as this; the errors are unchanged:

> IF YOU are in Distress of financial needs, dis-
> courage and unhappiness. Don't let it bother you
> because there is a sweeter and bright day tomorrow.
> A donation of $25.00 will bring you success and hap-
> piness.

A similar ad in the *New Pittsburgh Courier* asks for $37, but many others are content with as little as one. Other notices talk of sacred rituals, lucky charms, hands, and medals, love pills, of building "strong sex power," of "speedy" Mexican divorces, and of Spanish fly (in liquid or pill form—take your choice).

Black people say that aphrodisiac, charm, and fortune-telling advertising, as well as opportunities to play the numbers game through the papers, is important still because of the heritage of the race. Superstitions originating in Africa or the West Indies have not died. They point to whites who mount religious images, rabbits' feet or other symbols of luck on their auto dashboards or consult astrology columns as no different and can point as well to considerable editorial material, such as entire white magazines with such content as their support.

Use of such copy, particularly in leading publications not so economically pressed as are most small ones, is out of tune with the ideals expressed by publishers, who must realize that these ads merely trap the gullible. Vishnu V. Oak, a teacher at black colleges who specialized in the study of black press' business operations, pointed out in *The Negro Newspaper* that until the 1920's the papers were dependent for their advertising upon black businesses in their own area, a generally feeble source. Their income consequently has been both uncertain or low for a century. What advertising outside their own shopping areas they were able to obtain was almost entirely from white companies and only a few of these were large national firms. Among those few were tobacco, soap, bread, and motor car accounts.

The situation improved in the 1930's when a white agency took an interest in selling space for black publications. Within a decade some units of the press were selling to firms producing cosmetics, liquors, and food in addition to the earlier accounts. In two more decades the variety had increased greatly. To all the early advertisers were added more firms producing the same commodities as well as such new accounts as those for men's and women's clothing, musical instruments, travel services, records and tapes, and household equipment. In recent years an important type of advertising has been display space offering employment opportunities, placed by local, state, and federal government agencies as well as private industry.

Today advertising in the black newspapers, much more so than in the white, is still heavily local. A tabulation made by the author in 1970 shows that advertising occupies, on the average, 25 to 35 per cent of a newspaper's total space; of this, from 75 to 100 per cent is local in origin. Norman W. Powell, general sales manager of Amalgamated Newspapers, Inc., advertising representative for most of the larger papers, in 1970 estimated the national-to-local advertising to be about 35 to 40 per cent for national and 60 to 65 per cent for local. This figure was based on the seventy-two papers API then serviced. In contrast, the author found that the advertising in black magazines of all types had an enormous range, from 5 to 60 per cent of the total space of the consumer magazines, with an average of 38 per cent.

Change in Appeal. Along with the change in kinds of accounts has come altering of the appeal advertisers now make, especially in black magazines. A comparative study of the 1960 advertising in *Ebony* and *Life* made by Berkman in 1960 brought out the nature of that appeal at the time and continued in the decade that followed. He observed that a basic principle of communication, including advertising, was to address people in their own idiom, but also that "the idiom that a person considers his own may differ with the psychological setting in which the communication is perceived."[4] Thus, if copy appeals to the person's "aspiration to achieve higher status, it will address him not in the idiom of the present and lower situation but in the idiom appropriate to the status to which he aspires . . . ," he went on to explain.

Berkman found a great awareness of this condition among advertisers in both magazines. An example in *Ebony* was the presence of copy for lower-priced automobiles and not the higher-priced, although it frequently is thought that possession of a high-priced car confers upon a black owner a status he cannot achieve through home ownership or other symbols. To which might be added the view that when a black citizen is refused a house he wants to buy he enjoys buying what is not denied him: a car, a color television set, or some other commodity.

What has occurred in the decade that followed did not, however, confirm a prediction made by Berkman, a forecast resting upon a statement made also by *Ebony*'s owner, John H. Johnson. "It would seem," Berkman wrote, "that the advertising in Negro publications such as *Ebony* now, and for some time, will continue to reflect the socio-economic dichotomy which exists between the reality of the Negro's existence, and the status to which he aspires. But as the gulf narrows—as the dominant class status . . . tends to become the same middle-class status which predominates among whites—no longer will *Ebony* advertisements reflect the Negro's 'black reality' as opposed to his 'white aspirations.' "[5] Berkman went on to say that at the time this change occurs, the need for a distinctive Negro magazine will have disappeared and there won't even be an *Ebony*, as its owner himself had predicted.

What Berkman did not and could not anticipate, as did no other scholar or observer of the black press, was the rise of separatism and nationalism and with it a new interest and pride in blackness from which the press has benefitted in both advertising and circulation volume (the latter only among magazines). Berkman's "for some time" is sufficiently indefinite, however, to permit the prediction to be correct if the desire for separatism dies out after "some time." But if it persists, advertising in black publications may be greater than ever in both volume and revenue earned, and at last may sustain a powerful black journalism.

Selling the Space. Selling space in black publications is a matter of personal effort by individual publications and the assistance of a few agencies and representatives. The situation was discouraging until the early 1930's, when slight improvement was brought about by the W. B. Ziff Company, then a Chicago firm of advertising representatives but later a book and magazine publishing company, Ziff-Davis. It obtained space sales for a number of papers, supplementing what a few sold by their own efforts. The papers more successful in such individual efforts were several of those nationally known today, such as the New York *Amsterdam News*, Kansas City *Call*, Chicago *Defender*, and Norfolk *Journal and Guide*.

In another decade two Pittsburgh *Courier* executives launched what was to become one of the two major firms of advertising representatives serving the black press, Interstate United Newspapers, Inc., of New York. It made market studies and launched campaigns to obtain accounts for its clients, which, Oak reports, reached 135 newspapers and magazines in 1940, eight years after it was founded.[6] The Ziff accounts multiplied and new ones were added for soft drinks, liquor, sugar, and supermarkets.

The second major firm was founded four years after the first and called Associated Publishers. Interstate ceased in 1961, merging with Associated and the advertising sales activities of the *Defender* publications to become the present Amalgamated Publishers, Inc. At first the combined firm was called Consolidated Publishers; in 1962 the name became Amalgamated. At the time of the merger Interstate had thirty-two member papers, Associated twenty-four, and the *Defender* four. Amalgamated now is known as API, and has offices in New York and Chicago and a special Michigan and Ohio representative. Its officers in 1970 were headed by John H. Sengstacke, president of the papers bearing his name. Included in its staff then were a general manager, general sales manager, four account executives, and other officials. Its standards for representation require that a paper be in business a year or more, have an office and staff, apply for listing in Standard Rate and Data Service, and sign a two-year contract. In 1970 API had about seventy papers on its list.

Three nationally active advertising agencies were functioning in 1970: Vince Cullers Advertising, Inc., Chicago; Howard Sanders, Ltd., New York; and Zebra Associates, Inc., also of New York. These are dominantly black agencies. Formed in the late 1960's, the last named represents the present-day agency operation. It is called Zebra because of its integrated staff (blacks outnumber whites by three to two). But it is owned by blacks. A former account executive for J. Walter Thompson, a worldwide agency and one of the largest, and a New York television correspondent are the owners: Raymond League and Joan Murray. Within six months it had billings at an annual rate of $1,500,000, including such accounts as Fabergé, Clairol, and Fabricators, Inc. Associated with the agency have been Ossie Davis and Godfrey Cambridge, who appeared in a Zebra promotion film.

League told *Newsweek* that the inner city is a large, undeveloped market in which various ethnic groups, while of low income, together spend a total of one hundred billion a year. "But to reach them," he is quoted as saying, "You've got to speak inner city—and fluently."[7] So black dialect is used in the agency's copy. The nonblack staff members enable the firm to reach various other groups, such as Puerto Ricans, Italians, and Jews.

The sales efforts of such firms benefit at least half the black newspapers, but mainly the more substantial. Many a small community weekly or monthly magazine must depend upon one or two staff members, often not even a full-time person on advertising; whoever does the work often is the owner and editor as well. A large publication, on the other hand, has a sizable staff for such work. *Ebony*, as one would expect on a periodical well over the million mark in circulation, has ten advertising salesmen responsible for selling this magazine's space in a dozen cities where the black population is large. They work with the advertisers' local sales staffs, visit retailers, jobbers, brokers, and wholesalers.

Large or small, these publishing companies try to convince black as well as white advertisers that the black market is an important one and that the black media are needed if they are to reach this market (see Tables 13.1, 13.2, and 13.3).

Research and the Market. Little research has been done on either black publications or the black market; what results have been recorded are from advertising agencies, university teachers, and graduate students in schools of journalism, most of it conventional or traditional, with history predominating. Market research or product studies, readership or readability surveys, and content analyses on any large scale are few. Dr. Charles L. Allen, while assistant dean of the Medill School of Journalism at Northwestern University, in the early 1950's directed two advertising readership surveys, one of the Chicago *Defender* and another of the Baltimore *Afro-American.* The second study, issued in 1954, produced such findings as these: 82 per cent of the *Afro* buyers spent an hour or more reading the paper; small ads, vital statistics, and classified ads had high readership. These results were encouraging to the newspaper, which published them. With the realization of the billions of available dollars in the pockets of black families in the 1960's and 1970's more attention has been given to market studies. The results of several of the more important have been drawn upon for this chapter.

TABLE 13.1 ● Black and White Display Advertising Line Rates of Fifteen Black Newspapers

Newspaper	Open Rate
Atlanta *Daily World*	$ .25
Baltimore *Afro-American*[a]	.70
Chicago *Daily Defender*	.4025
Cleveland *Call and Post*	.40
Detroit *Michigan Chronicle*	.40
Kansas City *Call*	.25
Los Angeles *Sentinel*	.32
Louisville *Defender*	.18
Miami *Times*	.25
New Orleans *Louisiana Weekly*	.25
New York *Amsterdam News*	.80
Norfolk *Journal and Guide*	.30
Oklahoma *Black Dispatch*	.13
Philadelphia *Tribune*	.60
New Pittsburgh Courier[b]	.30

SOURCES: Standard Rate and Data Service reports, 1969; Amalgamated Publishers, Inc., 1970.
[a] All editions, $1.20.
[b] All editions, $.80.

TABLE 13.2 ● Location of U.S.A. Black Newspapers by States, 1969–70

Alabama	8	Iowa	1	New Jersey	3
Alaska	1	Kansas	1	New York	18
Arizona	1	Kentucky	1	North Carolina	6
Arkansas	1	Louisiana	7	Ohio	9
California	20	Maryland	1	Oklahoma	3
Colorado	1	Massachusetts	6	Oregon	1
Connecticut	2	Michigan	4	Pennsylvania	6
Delaware	1	Minnesota	5	South Carolina	4
District of Columbia	4	Mississippi	5	Tennessee	6
Florida	10	Missouri	9	Texas	15
Georgia	10	Nebraska	1	Virginia	4
Illinois	14	Nevada	1	Washington	1
Indiana	5			Wisconsin	3

SOURCES: Amalgamated Publishers, Inc., Representation List, 1969–70; *U.S. Negro World* Negro Press Editions, 1966, 1967; *Ayer Directory*, 1969, 1970; author's checklist based on newspapers identified.
NOTE: This table covers newspapers available for general public sale. It does not include periodicals or such specialized newspapers as those for colleges, churches and businesses. Regional editions have been counted separately. State with most black papers is California (20); regional distribution is: South, 63; Midwest, 54; East and West, 40 each.

But that there is a black market is not even agreed upon by all advertisers, advertising agency people, and some analysts of the black press. Louis E. Lomax, black author of several studies of the American black society, discussing the press in one of his books, said that the Negro market does not exist as such. "We respond to a product we already know about when we discover that the makers of that product have invested time and money to make certain that they attract our attention," he observed.[8] One of the leading black publishers calls the expression, *Negro market,* a misnomer. " . . . it does not mean a market for Negroes," W. Leonard Evans, Jr., president and editor of Tuesday Publications, said in 1967, "but rather it is an abnormal consumption in definable geographic areas of national brands at all economic and educational levels." The black market, in his view, is an economic and geographical rather than a racial matter.[9]

Taking another view about the same time was H. Naylor Fitzhugh, then vice president for special markets of the Pepsi Cola Company, and a former professor of marketing at Howard University as well as a black businessman. He said that there is a market and that

TABLE 13.3 ● States Lacking Black Newspapers, 1969–70

Hawaii	New Hampshire	Utah
Idaho	New Mexico	Vermont
Maine	North Dakota	West Virginia
Montana	Rhode Island	Wyoming
	South Dakota	

NOTE: The far West has more states without papers or states with only a few papers than any other region; California and Texas alone account for all but five in the West.

it has two aspects. The Negro, he said, is both a consumer and a Negro, " . . . and I am not sure the two can be separated. The Negro has to be addressed at both levels with both roles in mind."[10]

Two years later, *Media/scope* magazine examined the matter of advertising to blacks. It learned that "The Negro market means many things to many people." To some agencies and clients the black man is a consumer like anyone else but to others he is among many special markets in the demographic spectrum, it said. "But to an increasing number, he is one of several ethnic groups that deserve consideration, but not quite the same as the others." And Raymond League of Zebra Associates put it succinctly when he said in the same issue that "The black life style is completely different from the white middle-class life style." He also said, for the advertisers: "You can't play the numbers game to reach the Negro market." He went on to note the points made earlier in this book: that the black press serves a function not provided by the white, that is, status and recognition, thus creating a favorable climate for advertisers.[11]

Also not doubting the existence of a market is the Consumer Research Consortium, a small black-owned and staffed market research agency in Chicago begun in 1967. In 1970 it was setting up an all-black consumer mail panel in fourteen cities with large black populations.

D. Parke Gibson, president of a large firm engaged in conducting advertising campaigns and research for white firms interested in the black market, likewise has no doubts about the market being a reality. In a book, *The $30 Billion Negro,* he sets forth his argument, one which echoes statements made from time to time by various publication owners and publishers. The black people of the U.S.A. have a per capita income higher than that of the nations of Western Europe combined and much greater than that of Asia, Africa, and Latin America together. More than half the 6,000,000 black families, Gibson says, at the end of the 1960's owned automobiles, one out of every sixteen such families having two cars; 50 per cent of the families owned homes; 75 per cent had television sets. They constituted 92 per cent of the nonwhite market and 11 per cent of the population of the country, or 22,000,000 people, a society concentrated in seventy-eight cities.[12]

The nature of the market has been described in 1969 and 1970 by several reports. One of the most extensive was prepared by Young & Rubicam, a major advertising agency.[13] Its findings, announced in 1969, all were based on studies and reports made by various federal offices and publishing firms. Some of the delineations of the black market are these:

On population: The black population is increasing 64.3 per cent faster than the white. In 1969 the under-eighteen black population was 43.7 per cent, the eighteen to forty-four age group was 34.2 per cent, and the over forty-five was 22.1 per cent. The figures for whites were 33.6, 35.3, and 31.1 per cent. In 1810 the black population was 1,378,000; ninety years later it was 8,834,000; in another fifty it had almost doubled and by 1960 increased to 18,866,000. Black population migration between 1940 and 1968 was sharply to the North. The increase in the Northeast was 7 per cent, Northwest, 7 per cent, and North Central, 10 per cent (of the black population). The South and Southwest dropped 24 per cent. In contrast is the fact that in 1810 more than 90 per cent of the black population was in the South, a figure which dropped to 53 per cent by 1968. The West had scarcely any black population until 1930. Equally striking has been the movement of the black people into the urban areas; the report shows that in 1910 more than 27 per cent lived in cities; by 1960 the figure was 73.1 per cent or an increase of 167.2 percent (the whites, however, increased by only 42.9 per cent). By 1968 the twenty-five largest U.S. cities sheltered 38 per cent of the total black population.

On education: Of extreme importance to publishers of the printed word is the educational status of the people at which the publication is aimed. Today there is little difference between some comparable groups of blacks and whites, the Young & Rubicam report indicates. For example, those between twenty-five and twenty-nine years of age showed, for 1969, only 3.3 per cent difference on the median number of school years completed (12.1 for blacks, 12.6 for whites). In all except eight years of elementary, four years of high school and four of college, blacks had a higher percentage, i.e., a greater percentage of blacks had completed one to four years and five to seven years of elementary school than whites; similarly, a greater percentage of them had completed one to three years of high school.

On income: The report also shows that while the black family median income is increasing ($1,869 in 1950; $5,360 in 1968), the white income is still higher ($3,445 in 1950; $8,937 in 1968) but the rate of black increase is greater, 186.8 per cent to 159.4 per cent or increasing 17.2 per cent faster. The median white family income is higher by from $2,000 to $3,000 in all parts of the South.

Another comparison was reported in 1970 when *Chain Store Age* cited an *Ebony* study which said that blacks spend more than whites for shelter, food, necessities, and clothing (51.4 per cent of the black dollar, 45.2 per cent of the white) because the black family is larger.[14]

To these facts can be added the estimate of the U.S. Department of Commerce that the black market was to have reached forty billion dollars in 1970, a figure not realized, but that it may not be much delayed is indicated by the addition of two billion to Gibson's figure for 1968. And to this information should be added that the black population of the U.S.A. forms an ethnic group within the country larger than any single African nation except Nigeria. And economically and educationally it is a far more advanced group than that African nation. Gibson advised his white clients that if they wish to reach the black market they must do so through what he called the black-oriented media. "While it might have been possible at one time," he wrote, "business and industry can no longer lead Negro thinking through white-oriented media."

Joining Gibson in that view is William P. Grayson, executive vice-president of Johnson Publishing Company, the magazine firm. He points out that the nature of the market is favorable to advertising buyers today, since they are making a distinct attempt to appeal to younger consumers. He cites Commerce Department figures that show the black population to have had, in 1968, relatively more young people and fewer old than the white population. He reports that 44.7 per cent of the black group is under eighteen, but only 35.5 per cent of the white. Also, he notes a difference of eight years in the median age for blacks and whites, 21.7 as against 29.5.

Grayson summarized the nature of the black consumer of the late 1960's by saying, "The Negro of today is of a new breed. He is Black . . . and he is proud! He has more education, money and a sense of direction. He is ready to integrate into a bi-racial partnership on a basis of equality and mutual self-respect. He advocates joint cooperation with other ethnic groups to build a greater and more democratic America."[15]

Then there were the six prominent black marketing and media men who met at *Newsweek* in 1969 to discuss selling to the market. William Santos, director of market development, Fabergé, Inc., one of the panel, introduced the idea that "We can no longer say we are selling black because black is now taking on a new connotation. Black is soul, not color. They are people. It is not a race anymore. These young people that are thinking black now will soon become so confirmed in their minds that their buying habits are going to change. They are going to be looking for new symbols. And these symbols are going to take on a very new meaning, and the whites will do the same thing, too."[16]

But it should be noted that the few studies not sponsored by the publishing or advertising industry itself, such as those by Lyle, Bontrager, and other scholars reported earlier in this book, showed that black audiences preferred the white newspaper over the black and made more use of television than of any other medium and television is all white; white radio also predominates. Although not a major factor, influential militant blacks despise all the media except their own and a few sympathic publications.

The Attitude of White Advertisers. Perhaps the biggest obstacle to the financial stability of the black press, so far as advertising is concerned, is the attitude of white advertisers. If one riffles through files of back numbers or looks at microfilms of papers it is clear that most of the white advertisers have spent little money on black media (see Table 13.4). The reasons given usually are that the American blacks

TABLE 13.4 ● One Insertion Advertising Page Rates of Selected Consumer Magazines

Magazine	1 pg., b/w	½ pg.	1 pg., 1-color	½ pg.
Tuesday	$11,200	$6.790	$12,400	$7,460
Ebony	7,044	3,660	9,150	5,538
Miss Black America	3,500	2,770	4,000	2,600
Soul! Illustrated	1,750	1,000	1,950	1,200
Sepia	500	275	....	....
Tan	750	500[a]	1,000	+670
Philly Talk	600	360	700	....
Proud	500	300	....	....

Sources: Standard Rate and Data Service reports; publishers' rate cards.
[a] ⅔ page.

can be reached through the white media, that circulation is too low, ad budgets not big enough, or that the advertiser does not want to reach this particular market. Other reasons given are that the advertiser is convinced that black citizens buy too little or that they have special choices. Still others are that such advertising expenses pay only those who can cater to the black person's needs and that image or trade mark advertising is wasted on them. As if that were not enough there is also the assertion that the black press is not up to certain physical standards set up by agencies.

But some black advertising and marketing people, such as those who took part in a panel reported earlier or spoke in interviews for publication, while not agreed on whether there is or there is not a black market or whether it is or is not worthwhile to advertise in certain ways to it, agree that most advertising agencies have not tried to understand the market.

Several additional reasons for the lack of advertising were uncovered by a study made in 1968–69 by a Syracuse University advertising major.[17] They were noted by advertising agencies.

1. Fear of worsening an already poor image of an advertiser. For example, a company which has been struck can be accused of attempted bribery if it suddenly advertises its product heavily.
2. Reaction to implied threats of a few black media salesmen whose attitude is "Buy our paper—or else."
3. Fear of alienating white customers, especially in the South, with a resulting boycott.
4. Objection to the atmosphere created by the protest aim of some black papers and magazines; firms do not like to associate themselves with it.
5. Belief that the literacy rate of black readers is too low for certain types of advertising or kinds of commodities or services.

The researcher, Miss O'Connell, noted answers that she and others give to these objections and others more common reported earlier. A company's poor image can be erased only by fair and honest racial policies and a steady advertising program. Threats by salesmen are rare and do not come from major publication advertising staffers or representatives. Fear of offending white customers is realistic but boycotts have not materialized in any dangerous way. There are protest publications, to be sure, but most of the larger magazines and papers are not militant. The literacy rate is on the rise, as is the general educational level.

On the widely made point that white publications are enough or that radio and television are sufficient, a reply is that the publication issued for whites does not meet the needs of the black consumer, for it does not provide the right atmosphere. The message in the black publication is only for the black, a point about which he is ultraconscious at this time.

On some objections, however, there must be agreement. The black press, it is true, is not up to certain physical standards, particularly the newspapers. Even the larger papers, by comparison with white ones of the same importance, are not well printed: cuts reproduce badly; other work, such as page trimming, is inaccurate; printing of the body type often is blurred or smeary. Although it is doubtful that there is much solicitation of firms or organizations whose product or service is of little interest to blacks, where that does occur it is admittedly a misplacement of effort. Like all minority presses, this one has to some extent retained the idea that advertising money should be spent to sustain the press even if there is no direct return. But such reasons as low budgets, lack of purchasing power by blacks, or special choices being paramount in buying decisions appear to be excuses to cover either prejudice or lack of information.

A writer in *Advertising Age* in 1970 pointed out, however, that the objection of low quality printing is not taken so seriously any more. Now that there is a big, desirable market it is discovered, as noted by a Harvard report, "The Management of Racial Integration in Business," that "American advertisers stand to gain image within the Negro community, not only by their identification with the newspapers sincerely directed toward them; they also tend to place more confidence and trust in national advertising when carried in their own press."[18] In other words, more important than physical quality is the rapport between the reader and the paper. If the reader cares not at all if there are errors but is loyal to the paper for its community leadership the advertising will be taken seriously.

Proud as they are more and more in their blackness, there is reason to think that black citizens will continue to find it easier to use the predominant publications, for they are beginning to see a little more information about their race, more pictures of blacks in both reading matter and advertising, and more direct appeal to them from advertisers in white-owned and aimed publications. Until black newspapers and magazines are more readily available than now, the American black housewife or businessman is likely to turn to what is at hand. And this matter of availability is the problem of the circulation department.

● CIRCULATION

The closed-in-ness of the black society is dramatically demonstrated when one asks white persons about their knowledge of black publications. A well-educated white may know of the high-circulation *Ebony,* but rarely any other. A member of the white intelligentsia may know of one or two scholarly periodicals, such as *Journal of Negro History,* and of the militants' *Black Panther.* But a workingman of the orthodox variety—repairmen, drivers of delivery trucks, and factory workers—unless his job throws him into close relationship with Afro-Americans, knows vaguely that there are such publications and perhaps has seen a copy of *Jive* or *Jet* in the hands of a co-worker. Mr. and Mrs. White Citizen appear to be no more aware of the press of the black citizens than they are of the specialized journals for horologists or oculists. Yet these publications are molding opinions, influencing the minds of many members of a different race.

Shut as is the black society, despite the slight opening of doors in recent years but the shutting of some again in an era when determined separatism by certain groups is growing, the black citizen's knowledge of his own publications is only a little broader than that of the whites. The surveys made by researchers and the casual questioning by others show that most city blacks are aware of several publications intended for them, usually of one or two newspapers and two or three magazines. But beyond the limits of the consumer publication they rarely can go. White readers are either unaware of them or have little interest in their content. Consequently their circulations in general have been confined to the cities with large black populations. And those populations, if a statement by one prominent editor and publisher is correct, are only newly appreciative of the black newspaper. William O. Walker, of the Cleveland *Call and Post,* in his 1970 Negro Press Week statement, wrote: "As the Negro began to get sophisticated, there were some who did not want it known that they read Negro newspapers. Today, the Negro newspaper has been fully accepted in the Negro home. In fact, Negroes now take pride in letting it be known in public or private that they read their own papers."[19]

The lack of information among blacks about their own publications is not difficult to explain. In their history, American black citizens have had a low literacy rate. Their sparse incomes have kept down their purchases of publications even when they became literate in large numbers. The outlets or sources have been more limited than those for whites. A few newsstands in the black colonies are the typical sources; even there only a handful of the existing publications are sold.

The author has walked for many blocks on Chicago's South Side and in Harlem and found few opportunities to buy or see a black paper or magazine. In his own city of Syracuse, which has about 200,000 population, 10 per cent of it black, only two widely separated outlets sell more than two or three black publications. The larger stands on downtown streets or in shopping areas have on sale none of the newspapers and not more than two or three of the popular magazines. The black citizen, unless he happens to live within reach of a black college or university or a well-stocked library such as the Schomburg in Harlem, has little opportunity to see more than a few consumer publications. Such unavailability is built into the circulation system of the black press. It can be compared to the white little literary magazine or some other publication with a limited group of readers. Unless there is a considerable number of readers in each community the restricted interest publication will not sell and will be returned or become waste paper. The black press must base its circulation plans on realistic expectations. If there is insufficient or no demand, one hardly can blame a dealer for not displaying a given publication. The decision may be governed by other factors. In some geographical areas it clearly is prejudice. The dealer may not approve of the publications (it sometimes works in reverse, however). He may not want, if he is white, to encourage black patronage of his store. Nor does logic explain the decision. For example, a large stand in Albany, New York, stocks *Ebony, Sepia, Jet,* and *Tan,* but no black newspapers. Across the street is another stand; no black publications whatsoever are sold there.

Libraries are possibly the most consistent agencies for making black publications available to the public in any community, even when the number of black users of the institution is small. For libraries and library trustees are likely to have somewhat more sense of obligation to expose different viewpoints, an attitude that few newsstand operators seem to possess or perhaps can afford to hold even if they wished to do so. A small public library—the first free one in the nation—in Peterborough, New Hampshire, population about 3,000, takes *Ebony,* although only a handful of black residents are in the area. In the public library at Worcester, Massachusetts, a city of about 200,000, readers can see that popular monthly as well as *Journal of Negro History, Journal of Negro Education,* and the *Negro History Bulletin.* On the other hand, the library receives *Pravda,* the *Jewish Civic Leader,* and *Japan Times,* but not one black newspaper. The public library, main building, in Syracuse, a city similar in size to Worcester and with a large black population, receives the same scholarly magazines and *Ebony,* but also the national edition of the *New Pittsburgh Courier.* In Evanston, Illinois, a

Chicago suburb with about 10 per cent of its population black, the library receives the usual popular magazines and a local black community weekly. Not all these cities, to be sure, are cultural centers. What is obtained may depend upon budget, demand, space, and other factors.

Auditing and Other Problems. Oak, in describing the advertising situation among black publications, quoted a letter he had received from Joseph B. LaCour, some years ago manager of Amalgamated Publishers, Inc. He gave a clue to some of the circulation problems of black publications in the 1940's as well as today.

"Misrepresentation of circulation and lack of believable and authentic market data have . . . militated against the acceptance of media serving our market and the colored family as a consumer," he wrote. But he saw improvement. And his forecast was correct, for in the next two decades more publications, in proportion to the total number, now are audited, since without such attests some advertisers will not spend their money in a publication.[20]

The auditing picture has been clouded, to some extent, by the practice of some publishers of selling a portion of their circulation and giving away another; this latter, commonly known as controlled, enables them to keep their figures up and also uses such copies as promotional samples in the hope of converting their receivers into paid subscribers eventually. Since the reputable auditing firms and organizations, such as the Audit Bureau of Circulations, place limits on the number of free copies, such publishing houses cannot claim convincing audits. The problem is a sticky one especially for new firms, seeking to gain a foothold in a community or in some national field for which they are issuing a new specialized magazine which cannot hope to enjoy newsstand distribution.

Detweiler noted that in 1920 "only four papers in Ayer and Son's Newspaper Directory, out of a total of 217 listed for Negroes, make sworn statements of circulation." The vast improvement is reflected in the fact that most publications now listed in Ayer make such statements and that many are audited by the Audit Bureau of Circulations. About one-third of the papers serviced by Amalgamated Newspapers, Inc., are ABC members.

Pricing has been a troublesome aspect of circulation for some publications. Because of the lack of advertising revenue heretofore and the small possibilities of profits from substantial job printing contracts, in the life of this ethnic press, publications had to price themselves higher than nonwhite papers and magazines, often as much as double (the thoughtless reader, however, often did not realize that he was paying ten cents a week for a weekly and thirty cents or more a week for a daily). This necessary policy limited sales in a day of uniformly low pay for blacks. The differential is not so sharp today, although it persists in per copy sales.

Achieving dependability of circulation has been extremely difficult and damaging to circulation departments. Since the bulk of the distribution of newspapers is in the cities with concentrated black residential neighborhoods, many of which until recent years fairly could be described as substandard areas, the problems were great for distribution of all publications, black or white.

Costs of handling circulation in the central city areas are higher. Estimates, according to a report of the International Circulation Managers Association, in 1969 ran as high as 400 per cent in their increase over other sections. These charges result from difficulties in "making collections, high turn-over of carriers, and lack of parental influence and cooperation." Such difficulties are nothing new to black papers, but as shopping plazas and enlarged stores are set up in or near the black neighborhoods white publications are feeling them sharply for the first time.

Black magazines, except for a small number of community periodicals, are sold largely by subscription and distribution is left to the post office system. But the city or community publications, like the smallest local newspapers, must deliver copies to newsstands themselves and use the mail for distant subscribers. The small publication system of some is illustrated by the set-up at the *Star*, a New Haven, Connecticut, newspaper. Its various devices to produce circulation are common in the black press world. Late in 1969, when it was the fortnightly *Crow*, its circulation was about 7,000, on a mainly paid basis. Five thousand five hundred were distributed by mail; the others divided thus: dealers, 1,000; newsboys, 200; advertising checking copies and office copies, 500. In certain months as many as 1,500 special sales were made, as at a local parade; sometimes copies are given away for promotion purposes, as when 250 were distributed at a fraternity conference. The mail subscriptions of the *Crow* were so high because of special package deals with local church and other groups. The annual subscription price was $3.50 and was maintained at that figure even after a reorganization of the paper in 1970, including enlargement of its size in number of pages. Street sales were ten cents a copy until mid-1970, when the sale of the publishing organization to the staff made a doubling of the per copy price necessary.

● PRODUCTION

For years many of the early newspapers and virtually all magazines aimed at black readers were printed on presses owned by white proprietors. The nineteenth century publishers could not capitalize plants of their own, as did most of their white counterparts in the newspaper business because if they managed to raise the money for such an investment there was little likelihood that they would get enough general printing business to keep the equipment operating.

But a few owners, such as Douglass, did attempt to do their own printing. When that abolitionist orator opened the offices of his *North Star* in Rochester, New York, he was told by printing experts that he had the best printing equipment obtainable anywhere. Quarles, in his biography of Douglass, describes the plant. It was thought to have been the first possessed by a black citizen. Costing "between nine and ten hundred dollars" in 1848, it was all in one room. A small hand press, a type case, a work table, and a desk were in it. A white apprentice and Douglass' sons were his printing assistants.[21] With this meagre equipment, yet luxurious for its time, he and his helpers did all but print the paper, a four-page, seven-column paper much like the other Abolitionist publications. It actually was printed on the larger press of the Rochester *Democrat,* a white paper.[22] Douglass kept this paper, and its successor that carried his name, going for sixteen years. In 1850 a new press was bought as well as additional type and the paper improved in typography and production.

The production set-up of the Baltimore *Afro-American,* which was founded before the turn of the century, is in contrast to the small office used by Douglass. The *Afro* considers itself "the largest colored newspaper in the world operating its own plant."[23] In its three-story building at Druid Hill Avenue and Eutaw Street all the usual newspaper publishing departments are housed. Like other large companies, a composing room, an engraving plant, a photographers' studio, and paper storage rooms also are there. The production section has modern equipment, including a plate-making machine, a Varityper, a head-setter, and offset presses. In the composing room are a dozen typesetting machines. The paper uses six teletypesetters with them. The press room shelters a thirty-two-page Goss; it handles the plates made in the stereotyping department.

Development during the 1960's of the cold-type offset printing process using newsprint gave a boost to the small black newspapers which could not afford the big operation, such as that of the *Afro.* It is less expensive than the process of setting type, making up pages, and manufacturing lead plates for a press—the letterpress system long standard in U.S. publishing. It also is speedier, for the staff can paste onto sheets what it wants to reproduce—typed copy, clippings of printed matter of any sort from other publications, cartoons, photographs, the latter often reproducing better than by the old method of making an engraving on a plate first. The montage or assembled material is photographed; what the camera sees is transferred to a plate from which the final printing is done.

Whether printed on white-owned or black-owned presses and set by hand or by composing machine in whichever office, the production results, particularly of newspapers of any size and of small magazines, usually have been inferior. Although there has been improvement in recent years because of the bigger incomes of some newspa-

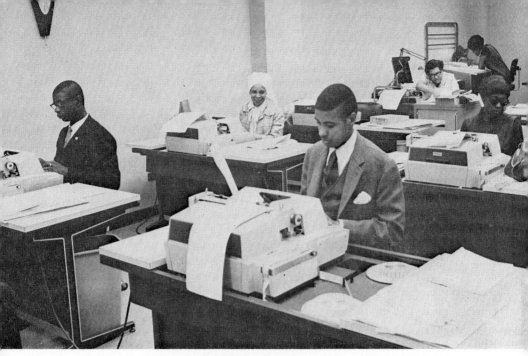

FIG. 13.1. **Muhammad Speaks,** the Muslim weekly published in Chicago, has one of the most modern plants in the world of the black press. Here type is being set in the composing room. (Chester Sheard photo)

pers and magazines, an examination of a large number of publications shows numerous areas where production improvement still is needed. What Oak wrote in 1948, and others before him, such as Detweiler, still is true of too many publications: "A study," he wrote, "of 66 representative newspapers revealed that, with the exception of a dozen papers, most of them are typographically inferior. . . . While an assortment of type faces is used for headlines and advertising displays, the quality of printing and typographical arrangement is so poorly done that they often look unattractive. An unbalanced and over-crowded appearance with pictures carelessly scattered everywhere seems to be the rule."[24]

Oak went on to say what he still could of numerous publications: the inking and press work of most newspapers are not of high quality. The appearance of many give evidence of worn-out presses. He complained that so few better-grade halftones were used by the more affluent papers and that line cuts were too sparingly used. Their appearance led him to conclude that the halftone engraving was poorly done.

Technical perfection is far from realized still, especially with the greater reliance on offset printing, which has led to numbers of small papers with disorderly looking pages produced by little more than a hasty paste up of material, much of it clipped from other publications. In some papers no thought is given to the clash of type faces, inappropriate typography, tilting columns of type, and unfinished stories cut in mid-sentence to make them fit space.

Perhaps a larger question should be raised: what standard did Oak and later critics use? What papers were compared? The unit of comparison doubtless was the white press, whose readers by and large were and still are better educated, more discriminating, and more demanding of the press than are black readers as a whole. Furthermore, perhaps the production refinements of white publications are unnecessary, as well as impractical for most black newspapers but definitely necessary for all black magazines. For, like white magazines, they cater to a more discriminating group of readers and advertisers, and their typographical effects, to be successful, depend upon excellent reproduction.

In bringing about change in production standards it is necessary to appeal to the publishers, not by pointing to the products of more affluent white firms but to note the arguments on a practical level of gaining more subscribers and advertisers and of more newsstand sales, showing, through research, that lack of better appearance and more careful makeup and better reproduction of halftones puts the black press second to the white, technically. Since it is clear that the trend among blacks is to depend upon television more than upon any other medium and that, in certain communities, as reported elsewhere in this book, black readers either prefer white papers (but not magazines) to black, or read as many white as black, it is necessary for black publishers to give more attention to production quality.

● THE POLICY OF IMITATING

A characteristic of much black publishing is its imitativeness, a practice not unknown in publications work by whites as well. Pride has observed that "Negro newspapers have usually taken on the fads and fashions of the moment in journalism. . . ." He cited the action in the early 1950's when a black paper in Los Angeles had its first page redesigned to be like that of a new daily established in the same city. A Miami weekly then followed suit. Another example was *People's Voice,* an imitation of *PM,* the adless daily of the 1930's.[25]

A classic instance was the long-existing typographical resemblance of the Chicago *Defender,* when it was not a tabloid daily, to the Chicago *Tribune.* When it became a daily it modeled itself on the New York *Daily News,* a highly successful tabloid. Pride could have included, as well, the New York *Amsterdam News,* which for years has looked like the now defunct New York *Journal-American.*

Black magazines have followed the same production policy, a notably successful strategy in the hands of the Johnson Publishing Company. The black trade journals and house publications follow the traditional format and typography for such publications in general. A few of the community weeklies are unconventional in format, *"In Sepia"* *Dallas* and *Bronze Texan News,* for example. Here and there a magazine stands out, as does *Essence* or *Freedomways.*

Unorthodoxy in format and typography is not necessarily a virtue; some experiments in American journalism have not been especially readable. Nor is great originality of design to be expected in a press which has had to struggle to survive and until recently had little reason to trust to design to gain support. The imitativeness certainly is understandable and pardonable. Although the black press has contributed little to developments in journalism, as Pride notes, it had neither time nor money for attempts at originality for originality's or art's sake. Furthermore, if a certain format is a factor in one publication's success it is only sensible and practical to learn from its experience. There were news magazines before *Time* and *Newsweek* and picture magazines before *Life* and *Look;* and white newspapers have looked much alike across the nation for many years.

But if the black newspaper in particular is to climb out of the position of being the second paper in the reader's fare it will more easily do so if it attains a personality of its own. And such personality is based heavily on a publication's physical appearance and quality.

● A SMALL OPERATION

The patterns of operation of black publications, in view especially of the need for the time being at least to be imitative in both appearance and production for the sake of efficiency and dependable economic results, are so much like those of any other, size for size, that it is unnecessary to review all the typical activities in managing the black press. To go a little behind the scenes of a small community publication may help gain understanding of what managerial problems must be faced and how they were being handled in the instance of one such paper. The sample paper selected is the *Star,* an offset-printed tabloid bi-weekly that grew out of a small newsletter begun in January, 1968, in New Haven, Connecticut, and called for nearly three years the *Crow.* Some details of its operations appear in the circulation section of this chapter. As one looks at copies of this neat and newsy paper, one has little sense of the financial uncertainties that still surround it. Newsier than many a larger community weekly because of the training of its editor (see Chapter 10), it carries a respectable amount of news that its little staff generates. Its news writing and headlining usually exhibit a professional tone. Its organization and operations are simple but businesslike.

After it left the newsletter stage the paper was owned by the Heritage Hall Corporation, also known as the Black Coalition, in New Haven, a city of about 150,000. The coalition, made up of

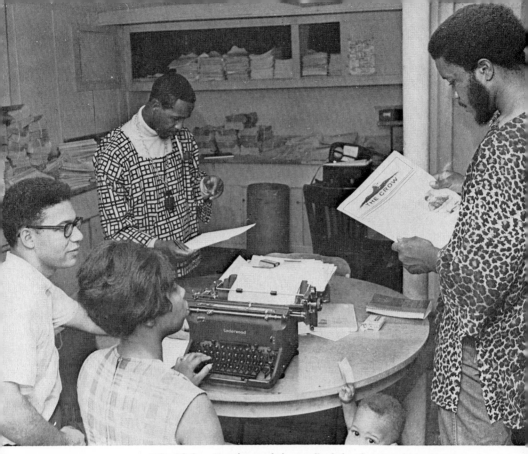

FIG. 13.2. Members of the staff of the **Crow**, a New Haven community biweekly (later the **Star**), working in a church kitchen in 1968. Mrs. Barbara Winters' editor, is at typewriter; Bob Greenlee, associate editor, is at left rear; Hugh Price, consultant, is at left foreground; J. Artis Yopp, ad salesman, is at right. (Evans photo)

about forty black groups, was formed right after Martin Luther King, Jr., was assassinated. Until mid-1970 it served as adviser or consultant and as a clearing house for New Haven's black residents. And it subsidized the paper.

The *Crow* was begun in a local neighborhood house, Dixie Community House. Volunteers produced the newsletter in their evening spare time. In August, 1968, it was moved to an old kitchen in the basement of St. Luke's Episcopal Church, remaining there until April, 1969, when it went to much larger quarters in a storefront building. The first three issues were given away to acquaint the city with it.

In Spring, 1970, the *Crow* staff bought the paper from the Black Coalition, incorporated the firm, increased the paper's size in number of pages, the price, and the staff, and issued a city as well as an out-of-town edition. It planned for weekly publication by 1971. In other words, from a subsidized, nonprofit venture the paper became a commercial enterprise, the staff convinced that it could make its own way.

The staff used Justowriters, a Varityper, and a headliner in preparing for offset reproduction of the tabloid by a printing firm in Hamden, ten miles from New Haven. Heading the staff was a young woman editor, Mrs. Barbara Winters, who brought training and practical experience in journalism to her job. She found that the weekly schedule followed at first (after going to printed form) was too costly. In summer, 1969, she put the paper on the new publishing schedule and increased pages from twelve to sixteen. In the early part of 1969 the advertising occupied a little over 32 per cent of the total space. At the end of the year it was up to 65 per cent.

Net, earned income in fall and early winter, 1968–69, was coming almost entirely from advertising, although financial conditions were improving steadily. Salaries then were being paid by the coalition but the printing and other bills were being met from the proceeds. That financial situation continued until the coalition authorized the formation of a separate corporation. But by fall, 1970, there was a setback. The city's residents began to feel the national economic pinch. Advertising fell off in volume. Unemployment rose in the community and subscribers decreased in number. The editors also cited as a cause of trouble the lack of cooperation from unnamed black leaders and opposition from segments of the black neighborhood. The final issue was dated December 3, 1970, and left New Haven without a black paper of its own. In early 1971 efforts to obtain refinancing succeeded and the paper was revived, with partly the same staff, and renamed the *Star*. It became one of a group of *Star* papers issued in New England. Most of its sales are through newsboys on New Haven streets. Mrs. Winters continued as editor.

14. AUXILIARIES AND COMPETITORS

THE THREE MAJOR AUXILIARIES of the black press examined in the preceding chapter—the departments or hired services devoted to advertising, circulation, and production—are only some of the aids. Less formally tied to publishing are news services, feature syndicates, and the output of those who do public relations, promotion, and publicity work.

Radio broadcasting is the one direct competitor to be examined in this chapter. White publications and broadcasts are the chief competitors for advertising and readers but they need no explication in this book.[1]

● THE NEWS SERVICES

The most important auxiliary outside those originating in the newspaper or magazine company's own precincts is the news service, since it provides copy that publication staffs cannot obtain for themselves without enormous expense. The black publications that use a commercial news service are the large city weeklies and dailies, and the press' one newsmagazine, *Jet*. Most national papers subscribe to United Press International, a white agency that sells its services on a commercial basis and one of the two largest in the world. The other general service in the U.S. is the Associated Press, also white, but out of reach of black papers because one franchise only is available in each city and that already is held by a white paper. (If two or more papers in a city are AP members they were part of it before the rule was agreed upon by the members of this cooperatively owned institution.) United Press International has correspondents throughout the world and provides news copy in several ways and grades for its clients, who are charged on a circulation-size basis.

Other services, all miniscule by comparison with UPI, also supply black publications with some copy; usually it is the small papers and magazines that sign contracts with Community News Service, Liberation News Service, and other specialized agencies.

Black news agencies, with the major exception of the one-time outstanding Associated Negro Press, have had an uncertain history, just as have many of the papers and magazines that have subscribed to their services. Detweiler reports that in 1921 a half-dozen services were available: the reciprocal service of the National Negro Press Association, Capital News Service, and the Negro Press Syndicate, all of Washington, D.C.; the NAACP and Exchange News Service of Boston and New York; and the Associated Negro Press of Chicago. To them he adds the Tuskegee Institute and Hampton Institute Press Services; probably the last two and the NAACP service were free and perhaps closer to publicity offices than objective news agencies.[2] Brooks has noted that in 1945 there were fourteen, attributing this information to the Bureau of the Census. He did not name them and added that he rarely saw any material in the black publications credited to them and surmised that most were highly specialized, dealing with sports, theatrical activities, and comics.[3] Perhaps either he or the Census Bureau confused news services with feature syndicates. Briefly there was a United Negro Press, mailing its service from Durham, North Carolina, beginning in the late 1940's; it specialized in news of blacks living in the southeastern section of the U.S., and later moved to New York City.

The NNPA service was an outgrowth, begun in 1947, of the desire and need of association members for less costly and better news coverage outside their own communities. Mutually owned and operated, it began with a bureau in Washington. Among the larger papers behind its operation were the Baltimore *Afro-American,* Kansas City *Call,* Norfolk *Journal and Guide,* and Atlanta *World.* Heading it was Louis Lautier, with correspondents in New York and Washington, two out-of-town columnists, and a sports editor in Philadelphia. The NNPA members, Brooks reports, did not respond heartily to the service, however. Some of the larger papers' owners believed that the service duplicated coverage they already were receiving from their own correspondents in Washington. Nevertheless, by 1948 it had thirty-three members. In a year this figure dropped to twenty. The service was ended in 1960. John H. Sengstacke, NNPA president in 1970, explained its cessation a decade later as the result of more local community coverage.

The original Associated Negro Press was founded in 1919 by Claude A. Barnett. News was supplied by mail, since virtually all black papers are published weekly. As with the white AP, this black agency was a cooperative, i.e., each member agreed to supply ANP with news of its own area and shared in its expenses. Barnett was joined by Nahum D. Brascher, the first editor-in-chief. He had worked for the Indianapolis *Recorder* and the Chicago *Defender.* P. O. Prattis, one-time editor of the Pittsburgh *Courier* and an early associate of Barnett, credits the founder with building and stabilizing the black press in his day through the service. His career was one of unusual devotion to black journalism and the black race. Widely known as he was to black journalists, he was little known to the world of journalism in general.

By training, Barnett was an engineer. Born in Sanford, Florida, in 1889, he went to public school in Oak Park, Illinois, and then to Tuskegee Institute, from which he received his engineering degree. But he entered journalism instead of that field, after nine years of working for the Chicago Post Office. He became an advertising salesman for the Chicago *Defender*.

Traveling around the U.S.A. for his paper, he realized that the black publications needed news of the black people, so he decided to form the Associated Negro Press.[4] He remained as its head until its cessation in 1964. During his career he was a special assistant to the Secretary of Agriculture during the third Roosevelt and Truman administrations, a director of the Supreme Life Insurance Company, and devoted to studying the African nations, in which he spent much time. He was particularly aroused by the demoralizing effects of segregation in the armed forces and is credited with having brought about some of the decrease in its practice.

After World War II Barnett traveled to Africa and added 100 publications to the list of ANP subscribers. He made fifteen trips to that continent for this purpose as well as to obtain information for his writing about the black society. He died in Chicago in 1967.

Lomax quotes him as having said: "It's a shame that we have a separate Negro society in this country and a separate wire service for Negro newspapers. We are working toward the end that some day there will be no more need for my news service and no need for anything else—including society—which at present the white community does not allow us to share."[5]

The highest number of domestic subscribers in any one year, according to Beard and Zoerner, was 112, in 1945. The African service in number of subscribers, in 1964, was large. More than 200 papers on that continent received it, some translating it into French, Portuguese, or other non-African languages. Of Africa's 158 daily papers, 108 received ANP material. During its last years under the original management the American services of ANP were used somewhat less. The drop occurred because the black press was losing advertising and circulation ground to television and the competition of white newspapers that began giving improved coverage to black news events in the realm of civil rights. In 1964 it was going to 101 papers, three magazines, two radio stations, and twenty-one private individuals. It was appearing in 90 per cent of the total circulation of black papers.[6]

Beard and Zoerner report that Barnett shut down ANP in July, 1964.[7] Considerable uncertainty seems to exist about just when it ceased and when it was revived. In its obituary of Barnett the New York *Times* gave the year of cessation as 1963.[8] But *Editor & Publisher* reported in 1965 the purchase of ANP by Alfred Duckett, who moved it to New York from Chicago, with plans to enlarge it.[9] It apparently functioned for several years thereafter but its logotype began to disappear from dispatches in black papers during 1968. Duckett has a long record of experience with black publications and in public relations work. Duckett in 1970 called the agency the Associated Negro Press International. It distributes occasional stories but Duckett's principal effort appears to be used in getting out Empire Features as a subsidiary.

During the completion of the agency's sale some staff members established another service, a feature agency called Negro Press International. In 1969 its logo was changed to Black Press International, the news service owned by *Muhammad Speaks* and issued from its Chicago offices. At this time the black press has no major news agency of its own comparable to what was once provided by ANP or NNPA.

News credits, when they appear in the black press, are to the publication's own staff writers or to stringers, to a black college free news service devoted to covering the college mainly, or to a small agency, like Liberation or Community.

Liberation News Service is used by only a few black publications, largely such advocacy organs as the *Black Panther* or some of the more militant small community papers, the latter tending merely to clip material from the larger papers that pay for it. Founded in 1967, the LNS stories or some distributed by the similar Underground Press Service are to be found chiefly in the white underground periodicals and papers, college papers, and magazines of the critics of society that consider themselves in the Third World or The Movement, as they put it. A typical report, datelined Saigon, detailed a crackdown on black market operators, concluding: "No wonder so many South Vietnamese people are siding with the revolutionaries. In liberated zones there's no black market—but also no inflation, no unemployment."

An incident, attributed to the *Christian Science Monitor,* is then related at length as evidence that the police may be joining the pro-revolutionary forces. It describes the plight of a policeman when it was learned that his wife was one of the persons whose black market goods had been confiscated. There was nothing whatever in the *Monitor* story, however, to indicate that the policeman might switch sides.[10]

Community News Service came into being after the Kerner Report indicated the lack of coverage of minority group events in New York City. "You've made your point. It's true. We are not doing a proper job of covering the communities and the neighborhoods. But, you see, we are not geared to do this well. We don't have the time or talent." In essence, this is what media people in the city said, making statements of this sort to people seeking a solution to the communication problem.[11] CNS was begun in 1968 with a Ford Foundation grant of $275,000. Since 1970 it has covered the black and Puerto Rican neighborhoods of the New York metropolitan area five days a week. The service is sold on a subscription basis not only to newspapers and broadcasting stations but also to organizations and businesses wanting information about trends, events, and issues in the ethnic living areas of New York. Administered by the Center for New York Affairs of the New School for Social Research, CNS is staffed by journalists experienced in either the black or white press. Its editor, George Barner, is a former New York *Amsterdam News* reporter. Its director, white Philip Horton, earlier was executive editor of the *Reporter*. Others have worked for the Louisville *Courier-Journal* and the *Saturday Evening Post*. Their staffers man district offices in Harlem, the Bronx, and Bedford-Stuyvesant, and a headquarters in lower Manhattan.

Most of New York's news organizations subscribe, paying up to $200 a week, with the fees smallest for poverty and neighborhood organizations. Among its newspaper charter subscribers were the New York *Times,* New York *Daily News,* New York *Amsterdam News,* and New York *Courier*. Stations WINS, WOR, WNBC-TV, and WCBS-TV were early broadcasting users. About five news stories, on the average, go to subscribers via motorcycle daily. An innovation is delivery of a daily community calendar so that assignments can be made for coverage of events. Typical story summaries from the CNS file include:

"Brownsville poverty agency demands seats on hospital board."

"400 Brooklyn seniors win college scholarships."

"Fund cut curtains two special New York Public Library projects in Harlem and the South Bronx."

"Planners of school complex in East New York reject charges of take-over by 'black separatists.' "[12]

CNS also serves as a training program for nonwhites interested in careers as journalists. And it has become a communication medium between the communities it covers, since the regular news agencies in New York do not report much of the news occurring in the boroughs where the various ethnic groups are concentrated.

The Need for Service. The need for a large scale black news-gathering service persists. Although the white media cover more news of the black society than before, it generally is only major events, particularly those that will have direct impact upon the white society, that get much attention: demonstrations, disturbances, honors for prominent blacks, political action, crime. The black press could use a large agency intended not as a political tool but as an attempt at reporting with a measure of objectivity those events and trends not observed and passed on to their subscribers by the other agencies. Such a service is needed for these reasons:

1. White news agency charges are too high for most black owners' budgets.

2. Black subscribers to white services receive much news not useful to them; furthermore, black papers are second papers to many readers, so they must concentrate on what the rest of the press does not contain; the black press also has no room for much of what is sent.

3. Only the major black news stories are received via the white-owned agencies. For example, most of the Richmond and Washington news in the Baltimore *Afro-American* would not come from such services. Even the *Black Panther* depends heavily upon the reports from the party's branches for news reports. The matter of emphasis also enters.

4. A black service is written by writers with an understanding of the readers and their interests that white writers for a black service do not possess. Even black wire service correspondents working for a white agency find that their copy has been filtered through white editorial minds.

● SYNDICATES

Closely related to these newsgathering services are the feature syndicates, in principle the same sort of operation, for they send material uniformly to their subscribers on different publications. These are firms that sell comic strips, panel cartoons, personal columns, and other content for release everywhere on the same date. In the white world they bear such names as King Features Syndicate and United Features Syndicate. Joining them in such business are the two major white news services, AP and UPI, for they too send out nonnews materials, as do various individual newspaper and magazine publishing companies, such as the *Saturday Review* and the Chicago *Daily News*. A few black writers appear in white papers via a white syndicate: Carl T. Rowan and Dick Gregory, each with a column bearing his name, are on the Allied Features Syndicate list.

A few independent black companies function similarly. Several newspapers offer their own features, so as to get more mileage from what their artists and writers prepare. Most black publications cannot afford to buy this auxiliary source of material. Consequently the white firms do little business with the black media and while the black syndicates fare better it still is a small operation for the majority.

Feature syndicates operate by mail, since much of their material does not require immediate publication. They provide mats or proofs for the purchasers needing illustrations—photographs, drawings, cartoons—and proofs that can be used in preparing material for offset printing. The latter is important today, since numerous black papers and magazines are printed by the photo-offset process.

Among the syndicates for the black press are Continental Features, the D. E. Scott Newspaper Service, and Empire Features. Scott supplies columns; Continental sells panel cartoons. "Tan Topics" and "Do's and Don'ts" and combination text and drawings in a feature called "Things You Should Know" are among its offerings. The latter is typified by one about George Washington Williams, a lawyer and historian who in 1882 published a two-volume history of the black race, and other works. A half-dozen lines about his life and a head-drawing constitute the feature. A sample of the panel cartoons is one with black characters in which a young wife says to her husband, about to start on a trip, "Write soon, dear, even if it's only a check."

Empire Features is a mail service that consists of sending its clients each week eight pages of material, printed on one side of tabloid-size sheets, for use in photo composition production or from which type can be set for letterpress printing. Begun in 1970, it reported fifty black newspaper subscribers within a month. The range of materials is wide and professionally prepared. A small paper that can afford it could offer its readers many of the standard nonlocal features of any newspaper, for there is column material on politics, personalities, television, books, Washington news, beauty, travel, poetry, and entertainment. Also included are a short story, several columns of news briefs, a panel cartoon, and illustrated feature stories as well as longer news accounts and feature photographs. The copy is concisely written and the photographs well produced. No editorials are provided; some political views are evident, such as Alfred Duckett's clear support of Martin Luther King, Jr., and his philosophy in his own "Big Mouth Says" column. This service has the same effect as any syndicate's offerings—it tends to standardize viewpoint and content and to dampen development of original, local material, since it is easy to clip and paste this readable and typographically well-dressed copy.

Various black organizations, such as the National Urban League, offer columns and other articles. For years NUL sent out each week an essay by the late Whitney M. Young, Jr., its national director. Such columns are among the most widely used writings by black leaders. Their authors usually are not professional journalists, but organization heads. Bayard Rustin and Roy Wilkins are among the regularly and most widely read; Wilkins is an exception, for he has been a professional newsman (see Chapter 10). A few now-working journalists write columns that go beyond the pages of their own papers. Usually these are handled by the originating publication itself and used in associated papers.

● CHANGING THE BLACK IMAGE

Public relations has been called the science of attitude control. Its practitioners are trained to use whatever psychological and communications tools are available to develop in various publics a favorable attitude toward the institution or person concerned. Some institutions in the black society have been aware of the power of such an activity but not many have had the money to use it in any nationally dramatic way. Publicity and promotion are simply tools of public relations, methods by which to influence a public to a view or an attitude; publicity using news releases to the press and broadcasters, for example; promotion turning out printed matter, films, and setting up special events which it publicizes. The distinction is largely a theoretical one today, for publicity promotes and promotion publicizes.

At its best, public relations wins understanding. Publicity helps, by spreading information. So does promotion, by calling attention to special efforts. The black press is at one and the same time the target, and the projector, of publicity and promotion; it is used to affect public opinion and it itself wishes to influence the public's opinion about itself and about the race it serves.

For years the black press was not much of a target nor much of a user of public relations techniques. Publicity offices of industry, government, and organizations, white or black, which prepare news releases, feature stories, take photographs and supply other free materials boosting their products, services, or aims either were not much interested in cooperation from the black press or saw little point outside the sports and entertainment worlds. Travel publicity is an example. Why should a steamship company operating luxury liners spend money on publicizing its service (including the purchase of paid advertising space) to a small group of readers most of whom could only dream of making such a journey? Not to overlook the fact that people of color might not be made welcome by some other passengers. Until the Caribbean, former family home for many an American black family or at least its forefathers, became a popular playground for Americans and within economic reach of an increasing number of black travelers, there was no point in having travel editors, travel columns, or making space for travel releases, especially if they were not tied into space that had been bought. The growing middle class in American black society is changing that, however, and travel agencies and airlines have another segment of the public to seek to influence. Black publication offices are finding more free copy coming to their desks and while they throw much of it away, more than ever before is being used, as an observant reading of almost any large black publication and many a small one reveals.

The Black Counselor. A black public relations firm seeking to go well beyond the commercial function of public relations, i.e., do more than soften up a public so that families will buy many packages of frozen soul food or women will invest in wigs, makes a social contribution. It comes on the scene at a time when the image of black America is changing and made up of sharply contrasting concepts. These images exist in the minds of all occupants of U.S. territory (beyond whose borders this study of black journalism does not venture). The black citizens have their images of the black people and the whites theirs; the Orientals, too, have their impressions of their fellow minority group. There no more is one black image than there is one white or yellow. And the black's concept of his fellows can be as erroneous as the white person's view of his black neighbors. To many a white a black person has certain characteristics. W. Leonard Evans, publisher of *Tuesday,* believes that one common stereotype is false ("lower mentality, a higher crime rate, think he's lazy, laughs a lot, steals chickens, and eats watermelons"). To others the black image is that of a gun- or knife-carrying, beret-wearing member of the Black Panther Party, potentially if not actually a revolutionist, or a young would-be political leader urging blacks to burn the banks.

The professional black publicist or public relations counsel is interested, outside the commercial area, in projecting what he deems a correct image of the American black society, whatever that may be, for it varies in different minds. He seeks to do so through black social organization channels, through white-sponsored enterprises working among blacks, and via church and educational institutions. The practice of public relations counseling under such circumstances is likely to resemble missionary work. In the commercial world, however, it is colored by the aims and purposes of all business. There it has been more scientifically and systematically carried out, for capital is available. Consequently, more and more public relations counsels are being called into service to advise dominantly white organizations, particularly government bodies, business corporations, and political groups, and individuals as well as others that may not have full rapport with the black people or simply want to spread their gospel to the black society. It is assumed by those that employ them that a black public relations firm has more entrée to the ghetto or black neighborhoods and organizations than a white firm doing such propaganda or opinion-molding work.

Stanley Penn, a *Wall Street Journal* reporter, in 1965 surveyed the development of black-run public relations firms. It is likely that what he discovered more than ever is so today. He traced the rise in business for black companies working for the business world to the civil rights movement, which resulted in what he called "the new awareness . . . of the importance of the Negro as a customer and an employe." Listing what firms are asked to do, he noted that they advise corporations on racial hiring practices, create contacts between black leaders and corporate executives, advise companies on participating in local civic movements, interpret the mood of the black community, arrange for company participation in conventions, and help determine the best advertising and merchandizing methods for cultivating the black market.[13]

These activities, it should be noted, illustrate the basic difference between public relations and publicity or promotion. Every assignment is a matter of giving advice, counsel, or guidance in some way, with a few adding research techniques to discover the facts that serve as a basis for later judgments, as in interpreting the mood of the community.

Penn estimated that at the time there were between fifteen and twenty public relations companies owned and run by blacks. Among the names he mentions are those of Joseph V. Baker Associates; D. Parke Gibson Associates, Inc.; and Louis-Rowe Enterprises. The present firms are spread widely in the country and not concentrated, as one might expect, in New York, but related to the population centers. Louis-Rowe added advertising counsulting services in 1969. Another development is the policy of Carl Byoir & Associates, Inc., one of the largest white firms in the nation, which affiliated itself with a black agency in High Point, North Carolina, so that Byoir could handle black accounts more easily. As do certain white agencies, some black ones undertake to issue publications financed by their clients, thus dealing directly in journalism. Penn cites as an example a magazine, *Caravan*, which Baker issued in behalf of three of its clients. It went to 35,000 black doctors, ministers, and other professionals as well as to college placement directors. It included feature stories and pictures of black people working in the offices and shops of the sponsoring firms.

Black personalities, particularly entertainers, more than ever are turning to counsels to manage their public problems as racial conflict becomes more acute. With the greater acceptance of nonwhites as television entertainers, actors, newscasters, interviewers, and behind-the-scenes managers, the black "p.r. man" as well as the white has more clients. The black press cannot escape the impact of these communicators.

Public Information Directors. When they practice outside of business circles, public relations counsels sometimes are called directors of public information. The aims are the same, whatever the title: to obtain greater empathy for the institutions they represent, be they churches, colleges, or hospitals. Black journalists at times start their communications careers in the public relations field, particularly for black colleges and universities. Such institutions have had to pay such low salaries for all staff that it has been difficult to fill the position, which frequently (as in many a white college as well), includes disseminating news, advising the student paper, teaching a journalism class or two, and running the alumni office. Thus bright students have been appointed, or new graduates, or young people just out of undergraduate journalism school, or newsmen with little or no practical experience or training in public relations work, which they reduce to writing news releases.

Usually these neophytes move on to jobs in the professional journalism field, but some remain as public relations or information directors, never having time to obtain the necessary media experience or any more special training than attending a workshop sponsored by the American College Public Relations Society. In the late 1930's, for example, a prominent black college had as its public relations director an eighteen-year-old who was not to be handed his first college degree (nor was it in journalism) for another decade. Several other black colleges later hired men without media experience of any sort. One began doing such work in 1946, and went successively from that college to two others, and has been at the third since the 1950's. He had published some magazine and newspaper articles but had no other practical media experience in his quarter of a century in public relations and publicity; in addition he has taught journalism classes at two of the colleges, relying wholly on uncompleted master's degree work in journalism. Some of these men and others like them have taught themselves much about media operations by spending time in newspaper, magazine, and broadcasting company offices and observing what is done and how. Others have sunk into the routines and exert little influence for their institutions except in a small local circle and are minor auxiliaries of the black press. Few such self-taught information executives are aware of the more sophisticated public information methods or the social contribution that public relations directors can make when at their best.

Another and far more professionally reputable area in which black communicators practice the art of opinion management and direction is in the government and social information office. Several black journalists have gained national attention for their work as government information specialists. Perhaps best known is Carl T. Rowan, who was head of USIA (see Chapter 10); others are William Gordon, who had American government information duties in Africa, Sweden, and the U.S.A., and Henry Burrell Woods. Before he became associate director, program development, of the USIA, Woods had a successful background of black newspaper and radio experience. He was with the St. Louis *Call* from 1935 to 1940, chief of the bureau there for the Chicago *Defender* from 1942 to 1949, a newscaster for WTMV between 1951 and 1954, and executive editor of the St. Louis

Argus for the next eleven years. During his news career he won various awards for news and editorial writing. Still other men and women, both with and without journalism training, have been sent by the State Department to Africa, Asia, and the West Indies as information officers. And all, as part of their duties, have worked with the press, either that of the country where they were or the black press, or along with the white, on the American continent, gaining understanding of the government body they represented.

For all such work is bound to affect the black press. It means visits from public relations representatives to editors seeking cooperation or vice versa. It means much more free copy—text as well as illustrations—coming into offices for use by editors. It means activities stimulated by public relations counsel which will lead to creation of news that must be reported by the media. It produces problems as well: where to draw the line between news and publicity or promotion, the risk of undue influence by publicists, and the demands of advertisers that they receive a given amount of space as "free readers" in addition to what they pay for, an attitude they often believe to be part of obtaining good public relations.

● PROMOTERS OF THE PRESS

Black publications have made little use of public relations skills in the larger sense. Usually they rely on proved promotion ideas only. These are not involved with applications of psychology's principles and often are mixed, instead, with human concerns, a natural consequence of seeking to serve a group of people facing multitudes of everyday problems. These plans and ideas may have a by-product of generating good will toward the publication. Like many other black activities, the publication must rely on its own community for support, although white interest sometimes is manifested via financial aid and personal participation.

As an example of one idea is Negro Press Week. Although not entered into with much zest in recent years, the press as a whole every February or March since 1941 has conducted, via the National Newspaper Publishers Association, such a week. Then, or just before or after, the papers print articles on heroes of black journalism—usually Cornish, Russworm, or Douglass—drawings, photographs, and special articles supplied by the NNPA committee that supervises the observance. Sometimes a radio program is included with outlets in cities served by black papers. Schools and colleges are asked to cooperate by drawing attention to the black press. Exhibits are staged also in schools and other public places. Like white publishers, black owners and managers appear to be convinced that the reader is indifferent to the publication per se and therefore bored by historical or laudatory articles about black journalism. Thus Negro Press Week often is allowed to go by with one brief article noting it or an editorial saying little beyond the customary.

The promotions staged or sponsored by individual publications at other times of the year are neither extremely costly nor inordinately fancy, mainly because the more elaborate, such as fashion shows and contests, usually are tied in with advertisers, who supply materials or awards. Newspaper and magazine staff people engaged in this aspect of publishing are busy with charity drives, scholarship programs, amateur photography and other contests, honor rolls, youth clubs, beauty queen competitions, and sports events. These goings-on often are responses to the needs of readers as much as to the desire of publishers to ingratiate themselves with those who buy the paper or magazine, as a brief review of some typical promotion enterprises indicates.

Perhaps the best known activity launched by a black magazine is *Ebony*'s "Fashion Fair" held in many parts of the nation. Sponsored by the National Council of Negro Women in conjunction with the magazine, it is staged in a local theater of a city with a substantial black population. Often it is an important annual women's social event in a community, especially since a scholarship fund benefits. *Ebony* representatives accompany the Fair, which seeks to tie into the fashion trends of the day. Displayed is everything from beach wear to wedding gowns; in recent years the interest in traditional African clothing has been rewarded.

When *New Lady* magazine was revived in 1969, parties were given to introduce its staff to important individuals in a black community and to interest women in becoming readers. In some West Coast papers (the magazine is published in California) the publicity ran to a full page of photographs of the event; some space was obtained even in white dailies.

A far different sort of promotion and perhaps more individually useful is the column run in a newspaper to which readers may send requests for assistance. For instance, a reader of the *Philadelphia Tribune* sent its "Mr. Help" column a complaint about a backing sewer. The paper arranged for the water commissioner's office to correct the situation. The Baltimore *Afro-American* offers a similar service, "Afro Line," in its local edition, describing it as "a community service to help you solve problems, whatever they may be." Readers send a postcard asking their question and identifying themselves. A typical question and answer:

> Q: My wife and I are separated. I have custody of our six children. I want to know, is there any place a broken man can get a divorce or legal separation. I can't afford a lawyer.
> A: At the Legal Aid Bureau, in People's Court Building, Fayette and Gay Sts., you can get helped.

The Detroit *Michigan Chronicle* service is called Chronicle Information Center. Much older than the "Life Line" type of service is that of the San Francisco *Sun-Reporter,* which has maintained a Public Affairs Bureau to call attention to "special aspects of new problems" as the newspaper explains. International as well as local matters are given attention. The late Tom Mboya, Sir Adetokunbo Adesnola, and other African leaders or American visitors to Africa have been lecturers or guests. This paper also sponsors an annual Merit Award Program which rewards local people for outstanding community service. That particular old reliable among promotions has been used also every year since 1939 by the Baltimore *Afro-American.* Pictures of the winners are printed in the paper. Related is a feature, the Good Neighbor of the Week, an article about someone in an area of the city, giving biographical and other facts, such as activities, interests, and hobbies.

Charity campaigns are among the oldest of the traditional plans. The *Philadelphia Tribune* has a public service program called Tribune Charities. Income from an annual public dinner is used to aid students wanting to go to college; the fund also gives assistance to persons needing financial help quickly. The *Afro-American* papers have Afro Charities. The Douglass Fellowships already described have a side value of being promotional. When the Richmond *Afro* won $1,000 for crusade reporting to fight racial inequities and an incurable disease largely found among black people the money was given to nonprofit organizations.

Special crusades, part of the black press since its founding, have a by-product of promotional value, even when not successful. As a crusading press, this one has a fine record which can be illustrated from the history of most newspapers and a few magazines. In recent years they have centered on eradicating slum housing, righting injustices practiced upon the individuals, opposing rent gouging tactics by landlords, and working for the hiring of blacks by firms doing business with them. Nor are these all only recent campaigns. P. Bernard Young, while editor of the Norfolk *Journal and Guide,* was looking out the window of his office, one day in 1933, when he saw the collapse of a decaying house used by black people. He took a picture of the ruins, wrote a story and an editorial demanding action on housing in that Virginia city. Later Young was appointed head of the Negro Housing Advisory Commission of the city; by 1949 Norfolk had four modern housing developments for black residents.[14] The paper was successful with other campaigns. *Time* reported in 1949 that it was responsible for the county floating a $750,000 bond issue to improve black schools and for changes in pay scales so black and white teachers were treated equally.

The Bud Billiken Club. One of the most effective promotions by a black publication was the early Bud Billiken Club of the Chicago

Defender, an activity still visible in smaller form. Begun in 1924, its major event was an annual parade and picnic in Chicago; the club was intended to attract and interest black children and perhaps eventually make them readers and possible advertisers. The plan centered on a club called The Defender Junior, with a regular page or two for children's writings and drawings, and reports of their activities. The staff member in charge called himself "Bud Billiken." As many as 150,000 youngsters came with their parents and friends to the mammoth picnic. Each member received a wallet card and an identification button; at one time membership totaled nearly 1,000,000. Chicago society women helped stage the affair.[15]

The first Bud Billiken was Willard Motley, later to become better known as the black novelist who wrote *Knock on Any Door*. Motley was only a ten-year-old at the time Robert S. Abbott, the publisher, selected him for the job. The club lives on today in an annual parade and picnic of smaller dimensions and in the paper's youth page. The plan has built incalculable good will for the paper.

Another *Defender* promotion device that was different, one which spread to other cities and became part of the language, was election of a mayor of what the paper called Bronzeville. Such mayors held unofficial conventions; the mayor became the official host to celebrities who visited the black neighborhoods.

Tons of literature are among the promotional materials issued by the black press over the years. The simplest are rate cards and leaflets describing the paper and its coverage, promotion letters, and booklets. *Negro Traveler and Conventioneer Magazine*, long established and alone in its field, in 1968 issued a variation and more elaborate mailing piece: a fifty-two-page duplicated presentation titled "Economic Impact of the Negro Traveler." Prepared by Clarence M. Markham, Jr., editor of the trade magazine, and his staff, it describes black people's conventions and also gives data on population characteristics, the black market, the disposable income, and other aspects and includes lists of publications, black colleges, and organizations that hold conventions.

● COMPETITORS OF THE BLACK PRESS

Every other medium, whatever the race or color of its owners, is a competitor for black publications: other newspapers and magazines, billboards, car cards in subways and buses, books (especially paperbacks), both television and radio, and what the advertising business calls point of purchase displays and direct mail. Such competition is at the usual two levels: for readers and for advertising accounts. Any revenue-producing form is competition. Any activity that consumes a potential reader's time is competition, even spectator sports and adless books. In this book, however, the concern is chiefly with the black-owned and operated radio. It directly affects the publications. Little information has been set down about it as a journalistic phenomenon.

Black radio so far has been the only electronic competitor from within the race for black publications, unless a piece of equipment that plays tapes or records is considered a journalistic communications medium. Black television stations are not yet operating, but may appear in a few years. Plans for such a station were announced in 1968 for Rochester, New York, but it has not materialized by this writing. Belafonte Enterprises, owned by the singer, Harry Belafonte, in 1970 also had plans to move into the video realm. High costs, such as a half-million to a million dollars, as reported by the Associated Press, may have hampered the Rochester venture. Inability to obtain a license is another obstacle. Dr. Carlton B. Goodlett, publisher of the San Farncisco *Sun-Reporter*, has described, for example, the efforts in 1965 of a black group to obtain a TV license. He was a member of Reporter Broadcasting Company, which was admitted to a Federal Communications Commission hearing. Competing also was the Bay Broadcasting Company, a white firm. The predominantly black company was not granted the license. Dr. Goodlett explained the reason:

"It goes without saying Reporter Broadcasting lost the license on the grounds that its application was submitted without the expertise of an FCC attorney; and the denial that community needs could be an issue indicated beyond a doubt that we were victims of a contest of wills between the nonprofessional and the professional."[16]

About a dozen radio stations are owned and operated by black citizens but several hundred more also devote their programs to black listeners. By all logic, if the black press, to be so considered, must be owned, operated, staffed, and aimed at the black race, with content about it, then black radio is genuinely black only when it also has a similar description. The reasons are much the same. And just as they are articulated for the press by black journalists so are they expressed by black broadcasters.

Dr. Haley Bell, co-owner of several black stations, told an interviewer that it establishes the atmosphere of trust with the black listener and that creates a better selling atmosphere. And Gregory Moses, vice president of James Brown Enterprises, said to the same writer that "there is a great pride factor" involved and that is why stations tell the listener that the operation is black. It "gives our people the feeling of voices, of someone looking out for their interests."[17] Bernard Howard, then president of a station advertising representative company bearing his name, called black radio "the only medium through which the Negro himself believes he can receive the happenings of the day as they happen, and he feels they should be reported. It gives him more of his side of the story, more of the internal facets non-Negro stations overlook; it gives him more of the editorials he likes to hear, delivered by announcers he knows are on his team, and it does this more consistently and more often than any other medium."[18]

As journalism, black radio is not yet socially significant in its everyday operations. Taking into consideration both its manifestations (as wholly or only partly black) it can be important in times of crisis, and has been in cities where disturbances have occurred, as for example after the assassination of Dr. King in 1968. Day in and day out it is competition for the community newspaper owner, for he knows that a radio station in his area is being listened to and can command thousands of dollars in advertising accounts. Such a publisher is perhaps not primarily concerned with the racial nature of the station's ownership. Unless he shares in the advertising budgets of local merchants, banks, and other businesses he has no illusions about his competitor's effectiveness.

The number of black and black-oriented radio stations has been increasing. Regardless of ownership, the black programming stations cover 93 per cent of the total U.S. black population of more than 22,000,000.[19] In 1968 the number of stations beaming all their programming at black listeners came to 108, double the number in 1963 and fifty times as many as in 1947, a contrast with the trend in the number of newspapers during the same period. Eight of the 108 stations were black-owned.[20] By 1970 the number of black-owned stations had increased to sixteen; in the interval nine had been bought or established and two of the older no longer were operating. The smallness of black radio can be realized when it is noted that in 1970 more than 7,350 commercial stations existed and only 118 had all-black programming. Black control accounted for less than one-tenth of one per cent of all stations.[21]

Consequently Dean Burch, while chairman of the Federal Communications Commission, was not exaggerating in 1969 when he said that blacks and other minorities are underrepresented in electronic media both as owners and communicators, "so far as certain parts of the industry are concerned. . . ." One of the other charges, he said, "which does have a great deal of factual basis is that very few blacks own any broadcasting facilities. . . . the way it's going to resolve itself is that black people will buy stations [because] there are no more television licenses [to distribute]. . . ."[22] Burch was asked if the FCC should perhaps favor black ownership, on the basis that the black community be represented, that is; that if all other things are equal should a black broadcast license applicant be granted a preference because he is black. He answered that he did not propose an FCC policy at the time and added ". . . but I think it would be relevant in a comparative hearing to know that 'Group A' consists of black people who propose to serve the black community and that it is not being served." This statement was interpreted by the Associated Press writer who was interviewing Burch as a hint that the FCC "might well consider favoring blacks in the competition for available licenses."

The Dominant Owners. Like black publishing, black radio has its dominant owners. The Johnson or Sengstacke of the radio world is James Brown, who is more familiar as an enormously popular singer than as a broadcasting mogul. His radio property, JB Broadcasting, is one of several units in James Brown Enterprises, which is engaged in record and music publishing and also is a restaurant franchise operator. The radio unit owns three of the fifteen black stations: WJBE, Knoxville, Tennessee; WRDW, Augusta, Georgia; and WEBB, Baltimore. Three dentists are chief owners of the other major radio group—Bell Broadcasting, Detroit. They own WCHB and WCHD, Detroit; and KWK, St. Louis. The principal owner is Dr. Haley Bell, the others are Dr. Wendell Cox and Dr. Robert Bass. Two whites owned 25 per cent of the firm early in 1970. The other black-owned stations as of then were KPRS, Kansas City; WGPR, Detroit; WMPP, Chicago Heights, Illinois; WEUP, Huntsville, Alabama; WTLC, Indianapolis; WORV, Hattiesburg, Mississippi; and WVPE, Chadbourn, North Carolina, all commercial stations, and three college-owned ones, WHOV-FM, Hampton, Virginia, WSHA-FM, Raleigh, North Carolina, and WTOP-FM, Washington, D.C.

Black Radio Programming. A guide to print and electronic media serving the U.S.A. black population reported in the late 1960's that programming by these stations divides into two types. Usually the northern ones broadcast news and rhythm or blues music and the southern send out news and gospel or folk music. Typically in both there are black disc jockeys who in time become community personalities.[23]

Talk programs have come into more favor in recent years, as tensions have increased in black communities. Other methods of having racial impact are to broadcast programs about black historical figures and editorials on social issues or interviews with leaders. Audience-response and phone shows also are popular. News programs are brief and limited largely to ethnic information. Station operators are divided over whether such newscasts should be made in the community's slang or in standard English.

Dr. Frederic Coonradt of the University of Southern California has described a station's electronic journalism when he told the story of KGFJ, Los Angeles, which had a disc jockey, Nathaniel Montague, who went as "The Magnificent Montague." His practice was to begin his program by shouting "Burn, Baby, Burn," a slogan he used for several years that became the battle cry during the August, 1965, disturbances in Watts. He had used the slogan while a rock and roll deejay in New York, Chicago, St. Louis, and San Francisco. But it ceased when taken up by people in the streets. Another member of the staff then was Roy Williams, who handled the news programs, using UPI radio and Los Angeles City News Service copy, but also giving time to an occasional documentary. Coonradt reported that the KGFJ newsroom had posted the order in which news stories were to be aired. The sequence was: civil rights story, civil rights story, top local story, national or international story, national or international story, local story, and local story. The researcher observed that a monitoring of sample broadcasts showed that this order was not always followed.[24]

Important exceptions to the practice of issuing only short newscasts are the occasions in the past decade when certain stations have remained on the air long past their regular broadcasting periods to give running accounts of events in disturbances in their communities.

Advertising on Black Radio. The vital competitive point of black radio is its ability to sell advertising time. Most studies of black radio have dealt on its success in reaching a market, affirming that it is an effective community medium from that standpoint. Especially is that true in towns and cities where there is no black publication. The existence of as many as three to five stations in one city, as in Washington and Atlanta, which have three each, Chicago and Detroit, with four apiece, and Baltimore, with five, would indicate eagerness to reach a lucrative market. The desirability of the market reached a height in the 1950's with the formation of a black radio network.

Before W. Leonard Evans was publisher of *Tuesday* magazine, he was president of the National Negro Network, Inc., launched in 1954. It included fifty stations and reported that it reached 12,000,000 black listeners. It operated from January, 1954, to fall, 1956, on a five-times-a-week frequency. The stations were in areas with large black populations. Offered were programs on a network basis to what were called Negro-appeal stations. The first output, a transcribed soap opera which Evans himself wrote (perhaps the first black story of this sort) was called "Ruby Valentine," starring Juanita Hall, who had won great popularity in "South Pacific." Advertising time was bought by Pet Milk and Philip Morris, among others. The NNN employed annually between 125 and 155 black actors and actresses, 10 to 15 musicians on a regular basis, 6 major writers, and a staff of about 18 in management and production. Because television's advent affected all radio, the network did not survive. Evans recently explained that it was discontinued also "primarily because of inability to resolve economic differences with a group of three radio chains that represented 11 of the 50 stations involved in network operations."[25]

Another black-owned radio network operated briefly in 1969, American Freedom Network. Stimulated by the demand for news after the assassination of Dr. King, coverage of that tragedy's aftermath was provided 240 stations in the U.S.A. and Canada. From thirty to thirty-five reporters provided news from throughout the nation for the new pool.[26]

Now black radio stations broadcast the usual kinds of commercials, with heavy accent on local accounts and sometimes in a strong vernacular accent in the announcing. Success in obtaining national advertising usually depends upon the rating of each station in relation to others in the community. They carry out promotion schemes somewhat like those of the black newspapers, hoping similarly to endear themselves to listeners and thus boost their ratings. Public service announcements are broadcast about lost articles and animals and the station acts as a job clearing house.

Competition in New Form. Black communications media now are experiencing a new turn in the competitive business world. Already noted is the situation wherein magazine publishers of long standing now see white foundations, banks, and periodical publishers combining to strengthen or launch black magazines that will seek to share in the budgets of their advertisers and appeal to their readers for subscriptions (see Chapters 7 and 12). Radio station owners learned in 1970 that two subunits of the large white denomination, the United Methodist Church, have provided resources that will go a long way to help black citizens own two radio stations, KOZN and KOWH, Omaha, Nebraska. Two grants totaling $11,000 and a loan of $150,000 were approved as seed money "to insure black ownership and operation of the stations."[27] All major stockholders are black Omaha residents; among them are Bob Gibson, of the St. Louis Cardinals, and Bob Booser, of the Seattle Sonics, as well as two doctors. The plan was to spread ownership of stock to the community by selling shares at a dollar each. The stations, one AM and the other FM, will serve also as training grounds for blacks. At this writing the FCC had not yet ruled on the purchase.

Newspapers will be affected by such support, if it should increase, more than magazines not only because listeners do not usually read at the same time but also because money spent on advertising over radio perhaps is that amount not devoted to the print media. The black press has enough problems without unexpected strength being given to its major competitor from within the racial ranks. Editors and publishers can take the view, however, that whatever improves the lot of black citizens is helpful to their papers and periodicals, for it can mean more purchasing power and better educated citizens, and therefore more readers.

That conclusion may not be based on an unfounded assumption if the position taken by the National Newspaper Publishers Association at its 1969 meeting is recalled. It endorsed "Black Journal," a National Educational Television program devoted to black community news and events and controlled and produced by blacks, for it was threatened with being taken off the air. Its retention was urged.[28]

Preferences of the People. Some advertising people believe that the black Americans are "more air than print oriented," as an anonymous writer put it in *Media/scope* magazine, some years back. It seems likely, because for so many years white papers and stations failed to cover local black news that members of the ethnic group turned to their own media. In recent times, because in so many communities there are no papers but there are radio stations, the latter sometimes are more important. *A Guide to Negro Media* lists numerous areas possessing black radio but no black print journalism.

Radio listeners constitute what the advertising profession calls the market. It is a segmented one, and made up of the same persons who are the targets for the black newspapers and magazines. This market, as John E. Allen, while executive vice president of Bob Dore Associates, in 1966, pointed out, "is completely different from any other. Different product uses, different brand preferences, different commercial response, different media habits, different population patterns."[29]

The place of radio in the preferences of a small sample of the black population is indicated in the Bontrager study of media use by the inner city inhabitants of Syracuse, New York, a city often used as a typical cross-section of the U.S.A. Most needed by these black inner city residents, they told him, was television (53.88 per cent). Daily newspapers were next, but far behind TV (20.16 per cent). Radio followed (18.10 per cent) and magazines were last (2.16 per cent). Television led all other media in "doing most to help the blacks" and providing fair treatment of them.[30]

Black radio broadcasting, in the full sense of major ownership by black people, is small but growing. If ownership is disregarded, such broadcasting is a far more substantial activity, with major stations, like WLIB, New York; WOOK, Washington; and WABQ, Cleveland, having large followings. Black broadcasting, especially if it involves television, as it is bound some day to do, will be a serious competitor to the publication of black newspapers and periodicals in both the advertising and readership areas.   ●

15. BLACK PHILOSOPHIES AND BLACK JOURNALISM

BLACK POWER . . . Black Nationalism . . . Black Rage . . . Black Capitalism . . . Black Revolution . . . Black is Beautiful.

Certain leading black newspapers and magazines have expressed themselves on these and other ideas that fill the air during the eighth decade of the century. What has been the reaction of black journalism in general toward them? What attitudes have been assumed by the black Americans who advance these ideas, surrounding themselves with despair or hope, or issuing threats of violent revolution in reprisals or pleas for peaceful reform through nonviolent means?

Few publications have been voices for the extremist views, such as going out into the streets, burning the cities, killing the whites, and other now familiar urgings to action by the most militant blacks and whites. Most papers and magazines that have tackled these issues have reported primarily, although neither consistently nor thoroughly, as a steady reading can reveal. In general, the press has asked for moderation as representing the attitude of the mass of the black citizens. Among the specialized publications—the trade journals, the fan magazines, and the confession periodicals, for example— little has been said about the social movements among the black people.

● SOME PHILOSOPHIES AND RESPONSES

Interpretation and analysis of the present-day ideas about race in the U.S.A. already have filled numerous books and been the subjects of hosts of articles. One idea, that of black power, is taken here as an example of the more complicated. There appear to be as many interpretations of it as interpreters. The editorialist, whether owner of the publication or employed to write its editorials, looks at it and sees concepts behind it. There are the viewpoints of LeRoi Jones, Malcolm X, Martin Luther King, Jr., Stokely Carmichael, James Baldwin, Eldridge Cleaver, Bayard Rustin, James Farmer, Whitney Young, Jr., Roy Innis, Huey Newton, Roy Wilkins, Charles Evers, Shirley Chisholm, Julis Lester, James Forman, and many others. Most have counseled their black brothers and sisters in recent years to follow one direction or another; some of these paths run in opposite directions.[1] And, as he looks more and more into black history, under the urging of educators as well as political leaders, the editorialist sees the source of some of these views in the life and work of certain older leaders. One was Marcus Garvey, who believed that black power should be used for settlement of the American black in Africa; another, W. E. B. Du Bois, concluded that the American social order had failed and that some other, specifically that of the Soviet Union, was superior.

S. E. Anderson, assistant editor of *Black Dialogue* magazine, divides the various views or philosophies into three groups. One asks the American blacks to allow themselves to be assimilated. Another urges them to withdraw, i.e., to take part in a new separatism or segregation or to leave the American shores altogether for the real homeland, Africa. The third tells them to take over the country by revolution, violently or by the ballot, urging speed because the race is headed for extinction by white conspirators.

President Richard M. Nixon in 1969 told the country that he believed the great mass of Americans to be a silent majority in sympathy with his policies about ending the Vietnam War. But the lack of expression by the large middle class was not considered, by certain of his critics, as proof positive of the approval of official policies. Not unlike the situation in the country as a whole has been the attitude of the rank and file black citizens toward black philosophies. Neither editors and publishers nor any others know whether their attitude is one of indifference toward leaders in the various groups or schools who think they have the key to the liberation of the black society or of quiet acceptance and support, more of one than another, but without public announcement.

The techniques of finding out what a public thinks or will do—or says it thinks or will do—have been developed but not to the point of complete reliability, as the 1970 British election forecasts showed. Even if completely dependable, and their use in consumer choice studies has been commercially successful, these surveys are costly. Gallup, Harris, and other pollsters rarely sound out black opinion on the appeals of various leaders or would-be leaders out of the wilderness. And few black publishing firms can afford to make them for anything but market studies which presumably will pay off eventually in increased advertising revenue. Black press executives must face a world of readers or potential readers with little knowledge of just who they are, what they are thinking, and how they will act. For the local publication rather than the national, the task of sounding out public opinion is not so important but still serious. As with any community publication, the owner-publisher-editor-advertising-salesman man-of-all-work comes to know most of his readers well. Yet he is likely to be so close to them that he finds it difficult to oppose them, a situation which for many years has explained the blandness of the American weekly community newspaper everywhere. It is difficult for one to support policies that will hurt friends. And his friends do not often tell an editor what they really believe unless he challenges them with his views.

● A NEW ELEMENT

Entering the situation is a new element, further complicating matters for people engaged in what already is a risky occupation. This new factor is the revolutionary spirit, growing steadily, whatever its methods or forms. In its time the black press has had to deal with opposition from the outside. It came from government, as during World War I, when it was unfairly accused of treasonous writings; it came from whites, as in the South for many years, where attempts were made to blast it out of existence and prohibit readers from having the papers in their hands; it came from within its own racial circle, as in the days of disagreement over the views of Booker T. Washington and W. E. B. Du Bois, when the newspapers and magazines were jammed between these two ideological enemies; and it came from outside again when in the late 1940's the press was accused of being communistic.[2]

In recent years it has been in a different type of crossfire. Whereas there always has been a revolutionary spirit among some people in the U.S.A., until the 1950's and 1960's it usually had been confined to a few leaders who rarely counseled the use of violent means to achieve the ends. Ottley quotes, for example, this passage from the Norfolk *Journal and Guide* of the early 1940's: ". . . Some Americans fail to recognize the distinction between righteous advocacy and what is called impolitic agitation. The Negro press is fundamentally an advocate." He then goes on to say that the black press is "the most loudly impatient agency for immediate, fundamental change in the status of the race. Possessed of no soft-talk policy, it is the Negro's most potent weapon of protest and propaganda. . . ."[3] And those papers that were loudly impatient "for immediate, fundamental change" gained little response from the masses except verbally. But in number and geographical spread, if not in intensity, certainly the disorders of the 1960's in the big cities were greater than at any time in American history.

Conditions reached the situation, at the midpoint of this century and soon thereafter, because of judicial decisions, the rise in education, and a developing social conscience among whites, where the black citizens had reason to hope for further improvement in their way of life, and began to work for a speedier accomplishment of it. In this effort there developed the variety of philosophies about the black society and the ways in which to improve its condition. These were represented by a variety of groups: the Black Muslims, the Congress of Racial Equality, the Black Panther Party, the National Association for the Advancement of Colored People, the Black Nationalists, the National Urban League, the Southern Christian Leadership Conference, the Student Non-Violent Coordinating Committee, US (a black revolutionary organization), the proponents of The Third World, and other local or regional organizations. They supported Pan-Africanism, or urged anarchism or nihilism, or recommended that the U.S.A. adopt the philosophies of Che Guevara, Mao Tse-tung, Karl Marx, Vladimir Lenin, and Fidel Castro, or, at the other extreme, Jesus of Nazareth or Mohandas K. Gandhi or some other social or political figure.

What exists, although to what breadth or depth no one knows, is what Nat Hentoff in 1968 described as "a swirling ferment of pride, increasingly disciplined rage, and very concrete programs. . . ."[4]

In the center of all this whirling stands the black press with the black population apparently either puzzled or indifferent, it is difficult to know which. The papers and magazines espouse a few of these organizations, here and there. The ones supported naturally are those most in accord with the policies of the publications' owners. The extremely militant groups issue their papers or magazines to further their positions, as does the Black Panther Party. The moderate organizations have their printed voices as well, such as *Crisis,* coming from the NAACP. Because they are older, perhaps, and their executives sometimes active in the publications work, the NAACP, Urban League, SCLC, and like bodies have had a measure of editorial support from some of the large as well as small general black publications. Black editors and publishers, on the other hand, often are affiliated with the larger national organizations and editorially bolster them of their own accord.

In general, the bulk of the black press has either given minimum attention to or opposed the extremist philosophies. Conservative as it has been and still is on almost all questions but the racial, the press could by its nature have little interest in what are considered the radical movements. Rooted firmly, of necessity, in the American business system, even though most of its life shunted to the side as of little importance, the press cannot afford and its owners have no inclination to challenge the social and economic order in any drastic, fundamental manner. That the troubles of the black race, in the U.S.A. and in other nations, are, or could be, linked with the way society is organized in any particular country is either not understood or is ignored by all but a handful of publications.

L. F. Palmer, Jr., a black journalist working in the white press, quotes an unnamed midwestern editor as saying: "The black revolu-

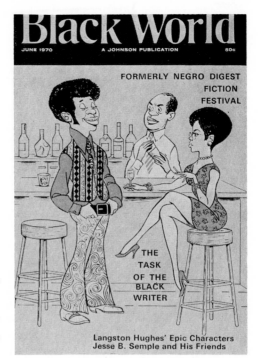

FIG. 15.1. An example of rising black pride is found in **Black World**. The magazine, formerly **Negro Digest**, was renamed in 1970 in response to reader urgings to bring it in harmony with the times.

tion has left the black press behind." The reason he gave is that advertising is picking up and publishers dare not become too revolutionary lest they lose "those new white accounts." Palmer summarizes what he calls the press' ambivalence on the Black Panther Party. At first, he says, it tried to ignore the Panthers. Then when the clashes with police occurred, these were covered but, avoiding the appearance of partisanship, no sides were taken. Palmer reports that the Illinois Panthers threatened the Chicago *Daily Defender* if it did not become "relevant." The paper then began covering such Panther activities as those beyond police encounters. After a Panther leader was killed in Chicago in 1969 the black press reviewed its concept of the party and the government attitude toward the group.[5]

● BLACK POWER

The key slogan of all those advanced by the forces seeking change in the past decade has been "black power." The varieties of interpretation and ambiguities of the term have made it difficult for the press to be clear in its attitude.

Stokely Carmichael, who is credited with originating the slogan while he was SNCC chairman in 1966, used it to arouse in black Americans pride in their ancestry, to urge them to return violence with violence, to gain political power, and to urge them to seek economic power as well. Usually his references to violent retaliation are all that whites know of his views, for conflict makes news and there is more news value in quoting "Burn, Baby, Burn" than in citing longer sentences explaining that economic opportunity is vital.

Both CORE and SNCC have undergone changes in their views on other matters, but continue to interpret the black power expression as meaning black nationalism and have resorted to vigorous language if not violent acts in the effort to achieve such power. To them it means separatism. Another interpretation, one which might be called constructive, is that typified by a statement from Joe Black, a vice-president of the Greyhound Corporation, who writes a column for a number of black newspapers that actually is a Greyhound advertisement.

"I am an advocate of Black Power," he wrote late in 1969. "Black Power through education and reform . . . not revolt. To me, Black Power must start with black pride and black dignity. Without those two ingredients . . . you've got black nothing."[6]

Martin Luther King, Jr., a disciple of Gandhi and a firm believer in nonviolent resistance to violence and as a force for social change, opposed black violence if it meant black militancy that depended upon force. His view still is implemented by SCLC: "We must never seek power exclusively for the Negro, but the sharing of power with white people," he said. He tried to make the point that "No one has ever heard the Jews publicly chant a slogan of Jewish power, but they have power. . . . We must work to build racial pride and refute the notion that black is evil and ugly. But this must come through a program, not merely through a slogan."[7]

From a prominent black publisher came still another meaning, far more personal. It is revealed through an incident. John H. Johnson once described to a magazine publishers' meeting his relations with his printer:

> Some years ago, about twenty now, after I'd been in business about four years, I owed my printer a great deal of money, and he would call my office, and he would say, "I would like to have you in my office tomorrow morning at nine o'clock." And I would say, "Yes, sir," whatever his name is (and I won't give it because I still deal with the same printer), "I will be in your office tomorrow morning at nine o'clock."
>
> Now, about five years passed, and I had paid all of my printing bills. I had a great deal of money in the bank and my printer knew it, my contract was about to expire, and this same man, without any coaching, without any speech-making, would call up and say, "Mr. Johnson? This is Charlie calling. I wonder if I may come over and see you tomorrow morning at your convenience at your office?" And I'd say, "Well, now, I don't know, Charles. We'll think about it." Now this was Black Power! This meant that I, as a black man, had power. . . .[8]

Other journalists have had their particular views. Adam Clayton Powell, the New York pastor and politician for whom the press has been a valuable tool as well as gadfly, called his version "audacious power." He defined black power as "a working philosophy for a new breed of cats—tough, proud of Negroes who categorically refuse to compromise or negotiate any longer for their rights. . . ." To this he added that it meant a "dynamic process of continuous change toward a society of true equals."[9] But he ruled out black supremacy and black nationalism.

● BLACK CAPITALISM

One would surmise that the black press would be enthusiastic about proposals for developing what has been called "black capitalism," i.e., making money available to black entrepreneurs so that they can enter or expand their business. But the press has been three-sided on the topic: restrained, some for it, or unenthusiastic. The expression black capitalism can have at least two meanings: It can mean a new or strengthened business in the black neighborhoods, on the one hand; or it can be an injection of dollar strength which gives the black businessman a fair chance at doing business with either or both the black and white worlds. Thus far it has meant chiefly the former. Thus it is not that the press fears new rivals, although there are some publishers who do, as noted in their uneasiness about the financing of new black magazines. Nor is it that the press fears government interference, although some owners find this a potentially dangerous association. But what the papers and magazines fear is that the present black capitalism plans are no way out of the economic bind, that it simply sets up small businesses in the ghetto. A cynic would say that small business is not much of an advertiser.

● SEPARATISM AND INTEGRATION

Publications of all racial groups are faced with the rise of desire for separatism; some begin on the crest of it, as did the foreign language publications of the U.S. in the nineteenth century after the great waves of immigration from Europe. Stephenson, after studying the response to black magazines in one city, put it: "If they properly capitalize on it they have an opportunity to foster 'black pride' as a constructive philosophy and facilitate eventual integration."[10]

The black Americans do not speak for separatism as one people by any means. But in their actions more and more are showing at least a partial acceptance of it. In any black community, a ghetto area, a new housing neighborhood, on a black college campus, or among blacks on a white campus, the separatism is obvious. The return of the "natural," the wearing of African types of clothing, the intense although not universal interest in all aspects of black culture and history, the plans of some leaders to gain community or even wider control, and the desire by all for recognition in the arts, entertainment, and sports worlds, among others, independent of white aid: all these are expressions of belief, in some measure, in separatism. Isolated or turned away for so many generations, the American black society now is itself tending to turn away from the rest of society.

Publishers and journalists are confronted with a living issue. For many years most of them have defended, and even fought for, the cause of integration of the races to one degree or another, few unwilling to include education as a minimum. Blacks and whites in other occupations who have thought integration a basic solution to racial problems similarly in recent years have had to adjust, to try to understand why integration must be put aside or delayed for a time. The believers in separatism, automatically becoming disbelievers in integration, are a highly vocal group that create news which the press should and usually does report, and sometimes editorializes upon. The editorial opinions expressed are written with caution. They are careful not to seem to offend the mounting pride of race in its readers while at the same time seeking to point out what they consider the disadvantages, say, of college dormitories solely for black students, black farms, black social colonies, and other activities which may cut members of the race off from the experiences and resources necessary for progress in competition with whites.

The editor finds himself in a dilemma if he is responsible for the formation of policy on his paper or periodical. What he says about separatism or black power or any other idea or movement within the black society must be handled delicately. Many publications are edited by their owners or publishers. Like the executives of many general papers and magazines, these men are businessmen first and rarely experienced or trained in editorial policymaking, so that views on these points are superficial. Or, nothing is said at all.

It is significant that Benjamin Muse, a former state senator in Virginia, a friendly historian of the Afro-American movements of the day, and author of numerous books and articles on the race problem, makes almost no mention of the part of the black press in what he calls, in a 1968 book, *The American Negro Revolution*. He covers the vital period from 1963 to 1967. Either he overlooked the press or decided its views were of no consequence. If the latter, it was not because of lack of sympathy with black America, for Muse has served on the board of directors of the Southern Regional Council and was given an award for his contribution to racial justice. When asked about this lack of reference to the black press he replied that in his 1968 book as well as in an earlier volume, *Ten Years of Prelude,* he did not recall "any situation in which Negro newspapers appeared to be a major factor." He added that "On the basic question pro-Negro matter in the Negro press was routine and taken for granted." He then employed a revealing clause: "pro-Negro matter in the white press—the flood of it in the early 1930's—was revolutionary."

Muse went on to say that "In retrospect I can see that some of the Negro editorial comment of recent years might have been of interest—particularly as it reflected differences of opinion within the Negro movement on such questions as that of 'separatism' vs. integration."[11]

Similarly, the press plays almost no part in *Black Political Power in America,* a situation that seems all the more strange since the author, Chuck Stone (C. Sumner Stone in his newspaper days) has been editor-in-chief of three leading black weeklies. It perhaps is a reflection of the absence of strong differences of opinion over the years, for the book is a study of black political leaders and political action over a long period. It might also be an admission that so often the black paper was for sale politically or lined up with a controlling party so obediently, in the past, that its part was routine and taken for granted, to use Muse's words.

Today, however, a unanimous point of view on the way in which Americans of the black race shall improve their circumstances is not to be expected of a press that exists in a democratic society so increasingly conscious of the demands of democracy. Such single-mindedness, however, is what the most ardent organization leaders seem to want, although most are realistic enough to realize how impossible it is that such accord could come about. The new publications being issued by fervent young men and women have no intentions of being organization men—if the organization represents the Establishment, as so much of the press unapologetically does.

Unanimity can be expected in goal if not in method, however. What black editor or publisher today would contend that Marcus Garvey was wrong when he wrote that "A race without authority and power is a race without respect"? This opinion appears to have been the motivation for much of the activities of the 1960's for the black citizens reaching in various ways to better their circumstances. They differ in interpretations, perhaps, of the key words, *authority* and *power,* just as they do in the means by which such authority and power are to be gained.

The effect of the black philosophies, then, has been to push the press to considering largely local issues or to be content with broad statements about national problems, with little guidance about the means by which the black citizens can sift one philosophy from the other and come to a decision about where they will stand and lend their strength. ●

16. PRO AND CON ON THE BLACK PRESS

Is BLACK JOURNALISM "good" journalism?

Before any answer can be given, other questions must be raised: What standards have been used? Who set up the criteria?

Black people, in defending certain attitudes and actions of this race, make the point at times that whites use white measuring sticks when assessing black performance and say that the requirements and ways of black people are not those of whites and need not be. Consequently they believe different standards should be used.

The criteria for judging the technical performance of the black press, however, have been color blind. Judgment of it should not be confused with past or present estimates of its efficacy as an advertising medium, its assertion of its right to exist, or the validity of the points of view expressed. Racial prejudice has been a factor in denying the press its share of advertising revenue and it also has operated against establishment of continuation of black publications in prejudiced communities (and is this, in America, not virtually all communities dominated by nonblacks?).

This chapter is concerned with evaluation of the black newspaper and magazine as a piece of journalism. The criteria generally applied admittedly have been set up by white people, but they are for the most part internationally accepted and respected in Africa and Asia as well as Europe and America. They are not necessarily American in origin, for the designers, typographers, editors, and writers of many countries contributed, over the years, to their formation, particularly the British. The criteria range from technological details like legibility of type to more debatable aspects like fairness in news coverage. What may be lacking in white criticism of the black press, in applying abstract standards, is understanding of why that press may not measure up at all times in all departments. Certainly in American journalism, and that of many other countries, the major standards—at least theoretically—are:

1. Integrity: being detached from political or commercial influ-

ence that might deny readers the truthful information they are led to expect.

2. Fairness, which in journalism means giving all sides (not just two) of a news event, restricting the paper's or magazine's opinions to the editorial columns, and avoiding printing opinions as news unless the source is clear.

3. Technical excellence, including legibility of printed matter, correctness of grammar and spelling, readability by the audience selected, originality in illustrations, suitability of subject matter for readers, professionalism in preparation of headings, layouts, and makeup.

To these could be added standards set up for noneditorial operations: advertising, circulation, promotion, and management. These standards were erected for the business world and apply to the business operations of the black press. They imply, for example, honesty in circulation statements, impartial treatment of advertisers in the rate structure, making only legitimate claims for a publication in its promotion material, and providing adequate working conditions, salaries, and fringe benefits for employes.

The first two standards for operation—integrity and fairness—are within the reach of publishers of all types of media. They are matters of policy rather than of technical expertise. Not that they are easy to attain or inexpensive. Covering all angles even of a fire story breaking out in a black neighborhood, for example, takes time and staff; similar coverage of a larger and more complicated event, such as a demonstration or strike, can be costly.

The third standard—technical excellence—often is much less attainable because it requires substantial capital investment, trained personnel, and high regular expense. Futhermore, in many communities, a black newspaper (and here the newspaper is more in question than the magazine) is quixotic if it spends large sums on achieving technical perfection which its audience is not interested in or perhaps even prepared to appreciate fully, a situation common in all shades and types of journalism.

Under what conditions, then, is it important that a black paper have the most highly recommended type dress, a horizontal rather than a vertical makeup, optically attractive page designs or tabloid instead of standard size, or some other technical characteristic? The answers are several: If: (1) it is economically no more costly than any other way; (2) competing papers are succeeding because of such practices and one's own is suffering as a result of not keeping pace; (3) readers demand but also respond; (4) advertisers respond more readily as a result; (5) the owner can afford it.

In this third area of technical excellence compromises are possible and sometimes necessary for survival. Failure to live up to this standard is understandable and to be preferred to the stilling of a printed voice in a community. The danger in compromise is that it can and does result in contentedness with slovenly reporting, careless writing, confusing make-up, and a generally mediocre publication, technically speaking, especially in a one-paper community where a white press is indifferent to the ethnic group.

In applying all such standards, ethical as well as technical, which have nothing to do with race per se, the black newspaper press of today as a whole comes off with a moderate grade only. As second newspapers and quasi-protest journalism, they, like their predecessors in the nineteenth century, can be considered possibly more successful as propaganda organs than as journalistic media devoted to offering their readers as much news as possible in the most objective way available. The early protest papers were influential and important not for their total content but for their value as outlets for opinion. As sermonizers, as exhorters, they were effective, but their readers still had to become informed of facts and strategies after the sermons were over. For those simpler times the protest papers performed a function, but it was not, and still is not, the sole function of a press that wants protection of its freedom. And, since then, papers have had to do more than supply such leadership and give their readers more nearly objective content.

Implicit in this assessment is the idea that the ideal black paper or magazine is one that informs its readers fully and also provides analysis, interpretation, and opinion material to help them comprehend the meaning and significance of events occuring in their own society and in the surrounding white society. On that basis, few black publications of today or the past score high. In proportion to number, neither do many white publications for that matter, a criticism made for many years by individuals and organizations. Insofar as the white press has to some extent overcome the faults of bias and exaggeration, it has made more progress toward meeting the standards than has the black press. But it must be remembered that it has been in a far better position to do so; in fact, it can be criticized adversely for not having made more progress by now.

That portion of the literature on black journalism in the U.S.A. that has attempted to evaluate the press has been predominantly adverse. One finds few defenders outside the writers of high-sounding, idealistic perorations published during Negro Press Week, the official time for praise. The whole American press, for that matter, has been a favorite whipping boy of politicians, reformers, and presidents throughout history. The serious students of the black publications—Frazier the sociologist, Sancton the journalist, Brown the public affairs scholar, and numbers of other black and white journalists discussing the profession—have had many faults to find. Those few who came to praise—Villard and Baldwin stand out—are outnumbered. The writers who sent down a balanced verdict—Myrdal is the best known of these few—generally are overlooked, as center-of-theroaders usually are, because partisans cannot use them. Furthermore, the evaluations have come at different times and on different aspects of the black press performance. For present purposes they sometimes are valueless because conditions have changed.

● THE CLASSIC ADVERSE CRITICISMS

Perhaps the most quoted critic of the black publications during any time in its history is the late E. Franklin Frazier, still regarded as one of the leading black sociologists, albeit somewhat outmoded. In *Black Bourgeoisie,* a book which the civil rights movement and later racial developments have made a landmark volume, he devoted a chapter to "The Negro Press and Wish-Fulfillment." It was an application of the volume's thesis: that the black, up to the early 1960's, was living in a make-believe world of his own creation; out of the black business and society world has arisen what he called a Negro bourgeoisie.

Frazier called the press "not only one of the most successful business enterprises owned and controlled by Negroes but also the "chief medium of communication which creates and perpetuates the world of make-believe. . . ."[1] He accused the press of representing only the bourgeoisie, not the black society as a whole, adding that it "promulgates the bourgeois values. . . ." He selects certain types of content to support his point, noting the stories of accomplishments of widely-known Negroes or prominent persons thought to have black blood (such as Pushkin and Dumas) but also the accomplishments of unknowns. These latter are exaggerated, he insists. A student who has a good college record is reported to be a genius; a black police magistrate is dubbed "judge." Such treatment of the news generates myths, he wrote.

But the darts thereafter in his chapter hit mainly at *Ebony,* as it was in the 1950's. Then it was emphasizing accounts of black men who became millionaires, with emphasis on their luxurious homes and cars; a few wealthy widows also were glorified. He reported that each month financially successful black businessmen were played up. The bourgeoisie and its press, Frazier insisted, ignore "the broader issues facing the modern world" because the black intelligentsia has developed an opportunistic philosophy.

His charges, which rested on now-outdated issues of publications, hold true today only on some points. The creation of a black world of society people continues in the large publications, especially the bigger newspapers. The reporting of relatively trivial accomplishments as significant goes on, particularly in the small weeklies (it is not their reporting but the way they report that is debatable). But the important issues facing and affecting all citizens, not blacks alone, are being dealt with somewhat more than before editorially. They may not strike hard but at least there is a group of papers with something to say. The problems of the rank and file black citizens, not the interests on the bourgeoisie mainly, are being reported in a substantial number of publications.

Few black publications, then or now, really qualified for his rating of being "one of the most successful Negro business enterprises," as the mortality rate and its owners' dependence upon outside enterprises (funeral parlors, banks, and insurance companies) shows. And too much of his writing about the black press is purely subjective. Sweeping generalizations are based on a few major publications. What is true applies to a handful, but at the time, as today, there were responsible publications not given to exaggerations of which all are accused.

After World War II was underway, attacks upon the black press began to mount, written by blacks and whites alike. Warren H. Brown, a black who at that time directed Negro relations for the Council for Democracy, late in 1942 published an article that drew fire. Some of the persons who objected to it did so particularly because it appeared in a then relatively small public affairs magazine and simultaneously in the *Reader's Digest,* with its multi-million circulation even in those days. Most newspapers are Negro first and American second, he charged, increasing segregation because they are race-conscious before being America-conscious. "They feed and prosper by sensationally playing up the Negro at his worst," he wrote. "When they publish news of the white community, it is generally an account of the white man at his worst . . . breeding ill-will between the races."[2]

In short, Brown's view was that the black press presented a dishonest picture of the U.S.A. and of the opportunity of the black man. He then went after Adam Clayton Powell, Jr., who was editing *People's Voice* at the time, and quoted some of the melodramatic editorial writing of that excitable minister-politician. There then followed numerous citations showing the headlines in various black papers that attacked the military establishment for its treatment of black troops, headlines that Brown considered "blatantly sensational and hate-making." He asked not for censorship but that the press not be "encouraged to run at a venemous, hate-making pace."

An article in reply appeared in *Saturday Review* but not in *Reader's Digest.* It was written by Vishnu V. Oak, a Wilberforce University professor of sociology and journalism, who some years later was to publish one of the few books on black journalism in this country. Oak, himself certainly a strong critic of the press, in his reply to Brown made the point that the American Negro would be unintelligent indeed if he did not, through his press, demand greater freedom for himself, "especially when he is fighting abroad for the preservation of democracy. . . ."

Several white writers joined in the criticism nevertheless. Two prominent southern journalists, John Temple Graves and Virginius Dabney, published articles. Graves' in the *Virginia Quarterly Review,* received much less attention than that of Dabney, then editor of the white Richmond (Va.) *Times-Dispatch,* for his appeared in several publications, including the *Atlantic Monthly.* He accused the press of stirring dissension between blacks and whites, publishing this view also in *Negro Digest* and the professional magazine for journalists, the *Quill.* He exhibited no such restraint as did Brown, but proposed that "the disturbing elements on both sides of the color line . . . be muzzled for the duration. . . ."[3]

Walter White, by then secretary of the NAACP, placed some of the blame for whatever truth such criticisms contained upon certain press weaknesses. These were the lack of staff or carelessness which led to publication of unverified copy and use of sensational headlines that gave the news a distorted emphasis. But, White declared in an autobiography, the fault was not all to be assigned to the black papers. They were doing only what white ones had begun to do long before, and to greater excess. Also, news of discrimination against blacks had long gone unpublished in the white press, and black readers wanted to know of it. White reported that he learned of pressure being brought upon President Franklin D. Roosevelt and the Department of Justice to indict some of the black newspaper editors. But the president discouraged that move. Then there were plans, White added, to deny newsprint to papers thought to be seditious. These, too, were discouraged. The NAACP early in 1943 called a meeting of editors of two dozen prominent black papers. The association's Washington office was made available for checking stories and the papers agreed to help each other in news verification. From this session came the National Newspaper Publishers Association.[4]

These actions were in response to wartime criticism of the press. But there were other charges. Brooks summarizes the major adverse criticisms generally leveled at mid-century. The newspapers were accused of sensationalism, questionable advertising policies, and overemphasis on the racial angles of the news. One coming from fewer sources was that certain unnamed leading journals were leftist or Communist inspired. It was this latter charge that Brooks studied, providing a quantitative report on the leading black papers of 1948. His findings were that these papers "reflect those values consistent with the American tradition rather than the espousal of doctrine alien to it," that they were fundamentally concerned with promoting civil liberties and other citizenship rights for the whole population, and that there was "uncompromising rejection of segregation and discrimination" as well as many another social practice "affecting adversely the status and role of colored minorities in American society." He also observed that these papers were not primarily organs of protest but were more journals of reform.[5]

About this same time Roi Ottley, later to be the biographer of

Robert S. Abbott and himself an experienced black newsman, attacked the commercialism of the papers. "Once the stuff of idealism is cut away," he wrote, "they are operated primarily for profit and in this sense are like their white contemporaries. What is good business in the judgment of the owners rarely is hampered by the nonsense about race."[6] Earl Conrad, the white man who left the white press to work in a black newsroom and wrote sympathetic and understanding articles about the black papers, in a 1946 article said that some publishers in the postwar period accepted money from the highest bidder for their political support. He thought the owners and other heads of these publishing companies hardly needed the dollars. Such selling out, he wrote, was a violation of trust. Conrad considered such blacks as quislings among their people. Nor did he exempt white leaders of the two major parties for making such deals. He pointed to the political stances taken in 1944 when Thomas E. Dewey and Franklin D. Roosevelt contended for the presidency. Some big, black papers supported Dewey but the black citizens in their communities voted overwhelmingly for FDR.[7] Whites similarly repudiated their press. In contrast to this was the 1968 election, when Hubert H. Humphrey was heavily supported by the black press as well as the black citizenry.

Now and again, in the next quarter of a century, came other adverse criticisms, these largely from within the fold. James Baldwin, the novelist, although in reality more of a defender than an adverse critic, did write in 1948 that the black press "supports any man, provided he is sufficiently dark and well known. . . . The Negro press has been accused of not helping much—as indeed, it has not, nor do I see how it could have. And it has been accused of being sensational, which it is."[8]

Enoc P. Waters, who was Associated Negro Press editor in the early 1960's, was unhappy about what he called the sameness of the black papers and the "narrow rut in which they operate." He called for more creativity and imagination. The reporting was "too prosaic and conventional." A crusading spirit was lacking; editors needed more of a sense of mission.[9]

Relative quiet prevailed until 1967, when Elaine Kendall, a magazine writer and author, writing in the unlikely snob-appeal *Holiday,* cast The Critical Eye department of the sophisticated magazine on the black press. Angry letters followed. She had analyzed mainly several of the larger magazines (those from Johnson and the now gone *Elegant*) and the usual national papers, generalizing about all from these. She saw these publications as not being realistic enough about the true condition of the black people of the country. "Moreover, the papers are disdained and unread by the young and impatient Negro leaders and intellectuals," she wrote. "When they do see them, they are dismayed and irritated by the galloping materialism they find there. . . ."[10]

Her opponents chastised her for accepting *Elegant*'s alleged circulation of 200,000, for omitting the New York *Amsterdam News* and *Tuesday* magazine, for comparing the black weeklies to the white dailies, and for holding views she actually did not express. Hoyt W. Fuller, managing editor of *Black World* (then *Negro Digest*), offended perhaps because Miss Kendall brushed off his magazine merely by saying it had the smallest circulation of the Johnson group, which was and still is correct, called the article names but gave no evidence and scolded *Holiday* for printing it.

Two years later appeared, during national Negro Press Week, ample substantiation of Miss Kendall's view about the disenchantment of the young black intellectuals with the press. It probably was as untypical a press week or month piece as can be found.

Dan Aldridge, in his "Serious Business" column for the *Michigan Chronicle,* the large Sengstacke paper in Detroit, commented on an editorial in his own paper which had praised the press. With that as a springboard he made these assertions:

". . . there are very few newspapers in the country that can rightly be called the 'black press.' The only two that come to mind are the papers put out by the Black Panther Party and the Nation of Islam." He admitted that there might be "a few others around the country." "Negro press," he said, was a better label for "our so-called printed media." He then called to his support the familiar views, referring to the press of two decades earlier, of Frazier the sociologist, already introduced in this chapter. Next he presented his own opinions, noting that "Too much of most Negro newspapers is concerned more with the social life of the few than with the political life of the many. Valuable space which could be used to educate, mobilize and guide our people is used to talk about cocktail parties, ski parties, and dating games. This misuse of valuable news space is more than naive. It is criminal."

He then observed that the Detroit *News,* a large white daily, although criticized for carrying so much crime news, "is no match for most Negro newspapers." Their front pages, he wrote, "are filled with the words rape, murder, kill, loot, rob, stab, shot, stomp, cut and blood." He labeled them "crime shooting journals."

Further objects of the attack were what the press omits (knowledge of Africa and leading Africans, what really is going on in China and Cuba, and other events), the press' practice of serving as "agents for cheating real estate dealers," even defending them, and its failure to take a position, on public issues, with specific examples.[11]

● **ON THE POSITIVE SIDE**

When it is not praised for its courage in fighting for the black American's rights, the positive criticism of the black press is more a matter of justifying or explaining its policies and viewpoints than compliments on its performance.

Praise for the press came in 1944 from Oswald Garrison Villard, grandson of William Lloyd Garrison and himself at one time editor of the New York *Evening Post* and owner and publisher of *Nation*. He also was a founder of the NAACP. The Negro press, as he called it, was the only one that had developed swiftly, in his view. Many of the editors, he believed, had shown and were then demonstrating great ability and power. Its growth in numbers and in the extent of its support by members of the race was astounding, he said, to many persons who had been unaware of the tensions from discontent and anger among the black people.

"Born of these bitter passions, the new Negro press speaks with vigor, and far too often with a violence, that have startled the whites who have suddenly been brought into contact with it." Viewing the same headlines as did Warren Brown, Villard saw them in a different light. "It is not cowed because this is war-time, it does not tremble before authority," he wrote. "It uses little or no restraint in discussing the refusal of this government to grant to our Negroes not only their constitutional privileges, but full equality in the army and the navy, the right to fight for their country on equal terms with white citizens. . . . These militant newspapers are both creators of the suddenly developed Negro sense of solidarity and themselves an index of a developing race consciousness and unwillingness to remain in a subordinate position, a helotry in a democracy."[12]

He recognized weakness, as well, adding that it was then unfortunately true that many Negro dailies and weeklies had to go to censurable excesses and injure their case by their unbridled attacks in what he considered an explosive period in the nation's history. He placed responsibility for these excesses mainly on those whites who believed that the U.S.A., as a democracy, could live part servile and part free. Villard thought that the white press might "similarly catch fire" after the war. He did not live to see this happen nor has it happened since his death in 1949.

James Baldwin, in one of his autobiographical essays, wrote in 1948 what is equally true today: "Negroes live violent lives, unavoidably; a Negro press without violence is therefore not possible; and, further, in every act of violence, particularly violence against white men, Negroes feel a certain thrill of self-identification, a wish to have done it themselves, a feeling that old scores are being settled at last."[13]

After describing Harlem as it existed in the late 1940's and noting that some steps were being taken to "make it less of a social liability," such as opening of a boys' club, a playground, and a housing project, he said that most of the projects were stimulated by Negro leaders and the Negro press [using *Negro*].[14] Baldwin added that it can be forgiven for its preoccupation considering the indifference and hostility of the white press. "The Negro press has been accused of not helping much—as indeed it has not, nor do I see how it could have," he wrote. He also did not hold it against the press of that time for being sensational. He also said that the terrible dilemma of the press is that it had to imitate the white, not having any other.

Baldwin seems to forget that the situation may have existed in the nineteenth century, but in this century, when the press was somewhat more oriented, there was less necessity for using white models. Even today, as noted in the discussion of production of black publications in the preceding chapters, little experimentation is taking place; like other American publishers, black ones evidently have found little or nothing to attract them in the press of other nations. Later Baldwin says that the critics of the press are irrational when they demand that "the nation's most oppressed minority" conduct itself with a skill and foresight not asked of Joseph Medill Patterson (founder of the New York *Daily News*) or of William Randolph Hearst, Sr.

What Baldwin calls the press' "innate desperation" is betrayed in its tone, he writes. He must be cheered to note today that with improvement in the condition of some blacks, at least, the press tone has changed. Its militancy is not so much born of desperation as of occasional victories and possibilities of more to come—blacks in high political office, such as mayors of large cities; in important educational posts (presidencies of black and white colleges), in government positions (senators, representatives, ambassadors), and in the sciences, arts, and letters.

A positive view of the black press can be obtained by noting certain of its actions in comparison to those of the white. C. Sumner Stone went into battle with Ben H. Bagdikian, one of the few published critics of the white press. In a *New Republic* article Bagdikian discussed the political views of American newspapers, saying at one point that President John F. Kennedy had no editorial support in certain cities, including Chicago. Stone accused him of racial myopia which, he said, characterizes the press of America, noting then that the Chicago *Daily Defender* (of which Stone once was chief editor) had supported Kennedy, as had many black weeklies.

"Negro newspapers simply are not recognized as co-equals or even respected for their editorial integrity and power," Stone wrote in his answering letter, "even if they are larger, far more wealthy, influential and professional than the smallest, most impoverished racist and editorially unkempt white rag."[15] Bagdikian in rebuttal wrote that "Negro newspapers are not the co-equals of papers like the Chicago *Tribune, Sun-Times, Daily News* or *American,* not because they are Negro, but because they are specialized papers, edited for the particular interest of one ethnic group."

His answer, in this author's view, was not adequate. The black to be sure are second papers, but not in the same sense as are the New York *Morning Telegraph* for racing fans, the Chicago *Journal of*

Commerce for financiers, or *Women's Wear Daily* for buyers and merchandisers. For these papers do not deal to any appreciable extent with social issues nor are they expected to take political positions. Racial problems today enter many areas: religion, employment, health, education, and government are only a few. But any of the large black national weeklies, and many of the moderate-size papers and the four dailies have their following, even though almost everyone in that following may read a white newspaper and some a white newsmagazine at the same time, for the followers do not see in their primary papers the social issues that concern them treated from the black viewpoint. Thus it is important for any politician gauging public opinion to be aware of what the black press is urging upon its readers or even exposing them to by way of news coverage. With black Americans more and more voting as a group their press is to be reckoned with.

Still another defense of the press came in 1969 from W. Leonard Evans, editor and president of *Tuesday.* Speaking in a panel on marketing he chided white advertisers and agencies when he said that " . . . the black newspapers, after being 100 years old, have never gotten their just dollars. Therefore, they are being criticized, they don't cover this news, or have this type of reproduction. How can they, when they have to live off circulation?"

The Myrdal study of the black people of America noted the charge that the black papers were sensational. It quoted the defense of their editors and publishers, i.e., they wanted to reach as many readers as possible so as to widen their chance of influencing them to improve and advance the race. Myrdal said that "the main factor" was that "the Negro community, compared with the white world, is so predominantly lower class." He also noted that the black paper was sensational because it was an "additional" paper.[16] Thirty years later it still was a second paper and yet it no longer relies so heavily on sensationalism, an indication of the belief among publishers that the economic condition of readers is improved, that the taste for sensationalism has lessened, that other media are gratifying it, or that to attract the best advertisers such sensationalism must be decreased.

● THE UNMENTIONED WEAKNESSES

Defenses and explanations have been entered for the faults usually mentioned by adverse critics: questionable advertising, inadequate facilities and low salaries for employes, technically low grade publications, accepting political bribery. These weaknesses are not attributed to all publications, although those resulting from inadequate and insufficient capitalization are general.

Several other weaknesses are not pointed out in the usual discussions of this press, possibly because they are to be found in portions of the American press of any color. They are: inadequate news coverage, blatant use of publicity copy to please advertisers or extend policy, lack of attribution of much material, plagiarism, outcroppings of racial bigotry, indifference to skilled workmanship, and self-promotion by owners and editors.

Few black papers, or few white ones, are free of many dozens of inches of promotional copy for new movies, packaged products, television programs, night club entertainers, recordings, and other advertised products and services. A respected black journalist, L. F. Palmer, Jr., has put it thus: "Black newspapers . . . are greedy for handouts." This attitude is explained by lack of qualified editorial personnel and the impossibility of covering the black communities in competition with the metropolitan dailies.

The entire special sections that deal with the new automobile models, real estate developments, and general business progress in a community contain largely articles praising or in some way publicizing local business enterprises. These pieces of copy help fill a few spaces on each page between the advertisements solicited especially to sustain these sections. In the black press such supplements are less common than in the white and are confined largely to the major papers and to areas in which advertising can be solicited: black educational institutions, local industry, and the national automobile companies. Such special sections, and the thousands of alleged news stories printed in the run of the paper are handled with little subtlety. Hardly any attempt is made to print only such free publicity as contains genuine news value. Publicity copy is not useless per se. The best of it contains genuine news elements. But the black press often shows little discrimination in its use of such handouts. On the second page of a leading, nationally circulated black paper appeared a typical example. Under a two-column photograph were these lines:

> IN A NEW BAG—As the leading all-time ground gainer in the history of the Los Angeles Rams, running back Dick Bass has already made a place for himself among football immortals. Now Bass, shown in Hollywood, has turned actor and will play a lead role in "The Young Lawyers," a two-hour movie for television.

One might expect to find this, if at all, on the entertainment or sports pages, where it is customary to provide such free advertising, but the *New Pittsburgh Courier* put it on its second page, which usually is reserved by papers for bona fide news.

On the women's page are the free publicity stories and pictures one has become accustomed to find in these pages of gratis space for advertisers. A fourteen-inch double-column story is all about the loveliness of Haiti—a land not known for its freedom from the conditions and restraints of which many blacks long have complained in the

U.S.A.—accompanied by a twenty-inch photograph of a girl tourist on a Haitian beach. Adjoining is a two-column of a girl cooking jellies, the picture provided by the firm that makes some of the ingredients mentioned in the recipes, although obviously trade names. And at the bottom of the page is a five-column spread of four pictures, all of whites, supplied by a firm that makes clothing materials; its name is mentioned five times in the underlines.

The women's magazine world has long been guilty of cooperating with advertisers or potential advertisers. A new high—or low—in such collaboration was reached by *Essence* in its first issue when the photograph of the girl on the cover was explained on the contents page thus:

"That great natural look of our cover girl is subtly encouraged by beauty aids from Yardley. Next to Nothing Bronze foundation and Next to Nothing Tawny Cake blusher light up her skin. Buttercup Green eye shadow and luscious black lashes by Lash Galore enhance her eyes. Fly-away Bronze livened her lips. Result? Muted, irresistible appeal."

Small, inadequately financed papers may be driven to this type of journalism, but the large, national papers and magazines that indulge in it are not so hard pressed. Typical of the practices of smaller papers are those to be found in a weekly published in the mid-South. An issue runs to six pages, almost 50 per cent of it advertising. Not one local story from its city, which has a population of nearly 100,000, appears. Except for two signed editorials, all copy is either local publicity, including pictures, or out-of-town stories lifted from other newspapers without credit.

The publicity material is blatant. Alongside an advertisement for a car repair shop is a picture of the proprietor and a story praising his enterprise. On the front page is a three-column picture of the proprietors of a local supper club, its name in capitals, having "an impromptu chat" with a "popular" representative of a brewing company, the latter's personality reported to be one of the chief reasons that his products are highly favored by many tavern patrons.

Insufficient News Content. Aside from the large national weeklies and certain middle-size city papers, the black newspaper publishers are engaged in producing many newspapers offering readers little news. This statement is not intended as a generalization about the black press. But in the author's possession are more than a score of current papers, the majority of them commercial ventures and not propaganda organs for groups defending causes, which present themselves to their readers as purveyors of news but actually contain little and make virtually no attempt at a systematic canvass of the black news sources, local, national, or international. He has seen as many more in libraries and in black publications offices, where they are received as exchanges. These publishers paste up material lifted from

the large white papers or from magazines, print publicity releases
without editing, and in other ways evade the responsibility for genuine local coverage and origination of news on their own. Usually
there is some local news, perhaps four or five stories, most of them
routine, but what actually is going on in the black community is only
skimmed over. In one community there were serious racial disturbances in several parts of the city. The local black paper not only left
the coverage to the white press (which published biased stories) but
failed to provide any interpretation of the events in an effort to clarify
causes.

As long ago as 1955 Simeon Booker pointed out that the surest
way for white dailies to gain black readers is to print news of all kinds
of black life. He noted that the Chicago *Tribune* outsold the more
liberal Chicago *Sun-Times* and the Chicago *Daily News* in the black
neighborhoods. "The *Trib*," a black told him, "was the first to pay
attention to Negro news. They not only attend our meetings and
affairs but they do feature stories on our leaders and outstanding
citizens."[17]

The same principle holds for black publications, as the failures
of some of the newsless cause papers should show as clearly as do the
failures of the more or less newsless commercial papers intent on
selling advertising space and pushing the news out of the columns to
make room for it.

The contention is that it takes too much staff and hence too
much money to cover the black community. But to go to press with
a paste-up consisting of an editorial, many columns of free publicity
stories containing few news elements, and nonlocal news filched from
other papers shows little serious interest in being a newspaper. It
shows only an interest in making money.

Failure to attribute the source of material occurs constantly in
both small and large publications, newspapers and magazines alike.
In many areas of the country are papers produced by the photocompo-
sition process, which requires that the staff mount on sheets corresponding to pages the copy they wish reproduced, including illustrations and advertising. Thus it is a temptation to lift whatever is
desirable from anywhere. A common practice is to clip wire service
stories from white dailies or other black papers that have paid for
such copy, and trim out the initials or name of the agency. This de-
liberate plagiarism is known to the agencies and papers thus being
robbed. But they are helpless to correct it, for the publications that
resort to such practices have no money and a legal case would be fruit-
less. A further complication is that news is perishable and in the
public domain the second day after it has been published. Damages
would be difficult to prove if a weekly or bi-weekly lifted copy originally published ten days earlier. Readers have no knowledge of this
background and credit such papers with being newsy. But alert readers remember having seen the identical material in the source publi-

cations and can draw their own conclusions about the initiative and integrity of the papers that clip and print so freely.

Even in some of the largest black weeklies many columns of news appear without indication of or even a clue to source. Some clearly is from the news bureaus of black institutions—colleges, National Urban League, and the NAACP. Many stories are matter-of-fact and are a service to an understaffed publication. But others are supposedly from the paper's own bureaus and stringers and are by no means impartial accounts of the news they allegedly report. When such stories come from small towns and large cities alike the implications are that the paper has its own sources there, but this is unlikely, considering the present absence of a national black news service and the limited use, at least officially, of a white service.

Related to this practice is injecting opinion into the news account, i.e., advancing policy by writing a story from an angle that conforms to the publication's viewpoint. Let it be clearly understood that white (and foreign language) papers do exactly the same thing. The malpractices of the white or other nonblack press are presumably not the standards of the black. It may result from overzealous campaigning or crusading or from the mistaken idea that interpretation and opinion are one and the same. Opinions disguised as news are not respected journalism under the American understanding of a medium's function. Yet a good many black publications either ignore, or are unaware of, this standard. Reads a streamer in a leading weekly: POWELL WINS SEAT AT A PRICE. Says another in a small weekly in a big city: POSTMEN'S LOW PAY SUBSIDIZES BULK MAIL. A large city paper backs into a slanted headline by using a device called a tag line above the main headline, which is in much larger type: *Dr. Allen Denies Rumor*—NIXON ADMINISTRA TION TO/BOOT ANOTHER 'LIBERAL.'

The view that skilled workmanship is of little importance on many publications is easily enough supported. Although it is lessening as a fault because of the training more easily available to potential and practising black journalists, it still is true that far too little concern is shown for correctness of grammar, rhetoric, and spelling, journalistic form, conciseness, and clarity in writing. Ted Poston, one of the most capable black journalists, a prizewinning and courageous writer long identified with the New York *Post,* said in an article on the black press that "the average news story is badly written, poorly edited, and often based on rumors which could be easily checked."[18] There has been improvement in the two decades since, but it is largely in some of the larger or exceptional middle-size papers. One can forgive such unprofessionalism in some small community paper conducted as a workshop experiment whose staff has no guidance or coaching, and which works as a group of volunteers. But in a major paper it is not rare for readers to encounter such a headline as this:

MAN ALLEGEDLY BEAT BY
COPS; BOOKED ON 6 COUNTS

Or this news story lead:

"Black power. . . . Brains not muscle flexing. Building not tearing down. That's power. Unbeatable power because it instills a feeling of respect. Of individuality. Of real strength." The story continues in this vein for two more paragraphs and then the reader learns that it is about Junior Achievement. Eight additional paragraphs praise that worthy group's work. It is an editorial, a feeble one at that, but dressed to look like news, and there is no news in it, just language.

A front-page story, with a four-column headline, begins: "The following telegram has been sent by the Memphis branch NAACP to Gen. L. F. Chapman, Commandant-Marine Corps, and to President Richard M. Nixon." (The telegram then is quoted in full.) Nothing more. No assistance is given to the reader in getting to the point of the telegram quickly.

Another type of unprofessionalism is encountered particularly in the numerous local voices springing up in the big cities: inner area or street corner newspapers, sponsored by self-help groups or government-supported agencies but others clear attempts at gaining a commercial foothold. In these latter, such amateurishness is encountered often. One can expect it with a group of neophytes, often teen-agers who lack training and whose paper makes no pretense at being a commercial competitor for the established publications. But ineptness should be rejected from a publication that takes subscribers' and advertisers' money. Two widely separated examples, geographically, are these:

In the Northeast a certain weekly not only is badly written and made up, without any idea of orderly and legible display of copy, but also contains in its masthead the statement that the advertising is obtained by a company of newspaper representatives. The firm has been defunct since the early 1960's. The paper also announces that it is a member of a certain black press organization. That, too, has been defunct for many years. The practice of such pretense is concious deception on the part of the owners, who made no reply when the matters were called to their attention.

In the Southwest is another weekly. It asked an organization for a news release, a document, and a photograph. The picture was used with the caption of a society photograph printed on another page. The document was the outline of a college course, literally in outline form. Instead of writing something about the course material the editor printed it verbatim. It had little meaning for the readers, who were not told why such an unjournalistic document should appear in the first place. The news release was printed on still another page, and headed merely "Lettter [*sic*] to the Editor." This, one might paraphrase, is no way to edit a newspaper.

The defenses are familiar. The alternative, the owners say, is to have no newspaper at all, for there is no time, between attempting to sell advertising space, obtain subscribers, write the copy, deal with the public, and do dozens of other jobs, to write headlines carefully, edit copy precisely, and plan artistic make-up. Especially if these are not crusading publications the reply to that might be that perhaps some of these badly written and poorly edited papers are not needed, that they do more damage than good in their communities and mar the influence and image of the black press as a whole.

● READERS' REACTIONS

The effort to learn what black Americans think of black journalism has been going on, in a small way, for some years. One of the more important attempts was made by the Chicago *Defender* and the National Non-Partisan League in 1945 when they polled blacks to ascertain their attitudes. The report of the results in the source used does not indicate the mechanics of the poll or how representative it was, nor how many persons were polled. Ninety-four per cent said they read black papers, 6 per cent said they did not. When asked why, 80 per cent of the former said they wished to find out what is going on that affects blacks. Another 15 per cent answered that other other papers do not give any news about blacks. Black papers, in the opinions of 97 per cent, are the "greatest influence in securing for the Negro first class citizenship."[19]

The few professional studies of response to this ethnic press made before the late 1960's deal with advertising content, as in the several completed by Dr. Charles L. Allen. The Department of Communications of the College of Communication Arts at Michigan State University in 1968 released studies concerning white-owned print and electronic media usage, attitudes and functions for low-income and middle-class teen-agers among residents of three low-income areas at Lansing. Among the finding were these:

Black teen-agers watch more television than whites, from the same economic environments. Lower economic class youngsters, black and white, were less likely to have gone to a movie in the preceding month or to have read as many magazines as the whites from both income levels.

When asked: "How often do you get a chance to read a newspaper?" the low income group (in this case whites and blacks) responded comparatively as in Table 16.1.

The report summary noted that 46 per cent of the black teenagers, 58 per cent of the white lower income teen-agers, and 69 per cent of the middle-class group reported some reading in a newspaper

TABLE 16.1 ● Frequency of Newspaper Reading Among Low-Income Teen-Agers

Weekly	Black Respondents	White Respondents
Every day	46%	58%
6 times	6	6
5 times	5	4
4 times	11	2
3 times	5	6
2 times	12	9
1 time	6	7
Less than once	7	6
Not at all	1	2

SOURCE: *Communication Among the Urban Poor,* Michigan State Reports, No. 1, Michigan State University, 1967.

every day. The implications of this study were presented thus:

"The young man or woman emerging from an environment that is below standard in economic and social aspects has been greatly dependent on a single mass medium—television—for his information and attitudes about the world outside his own neighborhood."[20]

This statement of the implications, however, overlooks the fact that these youth do read newspapers and thus while they are greatly dependent upon television are not uninformed by the press. Nor do we know from this study the relative extent of the dependence upon each medium.

The Bontrager Study. A somewhat more recent study made by Bontrager brought out, among other findings, several that reinforced the Lansing study. His random sample was 232 black inner city adults of American citizenship in Syracuse. Their median years of education completed was ten and generally they were of a low socio-economic level. Fifty-one did not read any newspapers; fifty-eight read both black and white, two read black only, and 121 read white papers exclusively. This finding confirmed Myrdal's and other observers' statements that the black paper is a second paper.[21] It differed, however, from the findings about a Pittsburgh group reported by Allen in 1967. He found 14 per cent of readership of white papers and 13 percent of the local black paper *(New Pittsburgh Courier).*[22] The difference from Syracuse might here be explained by the fact that the Pittsburgh weekly is among the older, prestigious publications of black journalism whereas Syracuse, at the time, had not seen a standard black paper for years. Furthermore, at the time the Bontrager study was being made, the two militant black weeklies, concentrating on opinion and carrying little news, were about to disappear from lack of support. Bontrager compared his findings also with those of Lyle in Los Angeles.[23] In the California city there was 70 per cent readership of the black Los Angeles *Sentinel,* also an established weekly, and 100 per cent readership of a white paper.

Differences in the natures of the three samples may to some extent explain the variations. They were not educationally parallel; also, housewives dominated the Syracuse response.

Despite their feebleness as news organs, the two Syracuse advocacy weeklies equaled or ranked ahead of any other black paper, in Bontrager's results. The *Home Town News* had forty-five readers. The *Liberated Voice* had twenty-nine. The Baltimore *Afro-American* also had twenty-nine. The *New Pittsburgh Courier* was next with nineteen, Chicago *Daily Defender* followed with twelve, New York *Amsterdam News,* nine, and *Muhammad Speaks,* one. It should be noted, however, that because of urban renewal, the chief black residential area of the city had by that time been dispersed and to some extent regrouped. One result was that there were fewer outlets for black newspapers and magazines than had existed five years earlier.

The readers responding to Bontrager's study, he learned, thought better of their black papers than of the white ones, although they read more of the latter. Using a rating scale of Excellent, Good, Fair, and Inferior, he was told that 15 per cent of the black papers were excellent and 3.4 per cent of the white. Black papers received a 33.6 per cent good rating, white 14.7 per cent. Fair was attached to 21.1 per cent of the black and 51.3 per cent of the white. An inferior grade went to 6.5 per cent of the black and 13.8 per cent of the white.

With magazines, however, the story was different. Black periodicals had a higher readership than white (fifty-three to thirty-five readers). On the other hand, seventy-nine of the 232 readers sampled read no magazines at all, a comment on both their cost and availability; the black papers, especially the two local weeklies, being more easily bought than the magazines, all of which were national and had no street selling plan.

The magazines preferred were *Ebony* and *Jet,* which had many readers in common. They not only led all black periodicals but also all white. Two-thirds of the magazine readers named *Ebony;* not quite one-fourth noted *Look,* the highest ranking white periodical. The next black magazine in line was *Sepia,* standing behind *Ebony, Jet, Look, Life,* and *TV Guide,* and with 14.37 per cent of the readers. *Tan* was the only other black periodical named, with six readers or 3.92 per cent. Bontrager points out that five of the first six are picture magazines.

The Michigan study provides some findings for comparison with Bontrager's at this point. The respondents were asked: "In the last week, how many magazines have you read or looked at?" The results are in Table 16.2.

Since all Bontrager's respondents were black, only the black column is comparable. Thirty-two per cent of his readers read no magazines at all, more than double the Michigan group, explainable by the fact that all the Michigan respondents were teen-agers and the Syracuse people were a cross section of a family.

TABLE 16.2 ● Magazine Readership Among Low-income Teen-Agers

More Than	Black Respondents	White Respondents
5	41%	31%
3	10	11
2	25	25
1	17	18
none	15	0

SOURCE: *Communication Among the Urban Poor.*

Another Syracuse researcher, Stephenson, was able to shed still more light on reader attitudes as revealed by reading choices, by using a quota sample "determined by the respondents' educational achievement." It presented facts about overall media usage, magazine readership, and attitudes toward changes in the mass media and white magazines.[24] As had other recent scholars, Stephenson learned that television was favored over other media. He also learned that virtually all his respondents (106 out of 109) read at least one magazine, with occasional readers far outnumbering the constant readers. Black magazines were most popular. Black pride was found to be "an increasingly important factor influencing the media choices of participants."[25]

Stephenson found only limited accessibility to black magazines. Weekly papers ranked low among the media chosen by the 109 respondents. Sixty-one or 56 per cent named television as the single medium most often used, nineteen or 17.4 per cent named daily papers, twelve or 11 per cent said radio, seven or 6.4 per cent black weekly papers, five or 4.6 per cent said churches and other organizations. Four or 3.7 per cent noted black and white magazines, and one or .9 per cent responded with informal, personal sources.

To be expected, therefore, is the finding that among the black or white periodicals the most popular was *TV Guide*. The general consumer magazines were, as before, led by *Ebony* and *Jet*. Stephenson compared his results with those of Colle, reported in 1965.[26] The Cornell scholar had used Rochester, New York, as his universe and an apparently better-educated group as his subjects than had Stephenson, who admitted that a weakness of his research was the diversity of his subjects' educational background and the lack of depth in numbers at most levels of education. Colle had divergent results. Television, while an important information source, was equaled by personal sources. Forty-two per cent of Colle's respondents said they did did not read any periodicals regularly; 75 per cent of the rest said they read at least one black magazine regularly. On the other hand, the Lyle study in Los Angeles (see Chapter 8) was confirmed by the Syracuse results on this point of magazine reading.

Such findings as these reveal a limited number of readers' evaluations of the black newspaper and magazine. Although economics and accessibility are important factors behind attitudes, a person who has an attachment for a publication or a great dependence upon it will find ways to get and read it despite cost or distance. Evidently, from the studies reported, there is little sacrificial buying and reading, an implied adverse criticism of the black press.

Individual Attitudes. Articulate members of the black race are more specific than these scholarly studies. Scientifically they have no validity, but individual reactions of blacks to their own press are worth noting. Conversations with them bring results that are interesting, if no more.

There was the woman to whom the black press had meant nothing in a life spanning more than sixty years. Always employed in desk work by white organizations, this press was never used or in evidence in her offices.

"Have you no interest, then, in the problems of the black race?" she was asked.

"On the contrary, indeed I have," she answered. "But the black papers never were needed in my work or my thinking about racial problems." The basic ones she depended upon, it turned out, were those produced by the Society of Friends (Quakers), never lacking in understanding and assistance to the black people.

On another occasion was the conversation with a college-trained man, in this instance one about to get a law degree. It essentially was like those with an engineer, a social worker, housewife, teacher, and businessman on other occasions.

"Now and then I look at *Ebony*," the about-to-be lawyer said. "And I see *Muhammad Speaks* as much as any."

"Anything else?"

"Johnson has other publications I am aware of." He seemed to be groping for the titles. He assented when they were named.

"Yes, that's right. But I don't read them. I've just heard of and seen them."

Of his own accord he went on to mention *Sepia*. "But I don't read it anymore," he said. "I read it when I lived in Miami. I also read the Miami *Times*, then. I lived on the West Coast for awhile and read one for teen-agers. Can't remember its name."

"*Elegant-Teen,* perhaps?"

"Sounds like it. I also used to read the Pittsburgh *Courier*. But I don't read black papers any more. Too much in them is of no interest to me now. Too much family stuff and I'm still single. *Ebony* has a lot of everything but doesn't stand for anything editorially. No editorials."

He was not taxed with the error about no editorials. Usually there is some such error about the black press in these replies (one young man insisted *Esquire* is a black magazine), showing little close acquaintance with certain periodicals or papers. From others, mainly militant students and organization workers, comes the view that most

black publications are Uncle Toms. The regular press, among the
well educated, seems less stimulating than that of the militant organizations. The frame of mind of those holding the latter view is
represented by a letter in a newsmagazine which had carried an
article about the black-run Zebra advertising agency.

"What America's black community does not need," the letter
writer said, "is advertising that, like all advertising, will sell them
$32 billion worth of generally useless and superfluous goods. I'm all
in favor of black entrepreneurs in the black community, but not
when they only turn out to be as destructive as the self-serving leeches
in the drugs and numbers racket—they may be more legal but they
are no more moral."[27]

● CONSTRUCTIVE EFFORTS

Although there seems to have been no follow-up, early in 1969
there was formed a Black Student Press Association whose purpose
was to improve the quality of the news media and to establish job opportunities for fellow college editors, as it was described.[28] Meeting
in Washington, the college editors announced:

"We don't necessarily want jobs in the mainstream of white
journalism; we would like to devote our energies to making the black
press a much more effective and relevant medium." The executive
director of the group then was Jay Harris, of Lincoln University
(Pennsylvania), who stressed the fact that the group intended to form
a network of news communications involving students from both black
and white schools. Although this plan appears to have petered out,
others on foot to strengthen black journalism education may bring
improvements such as were envisioned by BSPA (see Chapter 11).

Another scheme, to encourage publishers and owners of black
publications to conduct community service programs, is that of the
Coca Cola Company, long a big advertiser. Annually since 1968 the
firm has given an award to some paper during the NNPA convention.
Named for the late Carl Murphy, of the *Afro-American* papers, it
consists of a plaque and $1,000. Winners so far have been the Chicago
Daily Defender and the Norfolk *Journal and Guide*. Insofar as such
a plan makes the black papers more useful to their communities black
citizens may feel a little closer to the press and support it.

From time to time the black publications have been told, usually
by whites, that the black press needs to present a clearer image of
itself to the country's advertisers if it is to have favorable response
from them. The owners need to develop sound reasons why their
papers and magazines should be used as advertising tools, they were
told.

The events of recent years seem to have provided them with their
opportunity, as some elements in business, industry, and government

have made special efforts to employ blacks and have used both the display and classified advertising columns of the press to recruit. The moderate papers and magazines, which are the bulk of the journalism, have had such support and hence a way to keep an editorial message before their constituencies. And the backing has given them a new opportunity, in some instances, to offset the adverse criticisms which have surrounded the black press for many years, by correcting the faults so often attributed to the publications. A number of the older publications have made such efforts. But the publishers of the many new papers and magazines, often little more than neophytes, have failed to keep to the high standards. They cannot allege all the reasons which genuinely explained why the early protest press was journalistically unprofessional.

If the economic pressure to survive can be relaxed still further, the black press already possesses an agency through which editors and publishers can work if they seek to raise standards or bring about more interest in reaching existing standards. As with other press groups, it is the national organizations of those engaged in the work that can affect standards. And the black press has its National Newspaper Publishers Association. It might be preparing to launch other activities than its annual convention and its promotional plans in an effective effort to meet the kinds of unfavorable criticism being made now. It could do so through regional workshops, contests for greater technical excellence, community service and editorial courage, and the stimulation of research into the causes for the weaknesses and ways to eradicate them. But above all, it might help black journalists and publishers decide on their ever-important ideological positions in the light of developments toward the end of the twentieth century.   ●

17. THE FUTURE

IN THE LATE 1940's storms clearly were ahead for the American black press. Racial integration in education was on the move. This meant to some observers that in a few decades black newspapers and magazines would have little or no place. Newspaper circulations began dropping dramatically. Advertising space was as difficult to sell as at any time in the century, except for a few publications. Black consumer magazines were only just taking hold. Television was soon to become popular and to compete sharply with the print media.

Then, as the civil rights movement gained legal support, as there appeared a measure of popular backing for it from whites, and as the black Americans made known their desire for change in different ways, the future started to look less gloomy. A few consumer magazines became amazingly successful. Advertising dollars began to flow a little more easily. The purchasing power of some black citizens increased, as did their literacy. Race pride stirred; there was an eagerness for knowledge of the black past in Africa as well as in America. The outlook improved for the black press.

With the twentieth century only a few decades from its end, the question of survival of the black press is being raised again. Some of the same reasons for doubt or hope exist, but new conditions have been created that must be taken into account: a rebellious, and in some areas even a revolutionary, spirit has seized many black people. Government policies on both international and domestic affairs have polarized the American people regardless of race or color. Employment and income have improved for the black society at the same time that a minority of its members have opted for separatism and self-sufficiency. Television competition for the time of the audience has reached a new height. Integration of the races in education has been impeded in some quarters. New black groups have turned to an advocacy press with little dependence upon advertisers and turned away some readers of the standard black press, as reflected in lowering circulation figures (see Table 17.1).

321

TABLE 17.1 ● **Circulation Trends of Eight General Black Newspapers with 30,000 or More Circulation in 1965**

Newspaper[a]	1965	1966	1967	1968	1969	+ or —
Atlanta *Daily World*	30,400	30,400	30,300	30,100	30,100	—
Baltimore *Afro-American*[b]	36,023	33,089	33,901	35,139	33,687	—
Chicago *Daily Defender*	37,549	N S	36,541	33,320	33,320	—
Detroit *Michigan Chronicle*	54,744	49,123	47,233	47,233	45,788	—
Los Angeles *Sentinel*	38,612	34,284	39,084	41,482	38,084	—
New York *Amsterdam News*	67,662	74,213	75,664	82,123	77,708	+
Norfolk *Journal and Guide*	30,876	32,799	29,213	28,576	21,702	—
Philadelphia *Tribune*[b]	34,023	34,816	35,596	37,327	38,081	+

SOURCES: *Ayer Directory,* 1966–70; Standard Rate and Data Service Reports, 1966–70.
[a] Weekly except as noted.
[b] Semi-weekly

● A MORTAL PRESS

Always in danger of failure, the black press has survived despite great losses. No publication begun a century and a half ago has survived. Most of those of even fifty years ago are gone. Yet as an institution the press has continued, urged on by leaders who needed propaganda organs, by politicians who wanted voices, by white enemies who forced blacks to realize that their church and their press were their only outlets of expression.

At almost any point in its history it would have been reasonable to forecast the end of the press, either for economic or social reasons. In the late 1940's and early 1950's the speculators on the future of this press were in exactly opposite camps. One group, including Thomas W. Young, former president of the National Newspaper Publishers Association and business manager of the Norfolk *Journal and Guide,* thought that the black paper should see to its own disappearance by fighting against the injustices practiced against the black citizen, helping bring about democratic conditions that would make the papers unnecessary. Close to this school of thought were those who believed that racial integration would remove the need for a separate press. The author of this book, writing in 1949, observed that the press might be destined to remain a segregated one, and eventually would vanish as its readers lost their racial identity.[1]

The wrath produced by this prediction and similar ones was based more on fear of the implications to those connected with the press than on realization of the trends. Various side issues were introduced—whether the black people wanted segregation or were to blame for it, for example.

Subsequent events that no one had foreseen made the predictions of disappearance invalid in part. No one predicted that new social legislation would give blacks hope for just treatment. No one predicted a new rise to political power. Nor did anyone see that illegal wars would sharpen the contrast between an announced battle to the death for the rights of Asians to democratic freedoms and the treatment of minorities at home.

But the central idea persists: if there is racial amalgamation, a separate press may not be needed.

Simeon Booker, veteran black newsman and magazine writer, predicted in 1964 that "One of these days, the Negro press will be out of business. But it won't be for a generation or so. . . . It will continue to try to be the voice of the people inhabiting the ghettos in the cities with the poorest housing and the menial jobs. As long as the voice is strident, clear and militant, its function will be valued."[2] And in 1970 James D. Williams, a former editor of black newspapers and at the time director of the office of information and publication of the U.S. Commission on Civil Rights, wrote that "in a fully integrated society, the black press would shrink and eventually vanish, much in the manner of the foreign language press." He added, however: "Pending that . . . it is alive and well."[3] It should be noted, however, that the foreign language press has not vanished; because of the influx of Puerto Ricans and Cubans the Spanish segment has become one of the strongest, for example.

● THE MYRDAL VIEW

Gunnar Myrdal, the Swedish economist, in his landmark study of the American black society, however, interpreted the situation in the 1940's differently than did the prophets of doom. "The Negro press is bound to become even stronger as Negroes are increasingly educated and culturally assimilated but not given entrance to the white world," he wrote.[4] He was even more encouraging than that. He also said that better coverage of black activities by the white press would not substitute for the black publications. The news of blacks would continue, he believed, to have a relatively low news value to whites. An editor of a white paper, no matter how sympathetic to blacks, would reach a point where he could not satisfy the demand for black news without alienating whites. He would not have room for the news wanted by the white majority. The newspapers—and Myrdal concerned himself largely with them and not magazines—would grow as the level of education rose, the cultural differences between blacks and other Americans decreased, race consciousness and race solidarity were intensified, and the protests were stronger. Because circulations would be larger, more advertising would be obtained. The resulting income would produce material improvements—better equipment and enlarged and more capable staff. Weekly frequency would dominate, but a few dailies might succeed.

Earl Conrad was one of the few to contest Myrdal's views. He pointed out that the forecast was concerned with the press only as a business institution and that in effect Myrdal said that the press had to base its future on the continuance of segregation.[5]

A quarter of a century later some of Myrdal's predictions had been fulfilled, but some had not. The optimism still exists, but for other reasons than those he gave. Newspaper circulations grew, for a time, but then fell off badly. Advertising revenue increased, not because of larger circulations but because the white advertisers wanted a share of the black market, needed black personnel, or wished to support the moderate black press as a force against revolutionary elements. Some improvements in equipment resulted, but staff was not, on the whole, much enlarged or even professionally so much better trained, especially on the many new publications launched in the 1960's and so far in the 1970's. The papers did persist as weekly publications, a few became semi-weeklies and several were coming out four days a week.

What Myrdal and the contributors to his remarkable study did not foresee was the rise of the black consumer magazines, for mainly specialized ones were issued in those years. Only *Opportunity* and the *Crisis* were mentioned. Nor could they anticipate the establishment and growth of propaganda papers, notably *Muhammad Speaks* and the *Black Panther,* or the impact of television on newspaper advertising sales and reading and its domination of viewers' time.

● OTHER HOPEFUL PROPHETS

Myrdal was not the only optimist. Armistead S. Pride, chairman of the journalism department at Lincoln University; Louis E. Lomax, black author and journalist; and D. Parke Gibson, publicist, in subsequent years were among those who were hopeful of growth and strength. Pride, writing in 1951, wondered what the size and character of the black press would be fifty years later or at that great division year, 2000 A.D. He decided that "It seems reasonable to expect that Negro newspapers will be published for a long time to come," an opinion to be taken seriously, since it came from the still leading scholar of the history of the black newspaper. He relied for this view on "the momentum which the larger Negro papers have gained, their growing prestige and know-how, their knack of appealing to a special class as well as to an enlarging clientele of different races, and their role as special pleaders for the rights of minority groups. . . ."[6]

But Pride also said that this future depended upon their honesty in "throwing the spotlight on injustice, graft, lawlessness, discrimination, inferior educational facilities, hunger, lack of sanitary and healthful conditions. . . ." The rise of new protest papers, apparently at the expense of the standard weeklies, may indicate that enough of the black people do not believe the press is fighting their cause hard enough to support his prophecy. But there still are several decades to go.

Lomax, writing ten years later, said that at the time it was true that there was a separate group of readers with "special interests that can be appealed to and exploited." But he predicted that there would come a time when the Negro revolution will make it less true and "it is against this day that the Negro individual who is a publisher must begin now to make his plans."[7] He did not reckon, however, with the rise of separatism and the growth of pride in being black that led the black society, by the end of that decade, to be more loyal to what is its own, at least in the form of magazines and radio programs and books. But not newspapers.

He faced the idea, in a short-range forecast, of the black press becoming a general news medium. He feared that if it did it would be moving in "a market where new entries die like flies. The immediate future of the Negro press seems to be that of a community newspaper and its future to be tied to that of the Negro church and Negro social clubs."[8] The rise of small community papers, the great reliance of the large weeklies upon such church and club news to hold circulation, are evidence of the shrewdness of his forecast. In the long run, however, he was pessimistic. He noted that the other American ethnic groups at that time had their own newspapers, churches, and clubs. But the support of the institutions of these other groups was beginning to shrink, and he believed that that would happen to the black press and church, in time. "For, as housing and job barriers fall, Negroes will drift from the ghetto into general American life, where they will rise to positions of prominence and leadership in the general American community, as Americans rather than as Negroes."[9]

Gibson, with the optimism so typical of the public relations man who moves among advertising executives and marketing experts, in another decade wrote that he believed that the Negro market "will continue to exist for years to come" because of the factors that formed it, for they continue to exist. A market is available, therefore, to advertisers via either the black or white press; it is implied that a black press will be needed to service the advertisers. He saw population concentration going on, the birth rate continuing to exceed that of the whites, income on the increase. He also saw a new mood in the black community. That mood is "an increasing pride in blackness that for so long was denied. The Negro is becoming more self-conscious of being a Negro, and he is accepting this with pride," Gibson wrote.[10]

Two young black journalists, both experienced in white as well as black news work, in 1970 gave still other reasons for their view that the press will continue. L. F. Palmer, Jr., columnist and reporter for the white Chicago *Daily News*, wrote that the established black press will survive because, as Louis E. Martin, vice president of the Sengstacke Newspapers has said, so long as there is white racism there will be black papers. But Martin admitted that the black papers will have to become more relevant in point of view as well as in news presentation.[11] George M. Daniels, a former Associated Negro Press staffer and reporter for the Chicago *Defender*, later a church publicist, is optimistic about the future of the press. Speaking about it at Syracuse University, he said he believes it will remain a protest organ but politically moderate. It will continue to grow because, when measured by the number of new publications that continue rather than by the size of circulations, there is growth already evident in the early 1970's. This stability, he explained, is limited to the rise in advertising expenditures by black business, giving black publications less dependence upon white advertisers; especially, Daniels believes, is this true of the small community papers.

Other stabilizing trends he sees are the policy of diversifying their business being practiced by increasing numbers of publishing firms, the purchase of small papers by bigger ones to enlarge chain or group holdings, the raising of capital by companies going public, and the lower costs of production possible through technological developments such as offset printing.

"A black press always will be needed," Daniels said, "because the white cannot cover the black news in detail, such as marriages, births, and the activities of blacks in government." He predicted also resumption of a national black wire service and expansion of Washington coverage and foresaw more journalism education at black colleges.[12]

To all of which can be added a statistical point. The ratio of the black population to the total population, at the present rate of increase, by the year 2000 may place it at 25 per cent more than double the estimate for 1970 of 11 per cent to 12 per cent. If these new black Americans continue at least the present support of the black press it has considerable opportunity for continuation.

● INTERNAL HANDICAPS

Although the future of the black press is greatly dependent upon external developments such as acceptance or rejection by its natural audience or its success in selling advertising space to both black and white buyers, population growth, internal conditions, and attitudes are important also.

The press of the U.S.A., black and white alike, never has been known for its progressiveness, either in its social ideas or its technology. Except for a minority of newspapers and magazines, it generally has opposed social changes and defended the status quo.[13] For many years the nation's conservatives have been able to count on the consumer or general circulation newspapers and magazines for support. Democratic Party presidential candidates, from Franklin D. Roosevelt on, with the exception of Lyndon B. Johnson, have not gained the editorial backing of the bulk of the white newspaper owners, and most magazines, being highly specialized, have not raised their voices. Minority party candidates, such as Norman Thomas, Henry Wallace, and George Wallace, although at opposite poles ideologically, have had little support from the consumer press, including the black.

Such caution extends even to the physical aspects and management of the press itself, particularly the newspaper segment, for it has been slow to effect internal changes which would enable it to keep pace with the times. For that reason, and also for some lesser ones, some of the nation's most famous white dailies and periodicals disappeared in the 1950's and 1960's, including the New York *Herald Tribune,* the New York *World-Telegram,* the *Saturday Evening Post,* and *Collier's.*

The black press is no exception, although it never has been nor could it have been in a financial position to keep up with the times in techniques and methods. Thus it cannot be blamed for failing, since it could not be expected to try. But ideologically, by and large, it has played safe, earning for itself the condemnation of the black race's noted sociologists and of some of the few other scholars who have sought to evaluate it.

As the last third of the twentieth century begins, the standard American black press finds itself confronting a public split as never before in its history. Its potential black audience is, on the one hand, a large middle-class group of economically and educationally developing citizens still retaining their lower middle-class interests, chiefly entertainment from the mass media, black or white; and on the other, the small, potent group—the militant blacks who want change and want it at once and have among them leaders determined to get it by any means that will work. A third group, not part of its potential audience, is the lower economic and education population reminiscent of what virtually the nation's total black society once was and from whence the statistics about black poverty and illiteracy still are drawn.

The established black press also sees developing in the country a type of underground or advocacy press that is serving the militants and scorning the traditional publications or those who direct and edit them. The regular press is seeking to adjust, taking over some of the less disturbing causes on which there will be no weakening of the rapport with advertisers. It also is looking for ways, therefore, to keep its circulation from slipping away to the outright protest publications and yet retain journalistic respectability and a grasp upon the readers not yet won over to the militant press.

The slowness to improve their plants, forced upon them by low income and lack of capital, is being challenged by plans for new publishing projects. These come, for example, from the Black Economic Development Conference, the group which demanded a half-billion dollars from white churches in 1969. Although the program has not produced much of the money demanded, some grants have been made. One is from the Episcopal Church to underwrite a Black Star Press, one of four publishing firms in the total development plan. This project, supported by $200,000 from the denomination, was scheduled to be set up in Detroit under direction of the National Committee for Black Churchmen, according to Religious News Service and the New York *Times*. The first firm would be set up with $150,000 of the grant and issue a weekly newspaper, the *Inner City Voice*. The other firms are reported to be planned for Atlanta, Los Angeles, Chicago, Cleveland, and New York, if grants are obtained. Demands being made upon the United Methodist Church include one urging the board of publication to transfer ownership of one of its publishing facilities to the Black Economic Development group. With *Muhammad Speaks* having risen in a few years to the largest circulation of any black publication of newspaper format, other publishers cannot be indifferent to these somewhat similar ventures.

If such plans do not materialize or if they turn out, after all, to offer little competition to the existing print media, other mechanical developments may affect the black publications. These include the bringing of news from the newspaper office to the home via facsimile, cable television, or laser beam transmission, the latter using satellites. As John Tebbel points out, "the net effect would be to make newspapers directly competitive with television, and by means of dry-copying slave machines attached to the TV set, would make it possible for the viewer to have any part of the news or feature material being transmitted on a printed page instantly."[14]

The whole gamut of technological changes predicted during the 1950's and 1960's for the media eventually will affect the black press: publications projected on screens, prepared on tape or film for easy storage and repeated use, transmitted via radio and printed by facsimile receivers. Yet, as those decades went on, the country's newspapers still were being thrown on the porch or the apartment doorstep and the magazines continued to arrive by mail or crowd each other out of sight on newsstands, the technological miracles confined to using computers in typesetting and other behind-the-scenes operations, such as circulation list updating and selection of subscribers' names for special promotion schemes. Since little of such advance has as yet touched the black press it may be some time still before present-day publishers will gain the advantages or be faced with the necessity to scrap their present equipment to make way for new.

● CONTINUING AS PROTESTORS

Some observers of the black press, mainly of the newspaper, have said that to survive it must continue to fulfill its original mission as a protest press. Even so moderate a businessman at Kenneth O. Wilson, vice-president of the *Afro-American* papers, has been quoted as saying that the papers have the role of creating a climate in which business and industry can participate and that those black papers are strong that take up the great issues that affect the black consumer most, giving as examples the war on poverty, open housing, equal public accommodation, and representation at the very highest state, county, and municipal levels. The editors will keep their ears to the ground for the big story that affects Negroes one way or the other, he said.[15]

Similar advice has come from Simeon Booker. He believes that the press must be both a service and an entertainment institution at the same time. It must engage in what he calls "uplift projects, self-improvement and educational campaigns and inspirational stories to revive our discouraged populace." It also will need to continue giving attention to the lives of stars, personalities, society queens, and cultists.[16]

The likelihood of the black press becoming uniformly more outspoken in its protest function may be hampered by several circumstances. One is the climate of opinion existing at any one time in the nation. A black publication could hope to do little protesting in one of the notoriously repressive communities of the country, where even white protest journalism has hard going. Another danger, one that may seem remote at this time, is that as the black people more and more break out of their second-class citizenship and gain access to middle-class comforts and conveniences they will be captured by the hedonism so typical of the white society. The white press and broadcasting media have played a large part in firming up the philosophy of the worth of pleasure and ease for their own sakes.

Signs can be found that this tone is rising in the black press, particularly in certain of the magazines, which through their editorial and advertising matter treat as of paramount importance the achievement of status by possessions. It is made to seem significant that the black woman use the right shade of lipstick or see the merit of false eyelashes, and that she think it desirable to dress as does the reigning black queen of the television screen or Las Vegas night clubs. Such is not the atmosphere in which a fight for civil rights or social justice thrives.

Black publishers doubtless do not believe that the emphasis on luxury items like perfumes, furs, and extra television sets and record players is a contradiction in any program of crusades for social reform; when such items mean more advertising income it is difficult to denigrate them. But even if they do object, it is unlikely that they can do more than drift, as the white press has been drifting for years. All are dependent upon the economic order. Only correctives for that order, joined with a new moral concept that defies the hedonists and gives whites as well as blacks long-lasting goals, can arrest the trend.

The altruism and good will that have guided black Americans in the fight for justice may be dissipated in the pursuit of pleasure which seems to be the main occupation of many middle-class citizens of any race or color. And the black press, for the sake of its own survival, has an opportunity now to play an important part by providing leadership to its readers by its editorial emphasis.

● THE PLACE OF RACIAL HARMONY

Racial harmony is another factor in the black press' future. Some blacks have come to believe that they have a greater awareness of blackness by being among nonblacks than by being among persons of their own race. This view causes them sometimes to take positions in white institutions rather than in black. But others would reverse that—and they are the black segregationists. Two groups—those with a loyalty to the idea of blacks overriding their desire to be among whites and those who feel uncomfortable and in need of more self-confidence when not among black people—also will keep a black press alive. The press depends upon such racial harmony, limited as it may be.

But a larger harmony is possible: the harmony of the American people. And such harmony may, in the long run, benefit the black press more than the harmony of like minds about racial segregation to preserve the black heritage. If John W. Gardner, the former Health, Education and Welfare secretary, is right, the black press may someday play a larger part after an unhappy schism in American society. For in the 1960's he predicted that if no way was found to reverse the trend of that time—increasing conflict between the races—the U.S.A. would end up as two nations, "with an embittered and angry nation within a nation, with two peoples who don't know each other, don't mingle, and meet only to vent their hostility."[17]

It takes but little imagination to see the black press function as the militant press now operates: leading a nationalist movement and fighting for separatism. But it will come about only if there is one or the other kind of harmony: complete separatism or complete cooperation with other races. What is demanded of the black press is that it have the same zeal and devotion for harmony as the separatists have for their philosophy.

To sum up, it appears that in the future the black press may:

1. Survive and thrive because black Americans are proud of their race and are working for the survival of their culture. The press should benefit from that trend. But its owners must be alert, if they are to keep pace. They cannot fall behind the educational growth and cultural development of their readers nor do they dare move too much in advance of them. At the same time, they must solve the difficult problem of crusading for causes important to black people while not alienating the business interests upon which they depend. The publishers have the possibility of seeing the press grow slowly but firmly

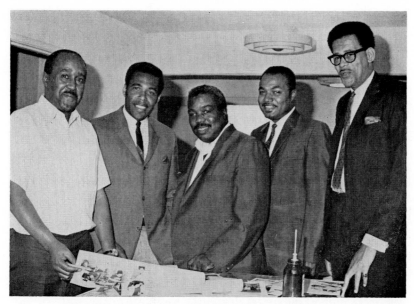

FIG. 17.1. The executive staff of **New Lady,** one of the new black publications launched with the aid of foundation grants and white business financing: Edward N. Evans, editor **(left);** J. Darnell Harvey, assistant publisher; W. Warner Beckett, publisher; David H. Wellington, general manager; and Robert O. Powell, advertising director.

in economic security, either because of the unity of separatism or the unity of cooperation between the races.

2. Fail because of the separatism desired by the growing number of black people—numerous intellectual leaders, such as teachers, authors, clergy, and students—and the possibility that it will be weak, with the result that integration of the races may resume in full strength and the press may be faced with the threat of the 1940's and 1950's once more. Unless it makes itself essential to the black people it might disappear as an unnecessary journalism.

3. Succeed because, at least for many generations still, there will be a black race, for the eventual amalgamation of the races will not occur as rapidly as integrationists desire. It will be a small press still. The success now seems to lie with the magazines, not the newspapers, for many of the latter, while increasing in number and advertising strength, are either standing still or losing in circulation, especially most of the important national and big city papers. That tends to limit their outreach and influence. The new newspapers are not all conventional business enterprises but often are advocacy papers supported by subsidy. The new magazines, on the other hand, are professional and commercial ventures for the most part, and dependent less upon an organization than on general public support—

readers and advertisers. The magazine's economic plan is a sounder and more independent one in a participatory democracy. As the white newspapers cover the black society more and more, the black magazine will supply readers with depth writing, fiction, and other materials for the ethnic group which will not, in sufficient quantity, be available through white periodicals and which cannot reasonably be expected to appear there.

Since the early 1960's the author has contended in various books and articles that the future of the magazine industry in the U.S.A. as a whole is with the specialized periodicals, not the giant consumer-aimed ones.[18] Events have borne out the prediction, for the *Saturday Evening Post* failed a few years after *Collier's* and a few other leaders, and in the early part of the present decade both *Life* and *Look* were having their economic troubles, as were some other large periodicals. That the future of the black magazine is in the hands of the special-ized periodical rather than the consumer is even more certain. The black population, even if it someday reaches the point where from the economic point of view it could support large consumer magazines, would be no more likely to do so than the general public. What is even more important, or at least less speculative, the costs of pro-duction and distribution, which are enormous portions of the large magazine's cost schedules, not only are likely to continue increasing but also will be even more difficult for the black magazine publisher to handle since, with the exception of *Ebony,* none ever has been able to command a volume of advertising comparable to that of the large white publications. The small, less costly operation aimed at a definable reader group can hope for survival. And that is the specialized magazine.

If the large black magazine survives it must win white as well as black readers to be of influence in the white world as well as the black. This effort can be motivated by both the desire for commercial success as well as the hope of bringing about greater understanding between the people of each race. It is dubious, however, that it can offset the economic hazards of mass circulation.

It is likely, therefore, that a black press of some sort always will be available in the U.S.A., unless *fully integrated* means the complete eradication of the black experience, culture, temperament, and per-sonality. Whether it will be an important and influential press de-pends upon the course of the black revolution now under way and the social changes occurring without respect to race.   ●

BIBLIOGRAPHY

■

No EXTENSIVE, readily obtainable, and annotated bibliographical guide exists as yet to assist the searcher for information about the black press of the U.S.A. Armistead S. Pride's *The Black Press: A Bibliography*, which he prepared for 1968 issuance in duplicated form by the Association for Education in Journalism, is helpful. But since Pride does not evaluate the entries the user is left to find his way in a maze of materials, mostly periodical articles or book chapters, many of which are not easily obtained, for they often are in obscure magazines, papers, and books.

The hunt becomes all the more complicated if the researcher wishes to find the work of black scholars. One cannot be sure, without additional investigation which may appear to be motivated by prejudice, which authors are or were of the black race. Furthermore, often their books were issued by small publishing firms no longer in business; a few, in fact, came from vanity firms, which not only makes them difficult to find but also casts doubts on their reliability as sources.

The literature of the black press is strongest in the area of biography. It is becoming richer as new works appear and as some of the earlier studies are reprinted. Much of the recent work, however, is about the already accepted figures, such as Douglass and Garvey. The work of Quarles, Foner, Cronon, Ottley, Broderick, Fox, and Rudwick in producing full-length biographies or analytical-biographical studies and of Bennett in publishing various magazine articles and book chapters so far has been the extent of reliable work in biography. Penn's history actually is more a melange of brief biographies than a sustained tracery of the life of the publications themselves.

By this writing Douglass and Du Bois had benefitted most from scholarly study. The outstanding biography of a black journalist is Philip S. Foner's four-volume *Life and Writings of Frederick Douglass;* it does not, of course, restrict itself to relating his journalistic activities. A convenient one-volume paperback version combining the strictly biographical sections of each volume has been brought out.

The important area of black press history, the richest about American journalism in general, is weak in the black press field. A few books and several dozen articles can lay claim to having been prepared according to high scholarly standards. Because nothing else is available, all writers on this press have had to rely on Penn's nineteenth century, adjective-laden attempt at recounting what took place and reporting on who was connected with the press. Wordy as it is, it nevertheless provides information no one else has assembled. The most reliable historical work has been done by Pride, for his dissertation, but this painstaking study concerns newspapers alone, is on microfilm only, and stops short at 1950. Another helpful book is Detweiler's, but it is limited by being half a century old and so taken up with space for quotations from the publications it discusses that various important facets of the subject are not handled.   ●

● **BOOKS AND MONOGRAPHS CONCERNED MAINLY WITH THE BLACK PRESS AND BLACK JOURNALISTS**

Broderick, Francis L. *W.E.B. Du Bois: Negro Leader in Time of Crisis.* Palo Alto, Calif.: Stanford University Press, 1959, 259pp.

Brooks, Maxwell R. *The Negro Press Re-examined.* Boston: Christopher, 1959, 125pp.

Bryan, Carter R. *Negro Journalism in America Before Emancipation. Journalism Monographs,* no. 12, September, 1969, 33pp.

Coonradt, Frederic C. *The Negro News Media and the Los Angeles Riots.* Los Angeles: School of Journalism, University of Southern California, 1965, 49pp (monograph).

Cronon, Edmund David. *Black Moses: The Story of Marcus Garvey and the Universal Negro Improvement Association.* Madison: University of Wisconsin Press, 1955, 278pp.

Dann, Martin E., ed. *The Black Press, 1827–1890.* New York: Putnam, 1971, 384pp. (anthology).

Detweiler, Frederick G. *The Negro Press in the United States.* Chicago: University of Chicago Press, 1922, 274pp.; reprinted, 1968, College Park, Md.: McGrath.

Douglass, Frederick. *My Bondage and My Freedom.* New York: Miller, Orton & Mulligan, 1885, 464pp.

Douglass, Frederick. *Narrative of the Life of Frederick Douglass.* New York: New American Library, 1968, 126pp.

Du Bois, W.E.B. *The Autobiography of W.E.B. Du Bois.* New York: International Publishers, 1968, 448pp.

Foner, Philip S. *Frederick Douglass.* New York: Citadel Press, 1963, 444pp.

Fox, Stephen R. *The Guardian of Boston: William Monroe Trotter.* New York: Atheneum Press, 1970, 307pp.

Franzen, Raymond. *Magazine Audiences in the Urban Negro Market.* New York: Our World Publishing Co., 1951, 63pp (brochure).

Garnett, Bernard E. *How Soulful is 'Soul' Radio?* Nashville, Tenn.: Race Relations Information Center, 1970, 61pp (monograph).

Gibson, D. Parke. *The $30 Billion Negro.* New York: Macmillan, 1969, 311pp.

Good News for You! The Afro-American Newspapers. Baltimore, Md.: The Afro-American Company, 1969, 64pp (brochure).

Graham, Shirley. *There Was Once a Slave . . .: The Heroic Story of Frederick Douglass*. New York: Messner, 1947, 310pp.

A Guide to Negro Media: Newspapers, Magazines, Radio and College. New York: Deutsch & Shea, Inc., 1968, 38pp.

Hill, Roy L. *Who's Who in the American Negro Press*. Dallas: Royal Publishing Co., c.1960, 80pp.

Holland, Frederick May. *Frederick Douglass: The Colored Orator*. Rev. ed. New York: Funk & Wagnalls, 1895, 430pp.

La Brie, Henry G. III, ed. *The Black Press in America: A Guide*. Iowa City: University of Iowa, 1970, 64pp.

Mathews, Basil. *Booker T. Washington: Educator and Interracial Interpreter*. Cambridge, Mass.: Harvard University Press, 1948, 350pp.

The Negro Market. New York: Department of Media Relations and Planning, Young & Rubicam, Inc., 1969, 164pp.

Oak, Vishnu V. *The Negro Newspaper*. Yellow Springs, Ohio: Author, 1948, 170pp.

Ottley, Roi. *The Lonely Warrior: The Life and Times of Robert S. Abbott*. Chicago: Regnery, 1955, 381pp.

Parks, Gordon. *A Choice of Weapons*. New York: Harper & Row, 1966, 274pp.

Penn, I. Garland. *The Afro-American Press and Its Editors*. Springfield, Mass.: Willey, 1891, 569pp.

Pride, Armistead S. *The Black Press: A Bibliography*. Madison, Wis.: Association for Education in Journalism, 1968, 37pp.

Quarles, Benjamin. *Frederick Douglass*. Washington, D.C.: Associated Publishers, 1948, 378pp.

Quarles, Benjamin, ed. *Frederick Douglass*. Englewood Cliffs, N.J.: Prentice-Hall, 1968, 184pp.

Rudwick, Elliott M. *W.E.B. Du Bois: Propagandist of the Negro Protest*. New York: Atheneum, 1968, 390pp.

Sawyer, Frank B., ed. *1966 Directory of U.S. Negro Newspapers, Magazines & Periodicals*. New York: U.S. Negro World, 1967, unpaged.

Sawyer, Frank B., ed. *1967 Directory of U.S. Negro Newspapers, Magazines & Periodicals in 42 States; The Negro Press—Past, Present and Future*. New York: U.S. Negro World, 1968, 40pp.

Sawyer, Frank B., ed. *Amalgamated Publishers Rate & Data List of 70 Black Newspapers in 28 States; Malcolm X Reference Section*. New York: U.S. Negro World, 1969, 87pp.

Schuyler, George S. *Black and Conservative*. New Rochelle, N.Y.: Arlington House, 1966, 362pp.

This is Our War: Selected Stories of Six Afro-American War Correspondents. Baltimore, Md.: Afro-American Publishing Company, 1945, 216pp.

● BOOKS AND MONOGRAPHS PARTLY CONCERNED WITH THE BLACK PRESS

Ainslie, Rosalynde. *The Press in Africa*. London: Gollancz, 1966, 256pp.

Baldwin, James. *Notes of a Native Son*. New York: Bantam Books, 1968, 149pp., pp. 49–53.

Bennett, Lerone, Jr. *Pioneers in Protest*. Baltimore, Md.: Penguin Books, 1969, 263pp., chaps. 5, 14–17.

Bontemps, Arna, and Conroy, Jack. *They Seek a City*. Garden City, N.Y.: Doubleday, Doran, 1945, 266pp.

Booker, Simeon. *Black Man's America*. Englewood Cliffs, N.J.: Prentice-Hall, 1964, 230pp., chap. 10.

Bray, Leonard, ed. *Directory of Newspapers and Periodicals.* Philadelphia:
  N. W. Ayer & Son, Inc., 1965–70 vols.
Clarke, John Henrik, ed. *Harlem, U.S.A.* Berlin, Germany: Seven Seas,
  1967, 361pp.
Conrad, Earl. *Jim Crow America.* New York: Duell, Sloan & Pearce, 1947,
  237pp., chap. 7.
Daly, Charles U., ed. *The Media and the Cities.* Chicago: University of
  Chicago Center for Policy Study, 1968, 90pp.
Drake, St. Clair, and Cayton, Horace R. *Black Metropolis.* New York: Har-
  court, Brace, 1945, 809pp., chap. 15.
Drotning, Phillip T. and Smith, Wesley W. *Up from the Ghetto.* New York:
  Cowles, 1970, 207pp.
Editors of *Ebony. The Negro Handbook.* Chicago: Johnson Publishing Co.,
  1966, 535pp., pp. 377–86.
Fisher, Paul L., and Lowenstein, Ralph L., eds. *Race and the News Media.*
  New York: Praeger, 1967, 158pp., pp. 123–40.
Frazier, E. Franklin. *Black Bourgeoisie.* Glencoe, Ill.: The Free Press, 1957,
  264pp.
Garnett, Bernard E. *Invaders From the Black Nation: The "Black Muslims"
  in 1970.* Nashville, Tenn.: Race Relations Information Center, 1970,
  32pp.
Garry, Leon, ed. *The Standard Periodical Directory.* New York: Oxbridge,
  1965, 1967, 1968, 1970.
Greenberg, Bradley S., and Dervin, Brenda. *Communications Among the
  Urban Poor.* Michigan State Reports, no. 1. Lansing: Michigan State
  University, 1967, 86pp.
Hughes, Langston. *Fight for Freedom: The Story of the NAACP.* New
  York: Norton, 1962, 224pp., pp. 40, 43, 46–48, 77, 95, 154, 203.
Johnson, James Weldon. *Along This Way.* New York: Viking, 1933, 418pp.
Kellogg, Charles Flint. *NAACP,* vol. 1. Baltimore: Johns Hopkins Press,
  1967, 332pp., chaps. 3,5,7.
Kinzer, Robert H., and Sagarin, Edward. *The Negro in American Business.*
  New York: Greenberg, 1950, 220pp.
Lincoln, C. Eric. *The Black Muslims in America.* Boston: Beacon Press,
  1961, 276pp.
Lomax, Louis E. *The Negro Revolt.* New York: Harper & Row, 1962,
  271pp.
Lyle, Jack. *The News in Megalopolis.* San Francisco: Chandler, 1967,
  208pp.
Malcolm X. *The Autobiography of Malcolm X.* New York: Grove Press,
  1968, 460pp., chap. 14.
Meier, August. *Negro Thought in America, 1880–1915.* Ann Arbor: Univer-
  sity of Michigan Press, 1963, 336pp.
Mott, Frank Luther. *American Journalism,* 3rd ed. New York: Macmillan,
  1962, 901pp., pp. 794–95, 821.
———. *A History of American Magazines.* Cambridge: Harvard University
  Press, 1957, 1958; vol. 2, p. 68; vol. 3, pp. 71, 63, 75, 283; vol. 4, p. 214.
Muse, Benjamin. *The American Negro Revolution: From Nonviolence to
  Black Power, 1963–1967.* Bloomington: Indiana University Press, 1968,
  345pp.
Myrdal, Gunnar. *An American Dilemma.* New York: Harper & Bros., 1944,
  1,483pp.
Ottley, Roi. *New World A'Coming.* New York: Literary Classics, 1943,
  364pp.
Porter, Dorothy B., comp. *The Negro in the United States: A Working
  Bibliography.* Ann Arbor, Mich.: Xerox, University Microfilms, 1969,
  202pp.

Pride, Armistead S. "Robert S. Abbott." In *Dictionary of American Biography*, supplement 2, edited by Edward T. James. New York: Scribner's, 1958, pp. 2–4.
Report of the Governor's Committee on Employment of Minority Groups in the News Media. Albany: State of New York, 1969, 38pp.
Report of the National Advisory Commission on Civil Disorders. New York: Bantam Books, 1968, 659pp.
Rohinsky, Merle, man. ed. *Ulrich's International Periodicals Directory*, 1969–70, vols. 1, 2. New York: Bowker, 1969.
Romm, Ethel Grodzins. *The Open Conspiracy.* Harrisburg, Pa.: Stackpole, 1970, 256pp.
Schoener, Allon, ed. *Harlem on My Mind: Cultural Capital of Black America, 1900–1968.* New York: Random House, 1968, 255pp.
Stone, Chuck. *Black Political Power in America.* Indianapolis: Bobbs-Merrill, 1968, 261pp.
Taft, William H. *American Journalism History.* Columbia, Mo.: Lucas Brothers, 1968, 94pp.
Villard, Oswald Garrison. *The Disappearing Daily.* New York: Knopf, 1944, 295pp.
Welsch, Erwin K., *The Negro in the United States.* Bloomington: Indiana University Press, 1968, 142pp.
West, Earle H., comp. *A Bibliography of Doctoral Research on the Negro, 1933–1966.* Ann Arbor, Mich.: Xerox, University Microfilms, 1969, 134pp.
White, Walter. *A Man Called White.* New York: Arno Press and the New York *Times*, 1969, 382pp.

● ARTICLES AND PAMPHLETS

Aldridge, Dan. "Black Press—Where Are You?" *Michigan Chronicle*, March 29, 1969.
Alexander, Charles T. "Is *Anything* Being Done To Interest Blacks in Journalism?" *Bulletin*, no. 535, American Society of Newspaper Editors, November, 1969, pp. 16–18.
Allen, John E. "More Media Planning at Client Level Is Needed for Negro Radio." *Media/scope* 10, no. 12 (December 1966): 162.
Anderson, S. E. "Review of Neo-African Literature" by Janheinz, Jahn, in *Black Scholar* 1, no. 3–4 (January-February 1970): 76,79.
Aronson, James. "The Inspiration of the Freedom Movement." *National Guardian*, Sept. 5, 1963, p. 3 (W. E. B. Du Bois).
"Baldwin Leaves Negro Monthly." New York *Times*, Feb. 28, 1967, p. 34.
Balk, Alfred. "Mr. Johnson Finds His Market." *Reporter* 21, no. 8 (Nov. 12, 1959): 34–35.
Bayton, James A., and Bell, Ernestine. "An Exploratory Study of the Role of the Negro Press." *Journal of Negro Education* 20 (Winter 1951): 8–15.
Beard, Richard L., and Zoerner, Cyril E. II. "Associated Negro Press: Its Founding, Ascendancy, and Demise." *Journalism Quarterly* 46, no. 1 (Spring 1969): 47–52.
Bennett, Lerone, Jr. "Founders of the Negro Press." *Ebony* 19, no. 9 (July 1964): 96–98, 100, 102.
———. "Frederick Douglass: Father of the Protest Movement." *Ebony* 18, no. 9 (September 1963): 50–51, 56.
Berkman, Dave. "Advertising in *Ebony* and *Life*: Negro Aspirations vs. Reality." *Journalism Quarterly* 40, no. 1 (Winter 1963): 53–64.
"The Birth, Death, and Resurrection of TLV." *Liberated Voice*, Dec. 11, 1968, pp. 1, 8–9.

"Black Is Beautiful But Maybe Not Profitable." *Media/scope* 13, no. 8 (August 1969): 31–37, 39, 65, 91, 95–96, 100.

"The Black Market." *Chain Store Age* 46, no. 5 (May 1970): 100–138.

"Black Press Does Its Own Thing, Spurs Readers' Heavy Buying." *Advertising Age* 41, no. 16 (April 20, 1970): 192–93.

Blank, Dennis M. "Integrated Comic Strives for Success." *Editor & Publisher* 100, no. 46 (November 1967): 13.

Booker, Simeon. "A Negro Reporter at the Till Trial." *Nieman Reports* 10, no. 1 (January 1956): 13–15.

———. "The New Frontier for Daily Newspapers." *Nieman Reports* 9, no. 1 (January 1955): 12–13.

Boyd, Dale E. "Black Radio: A Direct and Personal Invitation." *Media/scope* 13, no. 8 (August 1969): 14–15.

Braithwaite, William Stanley. "Negro America's First Magazine." *Negro Digest* 17, no. 2 (December 1947): 21–26.

Brown, Robert U. "Shop Talk at Thirty: The Negro Press." *Saturday Review of Literature* 25, no. 46 (November 1942): 5–6.

"Citations of Merit for Outstanding Performance in Journalism." Jefferson City, Mo.: Department of Journalism, Lincoln University, 1969, unpaged.

"Cartoonist and College Journalism Dean Will Speak at Press Institute." *Cleveland Press,* Oct. 9, 1969.

Cartwright, Marguerite. "The Big Wheel of the National Negro Network." Pittsburgh *Courier,* Aug. 16, 1954, pp. 13, 16.

———. "Magazines in Sepia." *Negro History Bulletin* 17, no. 4 (January 1954): 74, 94.

"Color Success Black." *Time* 92, no. 5 (August 1968): 32.

"Courting the Black Billionaire." *Media/scope* 11, no. 11 (November 1967): 41–42, 66, 69–70, 82.

Dabney, Virginius. "Nearer and Nearer the Precipice." *Atlantic Monthly* 171, no. 1 (January 1943): 94–100.

Dallos, Robert E. "Black Radio Stations Send Soul and Service to Millions." New York *Times,* Nov. 11, 1968, p. 64.

Draper, Theodore. "The Father of American Black Nationalism." *New York Review of Books* 14, no. 5 (March 1970): 33–41. (Martin R. Delaney).

Dunningan, Alice E. "Early History of Negro Women in Journalism." *Negro History Bulletin* 28 (May 1965): 178–79, 193, 197.

Eaton, Iris. "An Empire Built on a 'Magic Month.'" *News Workshop,* New York University, May, 1954, pp. 5–6.

Evans, W. Leonard Jr. "After 3 Years from Hope to Solution." *Tuesday* 4, no. 1 (September 1968): 5.

"Few Negroes Are Enrolled in J-Schools." *Editor & Publisher* 102, no. 18 (April 1969): 35.

Forkan, James P. "Black Ownership of Radio Grows—Slowly." *Advertising Age* 41, no. 6 (February 1970): 62–63.

"4.7% of Newspaper Workers Are Negro." *Guild Reporter* 25, no. 24 (Dec. 27, 1968).

Gerald, Carolyn. "The Measure and Meaning of the Sixties." *Negro Digest* 19, no. 1 (November 1969): 24–29.

"Good-by, Hambone." *Newsweek* 72, no. 4 (July 1968): 36.

Goodman, Walter. "Ebony: Biggest Negro Magazine." *Dissent* 15, no. 5 (September-October 1968): 403–9.

Greenlee, Rush, and Allen, Robert L. "The Black Press—An Interview With Hoyt Fuller." *Ball and Chain Review* 1, no. 2 (November 1969): 3.

Gross, Bella. "Freedom's Journal and the Rights of All." *Journal of Negro History* 17, no. 3 (July 1932): 241–86.

"Help Wanted: More Black Newsmen." Associated Press Managing Editor's Black News Committee, undated (c. 1969), 35pp.

Howard, Bernard. "Empathy: The Vital Plus of Negro Radio." *Sponsor,* Aug. 26, 1963, p. 61.

Hurley, Kay. "Gordon Parks: Shaper of Dreams." *This Week,* Oct. 19, 1969, pp. 10, 15.

Johnson, Charles S. "The Rise of the Negro Magazine." *Journal of Negro History* 13, no. 1 (January 1928): 7–21.

Kaiser, Ernest. "Five Years of *Freedomways*." *Freedomways* 6, no. 2 (Spring 1966): 103–17.

Kendall, Elaine. "The Negro Press." *Holiday* 41, no. 5 (May 1967): 82–84.

Klein, Woody. "News Media and Race Relations: A Self-Portrait." *Columbia Journalism Review* 7, no. 3 (Fall 1968): 42–49.

Kleinfeld, Ann, comp. and ed. *Negro Press Digest,* Feb. 7, 1966–March, 1968.

——. and Stevenson, Mrs. Louise, comps. and eds. *Negro Press Digest,* April 28, 1964–Dec. 31, 1965.

Koontz, E. C. "Pittsburgh Courier Leads Fight for American Negro Equality." *Quill* 54, no. 10 (October 1966): 44.

League, Raymond A. "Be Subjective in Evaluating Negro Media." *Media/scope* 13, no. 8 (August 1969): 18–19.

Lewis, David L., and Miao, Judy. "America's Greatest Negroes: A Survey." *Crisis* 77, no. 1 (January 1970): 17–21.

Mencher, Melvin. "Recruiting and Training Black Newsmen." *Quill* 57, no. 9 (September 1969): 22–25.

"Methodist Agencies Help Blacks Get Radio Stations." Baltimore *Afro-American,* March 28, 1970, p. 16.

Miles, Frank W. "Negro Magazines Come of Age." *Magazine World,* Part I, June 1, 1946, pp. 12–13, 18, 21; Part II, July 1, 1946, pp. 12–13, 18–20.

Moore, Trevor Wyatt. "Cool Cat With a Warm Message." *Ave Maria* 109, no. 11 (March 15, 1969): 17–20.

Morrison, Allan. "The Crusading Press." *Ebony* 18, no. 9 (September 1963): 204, 206–8, 210.

Moss, Elizabeth Murphy. "Black Newspapers Cover News Other Media Ignore." *Journalism Educator* 24, no. 3 (1969): 6–11.

"The Negro Market—Two Viewpoints." *Media/scope* 11, no. 11 (November 1967): 70–72, 74, 76, 78.

"Negroes Insist on Recognition by Advertisers and Newspapers." *Publishers' Auxiliary* 98, no. 34 (Sept. 28, 1963).

"Newspapers—Playing It Cool." *Time* 90, no. 4 (July 1967): 66.

Ottley, Roi. "The Negro Press Today." *Common Ground,* Spring, 1943, pp. 11–18.

"Our Black Guardians." *Afro-American* Magazine Section, Feb. 21, 1970, p. 1.

Palmer, L. F., Jr. "The Black Press in Transition." *Columbia Journalism Review* 9, no. 1 (Spring 1970): 31–36.

"The Pittsburgh *Courier*." *Tide,* Aug. 25, 1950, p. 68.

Poston, Ted. "The Negro Press." *Reporter* 1, no. 7 (December 1949): 14–16.

Powell, Adam Clayton. "Need for Militant Voice Led Powell into Journalism." *Lincoln Journalism Clipsheet,* February, 1945, p. 1.

Prattis, P. L. "Racial Segregation and Negro Journalism." *Phylon* 8, no. 4 (1947): 305–14.

"The Press." *Frontier,* June, 1955, pp. 14–15.

Pride, Armistead S. "America's Negro Newspapers." *Grassroots Editor* 2, no. 3 (July 1961): 9–10.

——. "The Negro Newspaper in the United States." *Gazette* 2, no. 3 (1956): 141–49.

Pride, Armistead S. "Negro Newspapers: Yesterday, Today and Tomorrow."
    Journalism Quarterly 28, no. 2 (Spring 1951): 179–88.
———. "Opening Doors for Minorities." *Quill* 56, no. 11 (November 1968):
    24–27.
Raymont, Henry. "Black Writers Win Literature Awards." New York *Times,*
    March 27, 1970, p. 22.
Reichley, A. James. "How John Johnson Made It." *Fortune* 77, no. 1 (January 1968): 152–53, 178, 180.
Ross, Irwin. "Roy Wilkins—'Mr. Civil Rights.'" *Reader's Digest* 92, no. 549
    (January 1968): 86–91.
Sale, J. Kirk. "The Amsterdam News." New York *Times Magazine,* Feb. 9,
    1969, pp. 30–31.
Sampson, Larry. "Chris Powell—'Drummer' for Revolution Edits Newspaper for Blacks." Syracuse University *Daily Orange,* Nov. 14, 1968, pp.
    1, 7.
Sancton, Thomas. "The Negro Press." *New Republic* 108, no. 17 (April
    1943): 557–60.
Schemmel, William. "Press—Black Voices Filling a Void." *Atlanta* 10, no. 1
    (May 1970): 48, 50, 52, 54.
Senna, Carl. "The Man Who Published 'The Guardian.'" Boston *Sunday
    Globe,* Dec. 1, 1968, pp. 58, 60–61.
Stevens, John D. "Conflict-Cooperation Content in 14 Black Newspapers."
    Journalism Quarterly 47, no. 3 (Autumn): 556–68.
"A Survey of the Mass Communications Areas in 66 Predominantly Black
    Four Year Accredited Colleges and Universities." New York: United
    Negro College Fund, Inc., 1969, 16pp (duplicated).
"Text of the Moynihan Memorandum on the Status of Negroes." New York
    Times, March 1, 1970, p. 69.
Tomkinson, Craig. "The Weekly Editor—New Orleans Weekly." *Editor &
    Publisher* 103, no. 23 (June 6, 1970): 68.
Townsley, Luther A. "ANP Provides International Coverage for 78 Member
    Papers in America." *Lincoln Journalism Clipsheet,* February, 1945, p. 1.
"Training of Blacks a Step Beyond Tokenism." *Media/scope* 13, no. 8
    (August 1969): 77–79.
Trayes, Edward J. "Black Newsmen." *Quill* 59, no. 9 (September 1970): 16–
    18.
———. "Still Few Blacks on Dailies but 50% More in J-Schools, Recent Surveys Indicate." *Journalism Quarterly* 47, no. 2 (Summer 1970): 356–60.
Twitty, John C. "150 Negro Papers and Their Fight for Civil Rights." *News
    Workshop,* New York University, Nov. 20, 1950, pp. 7–8.
"The Value of Grassroots Journalism." *College Management* 4, no. 6 (June
    1969): 40–42.
Van Breems, Arlene. "New Magazine Tries To Fill Void for the Black
    Woman." Los Angeles *Times,* Aug. 18, 1969, part iv, p. 8.
Walker, William O. "Anniversary of the Negro Press." Atlanta *Daily World,*
    March 12, 1970, p. 4.
Ward, Carl. "The Need for Black Journalists." *Tuesday* 4, no. 1 (September
    1968): 10, 22.
Waters, Enoc P. "The Negro Press: A Call for Change." *Editor & Publisher*
    95, no. 19 (May 1962): 67–68.
White, Jack E. "Color and the Comics." *Columbia Journalism Review* 8, no.
    4 (Winter 1969–70): 58–60.
Williams, James D. "Is the Black Press Needed?" *Civil Rights Digest* 3, no. 1
    (Winter 1970): 8–15.
Williamson, Lenora. "Specialists Cover Minority Communities for News
    Media." *Editor & Publisher* 106, no. 10 (May 1970): 13.

Winfrey, Carey. "Volume I, Number 1—Birth of a New Black Magazine."
    New York 3, no. 17 (April 1970): 58–60.
Witcover, Jules. "Washington's White Press Corps." *Columbia Journalism
    Review* 8, no. 4 (Winter 1969–70): 42–48.
Wolseley, Roland E. "The Vanishing Negro Press." *Negro Digest* 9, no. 2
    (December 1950): 64–68.
Young, A. S. (Doc). "The Black Sportswriter." *Ebony* 25, no. 12 (October
    1970): 56–58, 60–62, 64.

● UNPUBLISHED WORKS

Bontrager, Robert Devon. "An Investigation of Black Press and White Press
    Use Patterns in the Black Inner City of Syracuse, New York." Ph.D. dis-
    sertation, Syracuse University, 1969, 317pp.
Booker, James. "History of the New York Amsterdam News." New York
    Amsterdam News, 1967, 4pp.
Burd, Gene. "Magazines and the Minority Messages of Poets and Blacks."
    Text of address at Magazine Division meeting, Association for Education
    in Journalism, Aug. 27, 1969, 26pp.
Fleming, G. James. "The Negro Press." Manuscript prepared for Myrdal
    study, *An American Dilemma,* New York, 1942, New York Public
    Library, Microfilm Section.
Goodlett, Carlton B. Text of untitled address, Association of Afro-American
    Television Producers, Racine, Wis., Feb. 27, 1970, 13pp.
Grayson, William P. "Some of Your Best Customers Are Negro." Text of
    address, Second District Convention, American Advertising Federation,
    Nov. 8–10, 1968, Pocono Manor, Pa.
Jacobs, Louis. "White Awareness of the Black Press." Research paper, School
    of Journalism, Syracuse University, May, 1970.
Johnson, John H. "Understanding: The Key To Effective Communication."
    Text of address, International Magazine Conference, May 25–28, 1969,
    Williamsburg, Va., 6pp.
O'Connell, Sharyn. "Why Not the Black Press?" Research report, School of
    Journalism, Syracuse University, January, 1969, 13pp.
Pride, Armistead S. "A Register and History of Negro Newspapers in the
    United States: 1827–1950." Ph.D. dissertation, Northwestern University,
    1950, 426pp (microfilm).
Report of the Ad Hoc Coordinating Committee on Minority Group Educa-
    tion. Lionel C. Barrow, Jr., chairman, and William R. Stroud, secretary,
    Association for Education in Journalism, February, 1969, 12pp.
Report of the Ad Hoc Coordinating Committee on Minority Education.
    Lionel C. Barrow, Jr., chairman, and William R. Stroud, secretary, Asso-
    ciation for Education in Journalism, August, 1969, 13pp.
Stephenson, William David II. "Magazines and Black Americans: An Evolv-
    ing Relationship." Master's thesis, Syracuse University, 1969, 209pp.

NOTES

■

● 1 ● IS THERE A BLACK PRESS?

1. Felice, Kent de, "The Black Press Defined," School of Journalism, Syracuse University, January, 1969.
2. "Negro Paper Gives Backing to Wallace," *Press* State Service account in Cleveland *Press*, Nov. 17, 1968; "Whites Own Negro Paper for Wallace," Associated Press dispatch in Cleveland *Plain Dealer*, Nov. 22, 1968.
3. "Neutral Term," *Editor & Publisher* 101, no. 11 (March 1968): 7.
4. "Black Militants Flay D. C. Press Policies," *Guild Reporter*, June 20, 1969, p. 2.
5. Brooks, Maxwell R., *The Negro Press Re-examined*, pp. 13–14.
6. Moon, Henry Lee, "Beyond Objectivity: The 'Fighting Press,' " in Fisher, Paul L., and Lowenstein, Ralph R., eds., *Race and the News Media*, p. 139.
7. Miss Susan Rittenhouse, at Syracuse University.

● 2 ● THE BEGINNINGS

1. Conrad, Earl, *Jim Crow America*, p. 6.
2. Ainslie, Rosalynde, *The Press in Africa*, pp. 21–22.
3. Penn, I. Garland, *The Afro-American Press and Its Editors*, p. 28; see also Gross, Bella, "Freedom's Journal and the Rights of All."
4. Penn, p. 30.
5. Pride, Armistead S., "A Register and History of Negro Newspapers in the United States: 1827–1950," p. 4.
6. Bryan, Carter, "Negro Journalism in America Before the Emancipation," *Journalism Monographs*, no. 12 (September 1969): 30.
7. Ibid., p. 1.
8. Penn, p. 62.
9. Ibid., p. 67.
10. Draper, Theodore, "The Father of American Black Nationalism," p. 33.
11. Douglass, Frederick, *Narrative of the Life of Frederick Douglass*, pp. 21–22.
12. For discussion of the differences see Quarles, Benjamin, *Frederick Douglass*, pp. 70–79.
13. Foner, Philip S., *Frederick Douglass*, pp. 278–79, 311–12.
14. Douglass, Frederick, *My Bondage and My Freedom*, pp. 389–90.
15. Johnson, Charles S., "Rise of the Negro Magazine," p. 10.
16. Detweiler, Frederick G., *The Negro Press in the United States*, pp. 42–43.
17. Penn, pp. 78–79.
18. Detweiler, p. 44.
19. Pride, p. 97.
20. See Chapter 5 for discussion of black daily papers.
21. Pride, p. 71.
22. Penn, p. 114.
23. Pride, Armistead S., "Negro Newspapers: Yesterday, Today, and Tomorrow," pp. 180–81.

24. Conrad, Earl, "The Negro Press," p. 6.
25. Penn, p. 367.
26. Bontemps, Arna, and Conroy, Jack, *They Seek a City*, pp. 77–79.

● 3 ● BLACK JOURNALISM ENTERS THE 20TH CENTURY

1. The original Baltimore edition was founded in 1892. Other editions: Washington, 1933; Philadelphia, 1934; Richmond, 1939; New Jersey, 1940.
2. "Good News for You!" pp. 5–7.
3. Kellogg, Charles Flint, *NAACP*, p. 70.
4. Detweiler, Frederick G., *The Negro Press in the United States*, pp. 55–56; Penn, I. Garland, *The Afro-American Press and Its Editors*, pp. 133–38.
5. Detweiler, p. 56.
6. Lyle, Jack, *The News in Megalopolis*, p. 167.
7. Penn, pp. 133–38; *Lincoln Journalism Newsletter*, June 15, 1946, p. 7.
8. Detweiler, p. 55; the passage appeared originally in the Autumn, 1920, issue of *Favorite* magazine.
9. Du Bois, W. E. B., *The Autobiography of W. E. B. Du Bois*, p. 238.
10. Bennett, Lerone, Jr., *Pioneers in Protest*, p. 221.
11. Bennett has brought together the basic facts; Du Bois gives various personal glimpses; a useful supplement is Senna, Carl, "The Man Who Published 'The Guardian.'"
12. Ottley, Roi, *The Lonely Warrior*, p. 2; the major events in Abbott's life are summarized here; all other sources are brief passages in books or short articles.
13. Frazier, E. Franklin, *Black Bourgeoisie*, p. 149.
14. Du Bois. Material for this section was drawn not only from this autobiography but also from Broderick, Francis L., *W. E. B. Du Bois: Negro Leader in Time of Crisis;* Rudwick, Elliott M., *W. E. B. Du Bois: Propagandist of the Negro Protest;* and the chapter on Du Bois in Bennett.
15. Bennett, p. 249.
16. Detweiler, pp. 165–66.
17. Ibid., p. 171.
18. Ibid., p. 170.
19. Ottley, p. 291.
20. Miles, Frank W., "Negro Magazines Come of Age," pp. 12–13.
21. Rudwick, p. 88.
22. Ottley, p. 125.
23. Du Bois, p. 241.
24. Bennett, p. 237.
25. Cronon, *Black Moses*, p. 46.
26. Schoener, Allon, ed., *Harlem on My Mind*, p. 54.
27. "Publisher of Nation's First Negro Daily Is Dead," Buffalo *Evening News*, June 22, 1961.
28. Booker, James, "History of the New York *Amsterdam News*" (New York: *Amsterdam News*, 1967): 1–4.
29. Pride, Armistead S., "A Register and History of Negro Newspapers in the United States: 1827–1950," p. 161.
30. Ibid., pp. 138–39.
31. Detweiler, p. 68.
32. Ibid., p. 154.
33. Ibid., p. 155.
34. Ibid., p. 156.
35. Walker, William O., "Anniversary of the Negro Press," p. 4.
36. Conrad, Earl, "The Negro Press," p. 8.

● 4 ● WORLD WAR II AND AFTER

1. As quoted from a 1942 syndicated column in Brooks, Maxwell R., *The Negro Press Re-examined*, p. 24.
2. "Publishers: Owners of Negro Newspapers Are Hard-Headed, Farsighted, Race Conscious Businessmen," *Ebony*, November, 1949, pp. 47–51.

3. Ottley, Roi, *The Lonely Warrior*, p. 363.
4. "Clipsheet," Lincoln University School of Journalism, February, 1945, p. 1.
5. Stone, Chuck, *Black Political Power in America*, p. 189.
6. *Lincoln Journalism Newsletter*, February, 1945, p. 11.
7. New York *Times*, Dec. 19, 1947.
8. Baldwin, James, *Notes of a Native Son*, p. 50.
9. Parks, Gordon, *A Choice of Weapons*, p. 192.
10. As related to the author by Johnson in 1969.
11. Reichley, A. James, "How Johnson Made It," p. 152.
12. Ibid., p. 178.
13. Ibid.
14. Goodman, Walter, *"Ebony:* Biggest Negro Magazine," p. 404.
15. Institutional advertisement printed in various white newspapers and magazines at different times in the early 1960's.
16. Pride, Armistead S., "A Register and History of Negro Newspapers in the United States: 1827–1950," p. 3. Pride found 2,700 "racial news organs" in his search; an additional 300 for the two decades since 1950 is a conservative estimate.

● 5 ● TODAY'S NATIONAL NEWSPAPERS

1. A group consists of directly linked papers, each responsible to the same headquarters office; a chain is a series of more or less independent papers under a common ownership.
2. Bontrager, Robert D., "An Investigation of Black Press and White Press Use Patterns in the Black Inner City of Syracuse, N. Y.," p. 93.
3. Pride, Armistead S., "A Register and History of Negro Newspapers in the United States: 1827–1950," p. 24.
4. Lomax, Louis E., *The Negro Revolt*, p. 202.
5. Officially a six-day daily, in 1969 and 1970, because of a strike by employes, its frequency varied from three to four issues a week; it went on a 4-day schedule thereafter.
6. Sale, J. Kirk, "The *Amsterdam News* . . .," p. 40.
7. Baldwin, James, *Notes of a Native Son*, p. 50.
8. "What We Want/What We Believe," *Black Panther*, March 21, 1970, p. 23.
9. Ibid.
10. "What the Muslims Want/What the Muslims Believe," *Muhammad Speaks*, April 17, 1970, p. 32.
11. "The Black Mood," *Time* 95, no. 14 (April 1970): 29.
12. Malcolm X, *The Autobiography of Malcolm X*, pp. 237–38.
13. Lincoln, C. Eric, *The Black Muslims in America*, p. 133.
14. Kashif, Lonnie, "Nazi-Science Delves Into the Genes of the Black Man," *Muhammad Speaks*, Feb. 20, 1970, p. 3.
15. Palmer, L. F., Jr., "The Black Press in Transition," p. 36. In a letter to the author June 16, 1970, John Woodford, editor of *Muhammad Speaks*, writes: "Regarding our current circulation, the accurate figure nationwide is 600,000, and a recently expanded home delivery service is expected to increase that number." Bernard Garnett, in a 1970 report on the Muslims, says "close to 650,000 copies are produced weekly."
16. *Black Panther*, March 21, 1970, p. 5.
17. Ibid., Feb. 21, 1970, p. 28.
18. Letter to *Peace and Freedom* 30, no. 3 (February 1970): 2.
19. Ibid. 30, no. 4 (March 1970): 2.
20. Palmer, p. 32.
21. Ibid.
22. Pride, Armistead S., "The Negro Newspaper in the United States," p. 143.
23. Morrison, Allan, "The Crusading Press," p. 206.
24. Brown, Robert U., "Shop Talk at Thirty: The Negro Press," p. 54.

● 6 ● LOCAL NEWSPAPER VOICES

1. *Lincoln Journalism Newsletter*, September, 1955, pp. 1–2.
2. "Fresno State Hears Black Publisher," *Quill* 58, no. 5 (May 1970): 35.

3. "Text of the Moynihan Memorandum on the Status of Negroes," p. 69.
4. "Negroes' Gains Termed Uneven," New York *Times,* March 22, 1970, p. 55.
5. Moynihan Memorandum.
6. Gibson, D. Parke, *The $30 Billion Negro,* pp. 31–46.
7. "Publisher Is Slain in Jackson, Mich.," New York *Times,* Dec. 5, 1969
8. *New Pittsburgh Courier,* Dec. 20, 1969, p. 3.
9. Stephens, Gene, "Bogus Editorials Hit Negro Paper," Atlanta *Constitution,* Sept. 7, 1968, pp. 1, 8.
10. "Negro Paper Firebombed," Associated Press, April 30, 1969.
11. "The Jackson *Advocate* Story," Jackson *Advocate,* March 22, 1968, p. 8.
12. Cited by Sharyn Smith in a study of this and other black community papers made in 1968–69 at Syracuse University.
13. "The Value of Grassroots Journalism," pp. 40–42.
14. Sampson, Larry, "Chris Powell—'Drummer' for Revolution Edits Newspapers for Blacks," p. 1.
15. For much of the material about this newspaper the author is indebted to Linda Chiavaroli Rosenbloom of Rochester, who collected it while a graduate student at Syracuse University.
16. Letter to the Editor, Ft. Worth *Bronze Texan News,* Sept. 13, 1968.
17. Lyle, Jack, *The News in Megalopolis,* pp. 163–82.
18. Ibid., p. 163.
19. Ibid., p. 176.
20. Coonradt, Frederic C., *The Negro News Media and the Los Angeles Riots,* p. 47.
21. "Trade Winds," *Saturday Review* 51, no. 50 (December 1968): 16–17.
22. "College Aroused by Negro Paper/Revolutionaries Gain Control of Wayne State Daily," New York *Times,* Feb. 21, 1969.
23. "CSU Blacks Publish Own Paper," Cleveland *Plain Dealer,* Jan. 20, 1970.

● 7 ● THE BLACK MAGAZINES—THE FRONTRUNNERS

1. Franzen, Raymond, "Magazine Audiences in the Urban Negro Market," (New York: Our World Publishing Co., 1951): 9 (brochure).
2. "'Our World' Goes Bankrupt Owing 20 Ad Agencies," *Advertising* Age 16, no. 49 (December 1955): 109.
3. Goodman, Walter, "*Ebony:* Biggest Negro Magazine," p. 407.
4. Letter to the Editor, *Ebony* 23, no. 8 (June 1968): 21.
5. Ibid. 24, no. 3 (January 1969): 14.
6. *Lincoln Journalism Newsletter,* February, 1952, p. 3.
7. Balk, Alfred, "Mr. Johnson Finds His Market," p. 35.
8. Johnson, Robert E., "President Johnson Gives Views on Riot Report/Says Report Is 'Most Important,'" *Jet* 33, no. 26 (April 1968): 14.
9. Fuller, Hoyt W., "All in a Name," *Negro Digest* 19, no. 5 (March 1970): 98.
10. Evans, W. Leonard, Jr., "After 3 Years/From Hope to Solution," p. 5.
11. Letter to the Editor, *New Lady* 2, no. 3 (November 1969): 2.
12. Penn, I. Garland, *The Afro-American Press and Its Editors,* p. 120.
13. Letter to the author from Ken Jones, publisher of *Soul,* May 15, 1970.
14. Allen, Thomas H., "Mass Media Use Patterns in a Negro Ghetto," *Journalism Quarterly* 45, no. 3 (August 1968): 525.
15. Lyle, Jack, *The News in Megalopolis,* p. 178.
16. Stephenson, William David II, "Magazines and Black Americans: An Evolving Relationship," pp. 149–63; Bontrager, Robert D., "An Investigation of Black Press and White Press Use Patterns in the Black Inner City of Syracuse, N.Y.," pp. 197–203.
17. Hirsch, Paul M., "An Analysis of *Ebony:* The Magazine and Its Readers," *Journalism Quarterly* 45, no. 2 (Summer 1968): 261–70, 292.

● 8 ● THE BLACK MAGAZINES—THE SPECIALISTS

1. Kellogg, Charles Flint, *NAACP,* vol. 1, chap. 3.
2. Du Bois, W. E. B., *The Autobiography of W. E. B. Du Bois,* p. 259.

3. Rudwick, Elliott M., *W. E. B. Du Bois: Propagandist of the Negro Protest*, p. 151.
4. "Time To Speak Up," *Crisis* 75, no. 9 (November 1968): 312.
5. Gerald, Carolyn, "The Measure and Meaning of the Sixties," p. 27.
6. Ibid., p. 28.
7. "Minority Affairs," *Catholic Journalist* 20, no. 7 (July 1968): 5.
8. "E. Harlem Writing Center Publishes *Uptown Beat*," New York *Amsterdam News*, April 18, 1970, p. 18.
9. Kaiser, Ernest, "Five Years of *Freedomways*," p. 103.
10. Letter to the author, Feb. 19, 1970.
11. Raymont, Henry, "Black Writers Win Literary Awards," p. 22.
12. "Introduction," *Amistad* 1: vii.
13. Raymont, p. 22.
14. For background on *Black World* see the preceding chapter where it is discussed under its former name.
15. Friedlander, Paul J. C., "Blacks Are Ready To Travel, But—," New York *Times*, April 26, 1970, p. 39.
16. Letter to the author from B. J. Nolen, June 15, 1970.
17. Mott, Frank Luther, *A History of American Magazines,* vol. 2, p. 68.
18. Nolen letter.
19. Mott, vol. 3, p. 71.
20. Detweiler, Frederick G., *The Negro Press in the United States,* p. 127.
21. Letter to the author from Miss Mimi Reimel, assistant editor of *Philly Talk,* June 5, 1970.

● 9 ● WHAT IS IN THE BLACK PRESS?

1. Detweiler, Frederick G., *The Negro Press in the United States,* pp. 110–11.
2. Ibid., p. 126.
3. Ibid., p. 79.
4. Ibid., p. 106.
5. Pride, Armistead S., "The Negro Newspaper in the United States," pp. 141–49.
6. Moss, Elizabeth Murphy, "Black Newspapers Cover News Other Media Ignore," pp. 6–11.
7. Atlanta *Daily World,* March 12, 1970, p. 1.
8. "Man Beaten for Speeding," Milwaukee *Courier,* Jan. 3, 1970, p. 1.
9. "Pastor Hits Racist Headlines," *Greater Milwaukee Star,* June 7, 1969, p. 1.
10. Letter to the author, April 7, 1970.
11. "Cartoonist and College Journalism Dean Will Speak," Cleveland *Press,* Oct. 9, 1969, p. A-10.
12. Letter to the author, March 31, 1970.
13. Moore, Trevor Wyatt, "Cool Cat With a Warm Message," pp. 18–19.
14. White, Jack E., "Color and the Comics," p. 60.
15. Harrington, Ollie, "How Bootsie Was Born," in Clarke, John Henrik, ed., *Harlem, U.S.A.,* p. 90.
16. Ibid., p. 93.

● 10 ● THE BLACK JOURNALIST TODAY

1. *Lincoln Journalism Newsletter,* July, 1951, pp. 6–7.
2. "Press," *Time* 95, no. 14 (April 1970): 89.
3. Lewis, David L., and Miao, Judy, "America's Greatest Negroes: A Survey," p. 17.
4. *This Is Our War: Selected Stories of Six Afro-American War Correspondents.*
5. Pride, Armistead S., "Opening Doors for Minorities," p. 24.
6. Klein, Woody, "News Media and Race Relations," pp. 43–45.
7. White, Walter, *A Man Called White,* p. 209.
8. *Jet* 37, no. 9 (December 1969): 11.
9. Sancton, Thomas, "The Negro Press," p. 559.
10. Ibid.
11. Cronon, Edmund D., *Black Moses,* p. 181.

12. "Chuck Stone Quits TV Spot After 'Hate' Mail," Norfolk *Journal and Guide,*
    June 6, 1970, p. 14.
13. "*Jet* Editor Refuses To Censor Speech, Leaves Group," *Jet* 36, no. 4 (May
    1969): 8.
14. The author is indebted to Miss Mary Male for some of the information on
    Robert Johnson.
15. Letter to the author, March 10, 1970.
16. "New Black Journalists Group Backs Reporter," New York *Times,* June 29,
    1970, p. 24.
17. Advertisement in the New York *Amsterdam News,* Feb. 21, 1970, p. 22.
18. "*Times* Black Workers Unite for Security," New York *Amsterdam News,* Feb.
    21, 1970, p. 3.
19. Witcover, Jules, "Washington's White Press Corps," p. 43.

● 11 ● TRAINING AND EDUCATION

1. "Citations of Merit for Outstanding Performance in Journalism," (Jefferson
   City, Mo.: Lincoln University Department of Journalism, 1968): 15.
2. "Black Students See What News Job Is Like," *Editor & Publisher* 103, no. 7
   (February 1970): 16.
3. The author distinguishes between training and education thus: Training
   emphasizes learning of skills and procedures, often using workshops, practice
   sessions, and internships; education may include training but adds mental
   development and imparting knowledge (or guiding toward it) beyond the technical field, using standard classroom procedures, such as lectures and seminars.
4. "Program to Train Negro Journalists Recruits in Prison," New York *Times,*
   July 20, 1969; "*Afro* Gets $123,000 Grant from Ford to Train Writers," Balti-
   more *Afro-American,* March 8, 1969, p. 2; Becker, Jerome D., "13 Minority Fellows Receive Thorough Journalism Training," *Editor & Publisher* 102, no. 35
   (August 1969): 15.
5. "35 from Minorities in Columbia Course," *Editor & Publisher* 102, no. 25
   (June 1969): 10; Rock, Naomi, "Minority Group Journalists Are Being Trained
   by Crash Programs," Associated Press dispatch in Rome (N.Y.) *Sentinel,* April
   16, 1970, p. 4.
6. Rock, p. 4.
7. "Agency Course Set for Minorities," New York *Times,* Feb. 19, 1970.
8. "Help Wanted: More Black Newsmen," p. 19.
9. Ibid., pp. 5–8.
10. Ibid., p. 10.
11. "Journalism Awards Presented to Ten," Baltimore *Afro-American,* Dec. 20, 1969,
    p. 12; "The Washington Journalism Center Fellowships," brochure issued by
    the Center annually.
12. *ANPA Newspaper Information Service Newsletter* 8, no. 5 (May 1968): 4; "Help
    Wanted," pp. 26–27.
13. "Training for Minorities Set in Washington Pact," *Guild Reporter,* Dec. 12,
    1969, p. 7.
14. "For Young Negroes: Urban Journalism," *Gannetteer,* April, 1969, p. 7; "News-
    paper Fund Initiates Ghetto Summer J-Schools," *Editor & Publisher* 102, no.
    18 (May 1969): 35.
15. "Report of Ad Hoc Coordinating Committee on Minority Education to the
    Association for Education in Journalism," August, 1969, Foreword.
16. Ibid., p. 5.
17. Frazier, E. Franklin, *Black Bourgeoisie,* p. 159.
18. "Few Negroes Are Enrolled in J-Schools," p. 35; "Report of Governor's Com-
    mittee on Employment of Minority Groups in the News Media," (Albany: State
    of New York, 1969) brochure.
19. Booker, Simeon, *Black Man's America,* p. 143.
20. "A Survey of the Mass Communications Areas in 66 Predominately Black Four
    Year Accredited Colleges and Universities."
21. "Clark Establishing Programs in Mass Communications," Atlanta *Inquirer,*
    May 2, 1970.
22. Letter to the author, June 5, 1968.
23. Letter to the author, Jan. 12, 1970.

24. For discussion of some of these points see "Directions in Black Studies," *Massachusetts Review* 10, no. 4 (Autumn 1969): 701–56; Dunbar, Ernest, "The Black Studies Thing," New York *Times Magazine,* April 6, 1969, pp. 25–27, 60, 65, 68, 70, 75, 78; Dillon, Merton L., "White Faces and Black Studies," *Commonweal* 91, no. 17 (January 1970): 476–79; Roberts, Steven V., "Black Studies: More than 'Soul Courses,'" *Commonweal* 91, no. 17 (January 1970): 478–79.
25. Mencher, Melvin, "Recruiting and Training Black Newsmen," p. 22.
26. Such as Carl T. Rowan, Alex Poinsett, Era Bell Thompson, L. F. Palmer, Jr., Lahymond Robinson, Robert E. Johnson, Moneta Sleet, Jr., Roy Wilkins, John Britten, Consuelo Young, Lucile H. Bluford, Thelma Thurston Gorham, Lester H. Brownlee, Henry Lee Moon, George Daniels, Herbert Nipson.

● 12 ● PUBLISHERS AND THEIR PROBLEMS

1. See: MacDougall, Curtis D., *The Press and Its Problems* (Dubuque: Wm. C. Brown, 1964); Rucker, Frank W., and Williams, Herbert Lee, *Newspaper Organization and Management,* 2nd ed. (Ames: Iowa State University Press, 1965); Wolseley, Roland E., and Campbell, Laurance R., *Exploring Journalism,* 3rd ed. (New York: Prentice-Hall, 1957); Emery, Edwin, Ault, Phillip H., and Agee, Warren, *Introduction to Mass Communications,* 3rd ed. (New York: Dodd, Mead, 1970).
2. Johnson, John H., "Understanding: The Key to Effective Communication," address.
3. Sancton, Thomas, "The Negro Press," p. 560.
4. Daly, Charles U., ed., *The Media and the Cities,* p. 12.
5. Letter to the Editor, *Ebony* 25, no. 4 (February 1970): 16–17.
6. Ibid. 25, no. 6 (April 1970): 25.
7. "Negro Press Assays Role in Social Change," *Editor & Publisher* 101, no. 26 (June 1968): 19.
8. Lomax, Louis E., *The Negro Revolt,* p. 201.
9. *Lincoln Journalism Newsletter,* April, 1949, p. 6.
10. "News from the Ford Foundation," New York, May 20, 1969, p. 4.
11. Johnson address.
12. "Negro Press Advised To Analyze More," *Editor & Publisher* 89, no. 29 (July 1956): 60.
13. Biggart, Homer, "Baldwin Leaves Negro Monthly," New York *Times,* Feb. 28, 1967, p. 34.
14. *Muhammad Speaks,* Feb. 20, 1970.
15. White, Walter, *A Man Called White,* pp. 208–9.
16. *Lincoln Journalism Newsletter,* February, 1950, p. 2.

● 13 ● THE BUSINESS OPERATIONS

1. Kinzer, Robert H., and Sagarin, Edward, *The Negro in American Business,* p. 115.
2. "Black Is Beautiful But Maybe Not Profitable," p. 100.
3. Detweiler, Frederick G., *The Negro Press in the United States,* p. 116.
4. Berkman, David, "Advertising in *Ebony* and *Life*: Negro Aspirations vs. Reality," p. 53.
5. Ibid., p. 64.
6. Oak, Vishnu, V., *The Negro Newspaper,* pp. 114–16.
7. "The Zoo Story," *Newsweek* 75, no. 2 (January 1970): 58–59.
8. Lomax, Louis E., *The Negro Revolt,* p. 204.
9. "Courting the Black Billionaire," p. 70.
10. Ibid.
11. "Black Is Beautiful But Maybe Not Profitable," pp. 41–42.
12. Gibson, D. Parke, *The $30 Billion Negro,* pp. 7–8.
13. *The Negro Market* (New York: Department of Media Relations and Planning, Young & Rubicam, Inc., 1969): 1–3, 9, 15, 21, 23, 37, 39.
14. "The Black Market," p. 101.
15. Grayson, William P., "Some of Your Best Customers Are Negro," address.

16. "Courting the Black Billionaire," p. 70.
17. O'Connell, Sharyn, "Why Not the Black Press?"
18. "Black Press Does Its Own Thing, Spurs Readers' Heavy Buying," p. 192.
19. Walker, William O., "Anniversary of the Negro Press," p. 4.
20. Oak, p. 118.
21. Quarles, Benjamin, *Frederick Douglass,* p. 80; Foner, in his more detailed biography by the same name, relates that there were two white apprentices who helped with typesetting, wrapping, and other chores.
22. Foner, Philip S., *Frederick Douglass,* p. 84.
23. "Good News For You!" p. 14.
24. Oak, pp. 72–73.
25. Pride, Armistead S., "Negro Newspapers: Yesterday, Today, and Tomorrow," p. 186.

● 14 ● AUXILIARIES AND COMPETITORS

1. Readers wanting to consult books on white journalism may find several guides helpful, including: Price, Warren, *The Literature of Journalism* (Minneapolis: University of Minnesota Press, 1959); Wolseley, Roland E., *The Journalist's Bookshelf* (Philadelphia: Chilton, 1961); Taft, W. H., comp., *200 Books on American Journalism* (Columbia: University of Missouri School of Journalism, issued every two years).
2. Detweiler, Frederick G., *The Negro Press in the United States,* p. 28.
3. Brooks, Maxwell R., *The Negro Press Re-examined,* p. 82.
4. Townseley, Luther A., "ANP Provides International Coverage for 78 Member Papers in America," p. 1.
5. Lomax, Louis E., *The Negro Revolt,* p. 72.
6. Beard, Richard L., and Zoerner, Cyril E. II, "Associated Negro Press: Its Founding, Ascendancy, and Demise," p. 51; this account contains the commonly known facts about the ANP and Claude Barnett.
7. Ibid., p. 49; on p. 51, however, they also record the date as July, 1966.
8. "Claude Barnett Dies at 77; Founder of Negro News Agency," New York *Times,* Aug. 3, 1967.
9. "Duckett, P. R. Man, Buys Negro News Agency," *Editor & Publisher* 98, no. 6 (February 1965): 12.
10. "Saigon's Black Market: Screwing the Little Guys," *Black Panther,* Dec. 20, 1969, p. 29.
11. "Helping To Close the Communications Gap," Empire Features release, April 18, 1970, p. 5.
12. Williamson, Lenora, "Specialists Cover Minority Communities for News Media," p. 13; "Samples for CNS News File," *Editor & Publisher* 106, no. 10 (May 1970): 13.
13. Penn, Stanley, "Major Concerns Seek Help from Negro-run Public Relations Firms," *Wall Street Journal,* Nov. 12, 1965, p. 1.
14. *Lincoln Journalism Newsletter,* July, 1949, pp. 4–5.
15. "Chicago *Defender* Observes 50th Year of Service," *Editor & Publisher* 88, no. 34 (August 1955): 58.
16. Address to Afro-American Association of TV Producers, Feb. 27, 1970, Racine, Wis.; this group's membership is drawn from white television enterprises.
17. Forkan, James P., "Black Ownership of Radio Grows—Slowly," p. 63.
18. "Empathy: The Vital Plus of Negro Radio," *Sponsor,* Aug. 26, 1963, p. 61.
19. *A Guide to Negro Media,* p. 16.
20. Dallos, Robert E., "Black Radio Stations Send Soul and Service to Millions," p. 64.
21. Forkan, p. 10.
22. Associated Press dispatch datelined Washington D. C., Dec. 26, 1969.
23. *A Guide to Negro Media,* p. 16.
24. Coonradt, Frederic C., *The Negro News Media and the Los Angeles Riots,* pp. 22–23, 28.
25. Letter to the author from W. Leonard Evans, Feb. 2, 1970.
26. Garnett, Bernard E., "How Soulful Is 'Soul' Radio?" (Nashville, Tenn.: Race Relations Information Center, 1970): 12.
27. "Methodist Agencies Help Blacks Get Radio Stations," p. 16.

28. "Publishers Endorse 'Black Journal,'" New York *Amsterdam News,* July 5, 1969.
29. *Media/scope* 10, no. 12 (December 1966): 162.
30. Bontrager, Robert D., "An Investigation of Black Press and White Press Use Patterns in the Black Inner City of Syracuse, N.Y.," pp. 207–8.

● 15 ● BLACK PHILOSOPHIES AND BLACK JOURNALISM

1. See, for example, Lester Julius, *Look Out, Whitey! Black Power's Gon' Get Your Mama* (New York: Dial, 1968); King, Martin Luther, Jr., *Where Do We Go From Here?* (New York: Harper and Row, 1967); Malcolm X, *The Autobiography of Malcolm X;* Brooks, Thomas R., "A Strategist Without a Movement," New York *Times Magazine,* Feb. 16, 1969, pp. 24–25, 105–8, 111–12 (Bayard Rustin).
2. See Brooks, Maxwell R., *The Negro Press Re-examined,* which reports fully an analysis of the political content of several leading national black papers published in 1949.
3. Ottley, Roi, *New World A'Coming,* p. 268.
4. Hentoff, Nat, "Liberation—Not Frustration," *Nation* 207, no. 2 (July 1968): 53.
5. Palmer, L. F., Jr., "The Black Press in Transition," p. 34.
6. Advertisement in the *New Pittsburgh Courier,* Nov. 1, 1969.
7. Miller, William Robert, *Martin Luther King, Jr.* (New York: Avon, 1968): 258.
8. Johnson, John H., "Understanding: The Key to Effective Communication," address.
9. Muse, Benjamin, *The American Negro Revolution: From Nonviolence to Black Power, 1963–1967,* p. 175.
10. Stephenson, W. David II, "Blacks' Attitudes Toward Magazines," p. 175.
11. Letter to the author, Nov. 25, 1969.

● 16 ● PRO AND CON ON THE BLACK PRESS

1. Frazier, E. Franklin, *Black Bourgeoisie,* p. 146.
2. Brown, Warren H., "A Negro Looks at the Negro Press," pp. 5–6.
3. Dabney, Virginius, "Nearer and Nearer the Precipice," p. 100.
4. White, Walter, *A Man Called White,* p. 208.
5. Brooks, Maxwell R., *The Negro Press Re-examined,* pp. 15, 98–101.
6. Ottley, Roi, *New World A'Coming,* p. 280.
7. Conrad, Earl, "The Negro Press," pp. 5–8.
8. Baldwin, James, *Notes of a Native Son,* p. 49.
9. Waters, Enoc P., "The Negro Press: A Call for Change," pp. 67–68.
10. Kendall, Elaine, "The Negro Press," p. 84.
11. Aldridge, Dan, "Black Press—Where Are You?"
12. Villard, Oswald Garrison, *The Disappearing Daily,* pp. 24–25.
13. Baldwin, p. 53.
14. Ibid., p. 54.
15. Letter from C. Sumner Stone to *New Republic* 151, no. 18 (October 1964): 29–30.
16. Myrdal, Gunnar, *An American Dilemma,* p. 917.
17. Booker, Simeon, "The New Frontier for Daily Newspapers," p. 12.
18. Poston, Ted, "The Negro Press," p. 16.
19. *Lincoln Journalism Newsletter,* March, 1945, p. 15.
20. Greenberg, Bradley S., and Dervin, Brenda, *Communication Among the Urban Poor,* Michigan State Reports, no. 1 (Lansing: Michigan State University, 1967): 25.
21. Bontrager, Robert D., "An Investigation of Black Press and White Press Use Patterns in the Black Inner City of Syracuse, N.Y."
22. Allen, Thomas H., "Mass Media Use Patterns and Functions in a Negro Ghetto" (master's thesis, West Virginia University, 1967).
23. Lyle, Jack, *The News in Megalopolis.*
24. Stephenson, William David II, "Magazines and Black Americans," p. 121a.
25. Ibid., p. 4.
26. Colle, Royal, "The Negro Image and the Mass Media" (Ph.D. diss., Cornell University, 1967).
27. Letters, "Zebra Associates," *Newsweek* 75, no. 5 (February 1970): 9.

28. "Form Group To Make Black Press 'More Relevant,'" *Jet* 35, no. 24 (March 1969): 53.

● 17 ● THE FUTURE

1. Wolseley, Roland E., "The Vanishing Negro Press," pp. 64–68.
2. Booker, Simeon, *Black Man's America*, pp. 152–53.
3. Williams, James D., "Is the Black Press Needed?" p. 15.
4. Myrdal, Gunnar, *An American Dilemma*, p. 912.
5. Conrad, Earl, "The Negro Press," p. 8.
6. Pride, Armistead S., "Negro Newspapers: Yesterday, Today, and Tomorrow," p. 188.
7. Lomax, Louis E., *The Negro Revolt*, p. 204.
8. Ibid., p. 206.
9. Ibid.
10. Gibson, D. Parke, *The $30 Billion Negro*, p. 262.
11. Palmer, L. F., Jr., "The Black Press in Transition," p. 36.
12. Address to journalism students at Syracuse University, May 4, 1970.
13. See such discussions as Bird, George L., and Merwin, Frederic E., eds., *The Newspaper and Society* (New York: Prentice-Hall, 1942); Bird and Merwin, eds., *The Press and Society* (New York: Prentice-Hall, 1951); Liebling, A. J., *The Wayward Pressman* (New York: Doubleday, 1947); MacDougall, Curtis D., *Newsroom Problems and Policies* (New York: Macmillan, 1941); MacDougall, *The Press and Its Problems;* Villard, Oswald Garrison, *The Disappearing Daily;* Lindstrom, Carl E., *The Fading American Newspaper* (New York: Doubleday, 1960); Gerald, J. Edward, *The Social Responsibility of the Press* (Minneapolis: University of Minnesota Press, 1963); and Siebert, Fredrick S., Schramm, Wilbur, and Peterson, Theodore, *Four Theories of the Press* (Champaign: University of Illinois Press, 1956).
14. Tebbel, John, "So What About Our Own Credibility Gap?" *IPI Report* 17, no. 8 (December 1968): 8–9.
15. Quoted by Gibson, p. 160.
16. Booker, p. 156.
17. Gardner, John W., *No Easy Victories* (New York: Harper and Row, 1969): 17.
18. Wolseley, Roland E., *Understanding Magazines* (Ames: Iowa State University Press, 1965): 416.

INDEX

■